Introduction to Podopediatrics

Dedication

To my mother and father
PT

For my mother, Lydia whom I miss
For my father, Nick, upon whom I still depend
For my brothers, Nicholas and Robert, within whom I see our values
For my wife, Barbara, whom I love
For my children, Adam, Peter and Alec, whom I cherish
RGV

For Churchill Livingstone:

Editorial Director (Health Professions): Mary Law
Project Development Manager: Dinah Thom
Project Manager: Derek Robertson
Design Direction: George Ajayi

Introduction to Podopediatrics

Edited by

Peter Thomson BSc DPodM MChS
Senior Paediatric Podiatrist, Fife Primary Care NHS Trust, Dunfermline;
Private Practitioner, Dunfermline, UK

Russell G Volpe DPM
Professor and Chairman, Department of Pediatrics,
New York College of Podiatric Medicine, New York, USA

Foreword by

Justin Wernick DPM
Professor and Chair, Department of Orthopedics,
New York College of Podiatric Medicine, New York, USA

SECOND EDITION

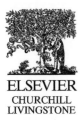

ELSEVIER
CHURCHILL
LIVINGSTONE

EDINBURGH LONDON NEW YORK OXFORD PHILADELPHIA ST LOUIS SYDNEY TORONTO 2001

CHURCHILL LIVINGSTONE
An imprint of Elsevier Limited

First edition 1993
Second edition 2001
    Reprinted 2004, 2005, 2006

ISBN 0 443 06208 0

British Library Cataloguing in Publication Data
A catalogue record for this book is available from the British Library

Library of Congress Cataloguing in Publication Data
A catalogue record for this book is available from the Library of
Congress

Note
Medical knowledge is constantly changing. As new information
becomes available, changes in treatment, procedures, equipment and
the use of drugs become necessary. The editors, contributor and the
publishers have taken care to ensure that the information given in this
text is accurate and up to date. However, readers are strongly advised
to confirm that the information, especially with regard to drug usage,
complies with the latest legislation and standards of practice.

The Publisher

ELSEVIER
your source for books,
journals and multimedia
in the health sciences

www.elsevierhealth.com

Working together to grow
libraries in developing countries
www.elsevier.com | www.bookaid.org | www.sabre.org

ELSEVIER   BOOK AID International   Sabre Foundation

The
publisher's
policy is to use
paper manufactured
from sustainable forests

Transferred to digital print 2007
Printed and bound by CPI Antony Rowe, Eastbourne

Contents

Contributors

Joseph C. D'Amico DPM
Professor and Past Chairman, Division of
Orthopedic Sciences; Professor, Department of
Pediatrics, New York College of Podiatric
Medicine; Private Practitioner, New York, USA

Jill Ferrari BSc(Hons) DPodM MChS
Lecturer, Department of Podiatry,
London Foot Hospital, London, UK

Edwin J. Harris DPM
Clinical Associate Professor of Orthopedics,
Layola University, Maywood, Illinois, USA

Alexandra M. John BSc MSc (Clin Psychol)
Head of Psychology Services, Sussex Weald and
Downs NHS Trust, Graylingwell Hospital,
Chichester, UK

Christopher Kelnar MA MD FRCPCH FRCP(Edin)
Consultant Paediatric Endocrinologist, Reader
in Child Health, Royal Hospital for Sick
Children, Edinburgh, UK

Linda Lang PhD
Associate Director of Medicine, AIDS Research
Director, Elmhurst Hospital Center, New York,
USA

Lawrence J. Lowy DPM
Assistant Professor, Department of Pediatrics,
New York College of Podiatric Medicine,
New York; Private Practitioner,
Bethel, Connecticut, USA

Iain W. McCall MB DhB DMRD FRCR
Consultant Radiologist, Robert Jones and
Agnes Hunt Orthopaedic Hospital, Oswestry,
UK

Malcolm Macnicol BSc(Hons) MBChB FRCS MCh
FRCP FRCSEd(Orth)
Consultant Orthopaedic Surgeon and
Senior Orthopaedic Lecturer,
The Royal Hospital for Sick Children and the
Princess Margaret Rose Orthopaedic Hospital,
Edinburgh, UK

Kevin Murray MBBS FRACP
Rheumatologist, Department of Rheumatology,
Great Ormond Street Hospital, London, UK

Kathryn Noyes MB ChB
Staff Grade Paediatrician (Diabetic Team),
Royal Hospital for Sick Children, Edinburgh,
UK

Jill Pickard MSc MCSP CertEd DipTp
Senior Lecturer, University College
Northampton, Northampton, UK

Barbara Resseque DPM
Associate Professor, New York College of
Podiatric Medicine, New York;
Private Practitioner, East Northport, New York,
USA

Christopher Steer BSc MB ChB DCH FRCPE FRCPCH
Consultant Paediatrician, Victoria Hospital,
Kirkcaldy, UK

Steven Subotnick DPM ND DC
Clinical Professor, Department of Biomechanics
and Surgery, California College of Podiatric
Medicine, San Francisco;
Adjunct Professor, Department of Kinesiology,
California State University, Hayward,
California, USA

John Thomson MD FRCP(Glas Edin) DObst RCOG
FChS
Consultant Dermatologist, The Royal Infirmary,
Glasgow, UK

Peter Thomson BSc DPodM MChS
Senior Paediatric Podiatrist, Fife Primary Care
NHS Trust, Dunfermline;
Private Practitioner, Dunfermline, UK

Ronald L. Valmassy DPM
Podiatrist, St Francis Memorial Hospital, San
Francisco, USA

Russell G. Volpe DPM
Professor and Chairman, Department of
Pediatrics, New York College of Podiatric
Medicine, New York, USA

Foreword

Having spent over 40 years studying and practising podopediatrics, I have learned the importance of keeping well-informed in this especially difficult field of medicine. Very often, the pediatric patient cannot give the information needed for the podiatrist to perform a thorough and comprehensive evaluation; it is up to the skill of the practitioner to know what to look for and how to assess this information.

The field of podopediatrics has expanded greatly over the past 10 years. Our knowledge base has broadened and the 'need to know' has become a priority in our everyday clinical experience. Both patients and parents expect the podiatrist to be on the cutting edge of the latest information and technology. *Introduction to Podopediatrics* addresses these matters in a well-organised and comprehensive manner.

This second edition is special and unique – it reflects the most recent knowledge and understanding of pediatric foot problems, considering not only the foot but the total patient as well. The addition of a chapter on normal child development, for example, functions as a benchmark in helping to understand the presence of pathology and its significance. The sections on the lower extremity in disease are outstanding and serve as an excellent reference for the practitioner.

The editors have assembled a diverse team of authors, each bringing their expertise from years of experience in their field. This team of authors not only comes from different professional backgrounds but also from different areas of the world. It is this diversity that provides such in-depth coverage of the subject.

I am very honored to have been asked to write the foreword for this book. It is a welcome addition to one's own library as it is a working document, ideal not only for the specialist but also as an essential text for the undergraduate, post-doctoral fellow and the non-specialist seeking enlightenment. You can rest assured that this book is going to be a key reference in the field.

Peter Thomson and Russell Volpe have generously offered their expertise and extraordinary talents in writing *Introduction to Podopediatrics*. They have years of experience, with solid backgrounds in both the academic and clinical arenas. Producing a text of this magnitude is a huge undertaking and this effort is acknowledged with appreciation for a worthy endeavour.

JW
New York, 2001

Preface

In the preface to the first edition of this book it was stated that the purpose of the book was to identify those lower limb problems in the pediatric population that could be managed by the podiatrist alone or as a member of a wider team. Similarly, many medical conditions were identified which, although they did not technically fall into the domain of podiatry, would nevertheless have an influence on the podiatrist's management of the child. This basic outline has been followed for this edition.

Deciding which subject areas to include and in what depth to cover them is one of the major challenges faced in planning an introductory text. In this edition the reader will find new or updated chapters on subjects of great relevance to the clinician seeking understanding of the child's leg and foot. This edition benefits considerably by the inclusion of a co-editor, which has allowed for this increase in the number of chapters. Five new chapters have been added, namely *History Taking and Physical Examination; Pediatric Gait; Growth and Development; Developmental Flatfoot* and *Serial Casting*. The book is organized by section, each representing a grouping of related chapters.

Section 1 is devoted to providing a foundation for approaching the child's lower extremity. It contains chapters on growth and development, psychological considerations and fundamental clinical chapters on the pediatric history and physical examination and the complexities of beginning to walk.

The second section introduces the major medical conditions that may involve the child's lower extremity. This includes a comprehensive chapter on a variety of medical problems of interest to the pediatric foot specialist, including diabetes, which is now included within the chapter *General Medicine*. It also includes chapters on three areas notably involved in childhood foot and leg dysfunction: rheumatology, neurology and cutaneous diseases.

Section 3 focuses on the lower extremity as a distinct entity covering various pathologies of the leg and foot. Included here are discussions of radiological evaluation of the child's foot and orthopedic conditions such as congenital deformities and fractures. The very important biomechanical conditions found in the child are discussed in chapters on torsional and frontal plane abnormalities and developmental flatfoot.

Finally, Section 4 covers the increasingly important topic of the pediatric athlete, as more children engage in organized sports at a young and vulnerable age. The remaining chapters in this section are on therapeutics of the child's foot and leg including physical therapy. Therapies frequently employed for the non-operative management of pediatric foot problems are discussed in chapters devoted to serial casting and orthotic management.

It is the editors' hope that this book will answer many of the reader's fundamental curiosities about the child's foot and leg as well as instill an appreciation of the complexities of the subject. We also hope it will leave the reader questing for greater depth and understanding of this specialized discipline in foot medicine, and under-appreciated component of pediatric medicine.

PT, RGV, 2001

Acknowledgments

The quality of any multi-author text is dependent upon the calibre of the authors contributing to the text. For this edition the editors were fortunate in being able to attract 17 people whose qualifications in their respective fields are without question. In addition, it may be seen from their contributions that as teachers they have no equal. Therefore the editors would like to thank all those clinicians who managed to create space in their busy schedules in order to take part in this work, some for the second time.

Once more the innocents who suffer most in such projects are the families. The editors would like to record their appreciation for the tolerance afforded by their long-suffering partners and to their children who, despite their young ages, stoically accepted the principle of distracted fathers and the subsequent lack of attention they might otherwise have expected. We hope the final product goes some way to redress the balance.

Our thanks also go to all those children who through their parents have allowed us to illustrate this textbook with clinical photographs. Their contribution is acknowledged as a fundamental teaching aid and one without which the book would be much the poorer.

PT would like to thank Dr Lowe for his critique on the section on fractures and also the Medical Illustration Department, Queen Margaret Hospital, Dunfermline.

Finally, the editors would like to thank the team at Harcourt Health Sciences for their support and guidance, especially Dinah Thom and Derek Robertson. Special thanks also to Mary Law.

PT, RGV, 2001

SECTION CONTENTS

1

Psychological considerations in the child patient

Alexandra M. John

The knowledge that a child requires hospital treatment whether for an acute or chronic illness can have a profound impact on both the child and the child's parents. The previously held beliefs concerning the wellbeing of the child are challenged and this raises concerns for both parents and children as to whether the child's health can be restored. The initial security and familiarity of the family doctor are exchanged for unfamiliar individuals and environments and the disruption of the daily routine such as attending school and carrying out housework or paid employment. The research into the prevalence of childhood chronic illness has revealed a rate of 10–15% and therefore indicates that this is not a rare occurrence in our society. It is important that health care professionals are aware of the physical and psychological issues that arise for both the family and the affected individual.

In this chapter a number of psychological issues are outlined and discussed in order to provide healthcare professionals with a framework which will aid them in their understanding of the impact that a chronic illness has on the individual and the family.

PARENT–PROFESSIONAL RELATIONSHIP

This relationship is a key concept in the process of communication between healthcare staff and the patient as the quality of the relationship will facilitate both the parents' and the child's understanding of the illness and as a result enhance the compliance with the treatment proposed.

3

When meeting parents and their children, healthcare professionals have choices in regard to how they interact with the family. Cunningham & Davis[1] proposed three models of interaction:

- professional as expert
- transplant
- the consumer.

The first model considers the *professional as the expert*. In such circumstances, the healthcare professional will hold all the expertise and will determine treatment and management of the case. There will be no attempt to involve the parents other than to inform them of the sequence of events. This model has some advantages to healthcare professionals as they are given a status and are rarely challenged. However, there coexists the potential for parents and children to become highly dependent on the professional as well as to be demanding. They consider themselves unable to make decisions and their parenting skills have been undermined.

In the *transplant model*, the expert role remains with the professional but this approach perceives the importance of transferring some of the skills to the parents in order to facilitate treatment. Physiotherapy and Portage home visiting are two good examples of this method of working. In order to facilitate this model, the healthcare professional needs to be able to instruct and teach the parents with sensitivity, to have good listening skills in order to record any feedback of the home treatment, and to have the ability to maintain a positive relationship with the parents.

Finally, *the consumer model* views the parents as having the right to choose between treatment options and to be given the necessary information to make informed decisions. Within the parent–professional relationship, it is the parents who have the power and influence. In this model, there is an acceptance that it is the parents who have the most knowledge and competence regarding their child's entire circumstances. The healthcare professional's role is to be a consultant and advisor and decision-making is through negotiation and is based on a mutually respectful relationship.

These three models provide potentially challenging methods of delivering services from an interpersonal perspective. The choice of approach will inevitably be dependent on the service context and the professional's own personal style.

COMMUNICATION

The initial concern for parents and children is their need for clarification concerning the meaning associated with the presenting symptomology. In order to ensure an appropriate diagnosis is made, patients and their families have to communicate the signs and symptoms to the medical and therapy staff. Their ability to communicate with professional staff regarding the problem may be more difficult than one might imagine. It is recognized that any anxiety experienced by the parents will affect their ability to listen and to provide complete, coherent answers to questions posed by the professionals. From the children's perspective, they will be in an environment where they will have little influence in ensuring that their voices are heard. Their own developmental level will impact on their ability to communicate their thoughts and feelings associated with the illness owing to a lack of expressive language skills. However, if children are not given the opportunity to express themselves verbally or non-verbally through facial and bodily gesture, they may become reliant on their parents to communicate on their behalf which can lead to a sense of helplessness and of not being understood.

Little research has been carried out on how accurately staff can identify the concerns of parents, let alone children. In the adult field, there are numerous studies that have explored how hospital staff diagnose emotional and psychiatric problems associated with physical health problems, with most studies significantly underrepresenting the difficulties.[2,3] The effect of this lack of appreciation of the concomitant difficulties experienced by parents and children results in those individuals not receiving the help they need. It has been proposed that the reason for poor communication from the hospital staff is due to a number of factors, e.g. limited time,[4] poor interviewing skills,[5] the assumption that the patient will disclose the problem without probing,[6] and the professionals' avoidance of strong emotions together with a wish to escape from awkward questions.[7] In addition, the environment in which the discussion takes place is important – open wards and clinical offices provide very different atmospheres for parents and children to raise concerns. For parents the office may provide the privacy to raise issues whereas for young to middle school-aged children the rough and tumble of the ward may seem a preferable place to raise their concerns.

Bradford & Singer[8] undertook a study in order to consider the medical and nursing staff's ability to predict accurately the concerns and anxieties of parents who had a child with a chronic illness. Their findings were salutary to those who work in the health context. They established that the staff were only able to predict 15–30% of the parents' concerns with regard to the amount of information that they received. Interestingly, the staff groups did not agree on what these concerns might be. Such evidence confirms that despite the knowledge that communication may be problematic and despite the wealth of literature available in order to facilitate improvements, healthcare staff still have difficulty in this area. There needs to be further attention given at the outset of a professional–patient relationship in order to ensure clarification and to derive open, direct communication between the two parties. Therefore, on seeing a child for the first time, it is important not to make assumptions regarding the child's response to podiatry. For children who may already have endured numerous hospital visits and medical/surgical procedures, to have their feet examined may be the last straw as they may associate previous examinations inappropriately with podiatry and as a result behave in an unexpected manner.

The impact of the diagnosis can be moderated and adjustment to it enhanced by the way in which parents and children are provided with the information, i.e. what they are told and when they are told. Occasionally, diagnosis may be made at birth but for others it is an evolving situation when there is no definitive time that the parents can be given a diagnosis. Therefore, the professional has to ensure that both parents and child are kept updated with emerging information and of the implications that such information may have for them. In a number of studies, parents have indicated that they wished to be told the truth early. The research also highlighted the importance of being told the truth in a sensitive manner rather than simply being given reassurance.

In hospitals, there are many potential barriers to communicating with children. The white coat is one of these and for many children prior to having to attend hospital on a regular basis the white coat will have been associated with pain and discomfort and authority where children are seen and perhaps not heard. In order to facilitate compliance with medical regimens, it is important that children have an age-appropriate understanding of their condition and what they can expect in order to prevent unnecessary worry and anxiety. The process of knowing to whom they can address their concerns will help children to be able to find ways to cope with their situation. This process may include talking to other children in the clinic, to parents or to hospital staff. Interestingly, it has been established that the process of worrying in anticipation enhances adjustment following the procedure.

When children are old enough to be aware of the illness and of the consequences to their daily life, it is necessary for the professional to speak with children at the appropriate cognitive level. This is important both at the time of initial diagnosis (when age appropriate) and at follow-up and review. However, to assess the children's cognitive level by their use of language alone may be misleading. Any mismatch between the manner in which children speak and their real abilities may be attributable to several factors, e.g. the unfamiliar setting or their own anxieties about what is happening. When children are very anxious they may regress both in the way in which they talk and how they behave. Another factor may be a child's own physical limitations. Certain children with cerebral palsy have great difficulty expressing their thoughts verbally because of their motor difficulties but they may well understand everything that is being said.

Therefore it is important to establish the child's level of understanding from those who know the child well before attempting to communicate. Frequently, young children will not talk to strangers and in fact are positively discouraged to do so in nursery and school settings ('stranger danger') and these children will look to their parents to provide permission to allow them to speak to the healthcare professional. Being aware of these issues will enable staff to understand that children are not being difficult and unresponsive but rather than they require reassurance and help in order to settle into the new situation.

Talking to parents about their child will facilitate better communication and thus better adherence and compliance to medical regimens. In addition, it is important to address the child patient: with the preschool child, reassurance about the reason for the admission or hospital appointment is appropriate. However, older children may well want to ask questions and therefore an open discussion is appropriate. At whatever age children initially learn about their condition, they will require more sophisticated explanations as they mature. Therefore, parents, carers and professionals must be prepared to provide varying amounts of information depending upon the child's maturity and the child's express wishes for further information. Inevitably, children will gather information from other children in the clinic or on the ward and will compare this information with the explanations that they have received from parents and other professionals. If the two do not match, the child will have to make inferential decisions as to why this information is different. Are the child's parents trying to protect the child? Do they find it so upsetting that they do not want to talk about it? Is the other child mistaken? Therefore to tell or not to tell requires careful consideration.

PREPARATION

Preparing children for hospital visits and procedures has been well documented and the research has highlighted that preparation can reduce the level of anxiety for some children and may have significant impact on the child's ability to make a good recovery.[9,10] Over the last 20 years, four main approaches have been utilized. Their purpose is to provide the child and/or parents with information. One approach provides parents with leaflets with a further reading list for parents to consult before the child enters hospital. The pamphlets contain information regarding the procedures that will be undertaken and usually provide some information concerning how the child will feel afterwards as well as giving information about the hospital environment itself. A second approach is more personal; parents and children are invited to the hospital to talk through the procedures and have the opportunity to have questions answered. The third approach is aimed at providing the child with some experiential experience through modeling on puppets or dolls. This is frequently used in cardiac catheterization and lumbar punctures as well as bone marrow transplantation. The final approach uses video or film material. Melamed & Siegel[11] in the 1970s undertook a series of experiments in order to establish which would be the most effective video for children. Their results demonstrated that in order to achieve the most effective outcome, the video should be of the hospital in which the procedure was to be undertaken. It should include the same staff, and it should show a child coping with the procedure rather than being in total control all the time. Eiser[12] and Miller & Green[13] have since replicated these findings.

The outpatient setting can be the venue for painful and difficult minor medical and surgical procedures and the sight of certain podiatric instruments and equipment may well be daunting to those unfamiliar to the clinic. Therefore, it may be useful to provide opportunities for children to examine equipment safely as this can defuse anxiety since it enables the child to gain some mastery over the proceedings. However, to create such opportunities for the child takes time from a busy clinic and therefore may not be practical. Under these circumstances, consideration may be given to setting up a specific time for new patients to attend when treatment is not the priority but the explanation of the forthcoming procedures and becoming familiar with the environment is.

Although certain children do benefit from these arrangements, there are some that do not. Unfortunately, such children become sensitized by these preparation procedures with the result that they become more anxious. A series of studies undertaken in the 1980s established that the effects of preparation were dependent upon its timing, the age of the child, the coping style, the anxiety of the parents and previous medical experience.[9,14] With regard to the child's coping style, it is important to discuss with the parents and child how the child has previously managed difficult and stressful situations. Such information will be useful as a guide but will not guarantee that a clear picture emerges as both children and adults have been found to use different approaches depending upon the circumstances.

DIAGNOSIS

How the family reacts to this initial stage will be affected by previous experiences of serious illness as well as the pre-morbid, psychological adjustment of individual family members. Separation from family and friends and the pain and anxiety associated with the diagnostic procedures make large demands on the coping skills of patients and of those of their families. The initial emotional reactions, which are considered similar to those associated with bereavement, should be accepted and should not be labeled as pathological.

Kübler-Ross's five-stage model[15] is useful in helping to understand the tasks parents have to face in adjusting to the diagnosis of chronic illness. First, there is denial and isolation; this stage shields individuals from the shock of the diagnosis and allows them to incorporate the news at their own pace. The second stage, anger, is frequently displayed erratically and results from a sense of helplessness and having to hand control over to others, thereby leaving the individual lacking any control over the situation. Bargaining is the third stage. Illness is viewed as being a punishment and the family may try to

strike a bargain in order to prolong life. The fourth stage, depression, occurs when there is a realization that bargaining cannot occur and that the child's condition has to be accepted. The final stage of acceptance occurs when the family has been able to acknowledge the implications of the chronic illness, to adapt to the new circumstance and to have established a means to reduce the level of interference with daily life to a minimum.

At one time, it was considered that individuals passed through each of these stages in a fixed and time-limited fashion and were then able to move on in their lives. However, more recent research has established that adjustment to loss is a much more variable process and will be subtly different for each individual experiencing the loss. It is not uncommon for parents and children to re-experience the loss at key moments in the life of the family. Such times are regarded as times of transition for the family, e.g. birth of another child, attendance at nursery or school for the first time, or leaving home. At these times, parents reconsider what might have been and have to learn to accept again what has occurred. This process equally applies to children who are old enough to have insight and awareness of their similarities and differences to their peer group.

A common experience, shared by many parents, is the increased emotional distress at the time when the family's second child enters mainstream school. This highlights the difference between the two children and the ongoing and pervasive nature of the needs of the child with chronic illness and the impact that this has had on each member of the family. Therefore, it is important not to view these stages as fixed since parents and siblings may be oscillating between any of the stages depending upon what is happening in the family life cycle. At such times, these families may require some professional support.

Impact of the diagnosis

To place the impact of being diagnosed with a chronic illness in context, it is helpful to consider a definition of a chronic illness and to consider the prevalence of such conditions in the community. A chronic illness refers to a disorder with a protracted course, which may be progressive and fatal, or the affected child may have a relatively normal lifespan despite impaired physical and/or mental functioning. It has been estimated that an approximate 10% prevalence rate of chronic illness is to be expected in the child population.

Early research on the psychological effects of chronic illness emphasized the negative consequences. Studies suggested that chronically ill children were at increased risk of emotional and behavioral problems and that the family in general suffered profound disruption to its normal functioning, resulting in significant psychological problems for its members.

Communication and relationship difficulties have also been reported as being common. Eiser[16] has written a comprehensive review in this area.

While it is clear that chronic illness can have such effects, not all research has demonstrated that the negative sequelae are inevitable. The impact of chronic illness is clearly not a single event, but a process that varies with the course of the illness. The risk factors for the children and their families experiencing particular difficulties or becoming caught up in the process of adjustment are poorly understood. There have been a number of psychological models proposed to provide explanations for how and why certain individuals adapt successfully and others do not.

Wallander et al[17] considered the interaction between risk and resistance factors. The risk factors associated with an increased chance of experiencing adjustment difficulties were the specific diagnosis itself, the severity of the condition, the visibility of the condition, whether poor bladder and bowel functioning were also involved, and finally cognitive functioning and neurological involvement. The resistance or protective factors were thought to be the individual's temperament, personal problem-solving skills, social support, the family's ability to adapt to new circumstances and how the individual copes with the stress associated with the condition.

Bradford[18] comprehensively reviewed this particular model and concluded that it did have certain useful features. However, it did not provide a complete explanation for the patient's responses to the illness. Leventhal's self-regulation model[19] considers the thoughts and beliefs concerning an illness of both the patient and the patient's family who will, as a result, develop theories and ideas about their illness as part of a three-stage process: initially, how the problem presents, e.g. the label it is given; the symptoms associated with it; and the duration of the illness. The second aspect is the development of the individual's own action plan to manage the presenting difficulty and the final stage is the patient's and the family's appraisal of the illness, i.e. whether they think they have the means or not to cope with the illness challenge. These three stages are interlinked and are constantly being modified as they are dependent on previous experience and how the latest experience fits or varies from the previously developed template of the illness. Leventhal considers five specific attributes as being important in shaping our understanding and our ability to manage the illness at each of these stages: illness identity, consequences, causes, time line and cure. Originally, the research was focused upon chronic illnesses in adult populations. More recently, however, Skinner & Hampson[20] moved the research into the areas of childhood and adolescent diabetes and found the conceptual framework to be useful.

When considering the individual factors highlighted above together with the other factors that are evident in the research literature, all of which have been identified to affect the psychological adjustment in children and their families, the reader needs to be aware that the conclusions drawn in the subsequent paragraphs are the result of several studies using differing methodological procedures. Therefore, it is difficult to provide unequivocal conclusions. However, despite this, it is useful to have a general framework to work from within a clinical context.

The first issue, age at onset of the illness has been highlighted as being important for psychological adjustment. A follow-up study of children with cancer noted that those children who had been diagnosed and treated in early life were less likely to experience adjustment problems in later life, when compared with those whose diagnosis occurred in middle childhood or adolescence. A second factor relates to the developmental stage of children and to their personal understanding of events.

Previous experience has also been established as having an important bearing on children's and adolescents' adjustment to their illness. Children who have had negative experiences are significantly more likely to experience future negative experiences and the associated psychological problems. Children enter the medical arena with preconceived ideas and attitudes about the staff, the hospital and the procedure. When these beliefs are not challenged, children are likely to attempt to prevent pain and suffering to themselves by responding with oppositional behavior and refusing to cooperate with procedures. Unfortunately, such actions result in a self-fulfilling prophecy as the clinical staff will resort to restraint in order to ensure the medical or nursing treatment is complied with. The result is that children have added another negative experience to their medical history and the prophecy is upheld.

Diseases with a high probability of fatality are associated with greater psychological disorder in both children and parents. There are a number of studies that indicate that there is an association between the increasing severity of the condition and the magnitude of psychological disturbance. Other studies have not established this finding. Children, who were severely affected with hemophilia, have been shown to be less affected than children with a milder form of the disease. The same trend also occurs in children who have juvenile arthritis or who have to live with the consequences of the side effects of thalidomide, and in those who have partial hearing or partial sight. In attempting to understand these results, it has been proposed that children who are severely affected recognize their limitations and do not attempt to compete with their able-bodied peers, while the mildly affected children try to compete in both worlds. The child's constant failure in the able-bodied world results in a poor self-image and poor adjustment.

Parental depression and ill health increase the risk for psychological difficulties in the child. Concurrent stress within family members as well as stress outside the family are associated with maladjustment in all family members to the diagnosis and subsequent treatment. In a more positive vein, social and/or emotional support is associated positively with adjustment as is increasing parental age.

The condition itself may also have a variable effect on stress levels. Donovan[21] studied two groups of families with adolescents aged between 10 and 21 years, who had a diagnosis of either autism or undifferentiated mental retardation. Mothers of children with autism reported higher level of stress, especially where behavioral difficulties were concerned, than the mothers of children with mental retardation.

While most research has focused understandably on the child patient's reaction to chronic illness and to treatment, it is important not to forget the impact on the siblings. It has been recognized that this group of children is particularly vulnerable to developing emotional and behavioral problems. A number of factors have been identified, namely the residual effects of parental distress owing to the care of the child with a handicap; to an increased responsibility at home; to decreased parental attention and resources; and, finally, to a pathological identification with the sibling with the handicap. However, the research literature also produced a variety of positive as well as negative outcomes. The conflicting results are partly attributable to the methodological weakness of the studies, e.g. no control groups; indirect measures based on parental interview, which may well be biased; and a reliance on single measures, such as the current psychological state of the child. This last issue may easily misrepresent how the sibling is adjusting, as adjustment will inevitably vary over time as different demands are placed on the child.

One study found that brothers and sisters were not embarrassed by having a sibling with a handicap but were embarrassed by having to cope with problem behavior in a public place, especially when they were in charge and when they felt unsure as to how to cope.

Factors, such as a small family, a small age gap between the sibling and the child with the handicap, younger siblings and a handicapping condition that is not obvious, have been associated with greater problems for the siblings.

Dyson[22] compared 55 older siblings in Canada (aged 7.5 to 15 years) of younger children with a handicap (aged 1 to 7 years) with 55 matched siblings of children without a handicap. Dyson found that there was no difference in level of self-concept, behavior problems and social competence between the two groups. The study also supported previous studies showing that there was no higher incidence of psychopathological behavior.

Dyson also looked at the personal attributes that related to adjustment in siblings of handicapped children. Generally, siblings of children with a mental handicap showed better behavioral adjustment and a higher social competence than the siblings of children with a sensory or physical handicap and other milder handicapping conditions. The author considered that the discrepancy was due to differential social consequences. It was thought that a mental delay might encourage an earlier social and family acceptance than other disabilities such as sensory or physical handicaps, speech disorders or learning disabilities. It is possible that some of these conditions are ill-defined and therefore might produce a sense of frustration in the family, which could affect sibling adjustment.

Suelzle & Keenan[23] considered that families of children with a handicap became more isolated as the children became older. Dyson also reported that there was an increase in behavioral problems in the sibling as the child with the handicap became older. Such changes may occur because there are more clubs and organized activities for younger children with a handicap. School also acts as a social network for the family, but as the children outgrow these there are very few new networks to replace them for the adolescent in the adult world. This may result in the families becoming more internally dependent

upon one another for care and entertainment than able-bodied counterparts.

Siblings also reported that their parents were being overly involved in the protection of the ill child. The research also noted that siblings were reluctant to express their feelings of dissatisfaction as well as their negative feelings to the family. Other studies have noted that adjustment was poorest when the parents' health was deteriorating but that their needs were also unmet when the parents were feeling well.

TREATMENT

Frequently, the commencement of treatment is perceived by parents as a time both of relief and of optimism. The focus is on the concrete tasks at hand such as daily injections, physiotherapy, speech therapy and other medication schedules. Despite these treatments, the illness may require repeated admission to hospital, resulting in separation from the family and disruption in schooling and peer relationships. A parent may have to give up work to look after the child and suffer extra expenses involved in living in hospital, in travel and providing special diets. This focus on the 'here and now' enables the family not to consider the long-term implications of the illness or disability but rather to pace the integration of the information associated with diagnosis and treatment.

CONCEPTS OF ILLNESS

A clear knowledge of the developmental milestones of childhood and adolescence is essential as this allows the healthcare professional to have an awareness of the cognitive level of the child and therefore to know how much information the child can understand and in which way to best present the information.

Studies into children's concepts of illness and health were pioneered by Nagy in the late 1940s and developed in the 1980s by Bibace & Walsh.[24] These researchers suggested that the understanding of children of the cause of illness is related to the three stages of the knowledge development of illness and to their personal experience of illness. Between the ages of 0 and 7 years, children are confused between internal and external organs. Between the ages of 7 and 9 years, children are confused about organ function and their relationship but are aware that there are a number of organs. Finally, between the ages of 9 and 18 years, there is the development of the cognitive skills that allow for a mature appreciation of the organs and that there is a relationship between organs and their function.

Bibace & Walsh[24] used a Piagetian model in order to describe six stages in the children's understanding about illness etiology. Under the age of 4 years, children pass through the stages of incomprehension and phenomenism. The latter stage refers to the fact that children think that illness is due to some magical, global or circular response, e.g.

Adult: How do people get a cough?
Child: From the wind.
Adult: How does the wind give you a cough?
Child: It just does.

Between the ages of 4 and 7 years, children pass through the stages of contagion and contamination. Children believe that illness in the contagion phase is due to objects or people being near them but not touching them. They then progress in their understanding by being able to distinguish the cause of the illness and how it is effective. The child perceives that the harmful causative object is outside the body and that the individual becomes ill by bodies being in contact.

Children between the ages of 7 and 11 years will pass through the stages of internalization thereby gaining an understanding that illness is located in the body but that the cause may be external. Children become aware that the illness may be contracted from another individual and they are likely to believe that illness is contracted by touching another person or animal. They are also likely to believe that non-contagious illnesses may be contracted.

At the ages of 11 years and older, physiological and psychophysiological are the two relevant stages of explanation. Children understand illness is due to a malfunctioning organ, e.g. bronchospasm, where the bronchioles and bronchi experience spasm because of an allergen. In the most mature conceptions, children understand that illness is due to internal physiological processes but in addition they also perceive that there could be a psychological explanation for the illness. In order for the child to be adequately informed, the clinician requires a knowledge and an awareness of these concepts of illness when talking to children in order that appropriate explanations can be provided.

The child's cognitive ability is also important since with increasing maturity the child develops a greater understanding of the implications of the illness and the potential restrictions that these will place on the child's life. A child with diabetes quickly becomes aware of the daily routines of insulin injections, of measuring blood sugar levels and of dietary restrictions. The difference between the child's peer group and the child also gradually emerges. Cognitively more mature children begin to understand the underlying cause for the diabetes mellitus and how the insulin injections prevent hyperglycemia. It is at this time that children should be helped to find ways of incorporating treatment routines into their lives so that the level of intrusion is minimized. It is important that children and their families find the right balance between spending time on therapy and other age-appropriate activities, as it is very easy for families to become preoccupied with only one aspect of a child's development. Realistic goals should be set and emphasis placed on ensuring that children continue to be involved in activities that are appropriate to their age.

ATTACHMENT

Another important psychological element to how children and families cope with hospitalization is associated with children's attachment to their parents. The theory on attachment was developed from the work of Robertson[25] and Bowlby[26,27] who observed children in hospital during protracted periods of separation from their parents. In the 1950s such separations were the norm and were the way in which hospital care was delivered to children.

Bowlby described the initial behavioral and psychological disturbance of these children as protest. This was displayed by children who cried excessively, would call out and constantly seek their parents. Following this stage, children would demonstrate behavior that became known as despair. They would exhibit reduced activity levels, be withdrawn and appear hopeless. Finally, if the separation was long, or permanent as when a parent dies or a child is adopted, children return to their usual old behaviours. However, if parents return, then the child appears to reject them and no longer seeks contact or interaction with them. Such profound observations have made a significant impact on pediatric practice, with parents being actively encouraged to stay with their children. On those occasions when the child is required to stay in hospital for weeks at a time, e.g. during treatment for leukemia, aplastic anemia or organ transplantation, beds have been made available for parents on the ward.

Secure attachment between children and their parents/carers is imperative to the emotional and psychological wellbeing of all children. However, for children with chronic health difficulties, there is an increased risk of their attachment being hampered owing to the demands of the treatment process on both the child and parents. Prematurity, which occurs more frequently in children who have enduring physical health problems, such as a child who is diagnosed as having cerebral palsy, poses a risk for preventing or delaying the attachment process. Parents may find it harder to emotionally invest in their child as the infant is less responsive and there may be a risk of the child dying. The infant may also be connected to various pieces of medical equipment such as ventilators, drains and injection pumps, which may hinder parents in their ability to provide physical care and comfort for the child. It is not uncommon for parents to think that they are unable to care for their child as well as the healthcare professionals and will prefer to hand over responsibility to them, as they lose confidence in their own abilities to parent. This early experience can have ongoing impact with parents not feeling emo-

tionally attached to their child months or years after the event. The fact that attachment does not occur in the early weeks/months is, however, not the catastrophe that it was once thought. Attachment is a lifelong process, with the result that if an infant misses the early opportunities the parent can form a bond with the child later and aid the development of internal representation of the parental figure at this later stage of the child's development. Children's attachment to their parents continually undergoes transformations through childhood and adult life in order to cope with the developmental accomplishments that each individual acquires. The emergence of autonomy and relationships with a peer group outside the family is an example of when attachments have to be modified in order to incorporate a greater sense of self and belonging with others.

When a child has a chronic illness, attachment with the main carer may be moderated by the experience. This is particularly frequent if the child is between 6 and 18 months and the parent is unable to stay with the child in hospital. In these circumstances, Bowlby's research demonstrated that children could experience acute stress responses. He described three stages of acute distress that children experience when they are separated from their carers (see above). Therefore, it is important to enable carers to stay with their child. In addition, repeated admissions to hospital for children under the age of 4 are associated with marked adjustment problems in the longer term, specifically in terms of behavioral problems and reading problems at adolescence. In the light of this research, it is important to admit children to hospital only when it is absolutely necessary and to ensure primary care is always available to support the child and the family later.

Unfortunately, a well-attached infant does not necessarily become a well-attached preschool child or adolescent. Given that the attachment process is dynamic this should not be a surprise. Sroufe[28] has stated that quality of the attachments in preschool children is influenced equally by how the parents manage the child's aggressive influences and feelings during the transition between infancy and the preschool years as by the quality of the early care. The admission to hospital of a child may result in the expression of aggressive and demanding feelings and behavior that has to be managed and contained in order to ensure the child's emotional security. The development or acquisition of a chronic problem may therefore contribute to attachment difficulties depending on how parents and children adapt individually and as a family system.

Children show signs of being 'attached' to their parents when they demonstrate that they are able to explore the world around them but use their parents as a secure base.[29] When the parents leave, the child becomes highly distressed and clingy and on their return will greet the parents positively and will approach them for comfort if the child has been distressed and will then resettle to the play activities. The poorly attached child will show one of two responses,[29] either insecure avoidant or insecure resistant attachment.

In the first response, the child's attachment is characterized by being minimally distressed when the parents leave and by avoiding the parents on their return. Such children appear to be preoccupied with play and exploring their environment but are in fact very aware of their parents' presence.

Children showing the second alternative response, insecure resistant attachment, explore their environment in a very limited manner even when their parents are present and become highly distressed by their departure and on their return seek contact but do not settle readily.

More recently, Main & Salomon[30] have added an additional classification of insecure infants who display disorganized/disorientated behavior. Such children demonstrate a sequential display of contradictory behavior patterns, e.g. a child in the middle of a display of anger becomes devoid of affect and moves away from the parents. These children also demonstrate simultaneous contradictory behavior patterns, e.g. sitting on a parent's lap for extended periods of time but with their eyes averted and ignoring their parent's verbal attempts at interaction. Other facets of this group are incomplete or undirected movements and expression, including stereo-types, direct indices of confusion and apprehension and behavioral stilling.

When evaluating the child's response in hospital it is important to consider the overt stressful triggers. In addition to already being frightened of strangers, of being in a dark room and of loud noises, which are normal fearful reactions of children between the ages of 4 and 7 years, temporary loss of a parent while undergoing a magnetic resonance imaging scan, or even an X-ray if the mother is pregnant, can be acutely stressful. Discussions with the child prior to coming into hospital will have elicited the child's anxieties and, as a result, appropriate strategies can be adopted in order to minimize the psychological impact on the child.

The same principle is important for outpatient appointments, as children may have all kinds of thoughts about why they are having to come to the hospital. A young child may think that it is a punishment for being naughty. Slightly older children (7 to 10 years) know that the purpose of the treatment is to make them better. Adolescents may experience difficulties as they may have concerns about their physical appearance, their sexuality and enforced dependency. Although children with handicapping conditions are familiar with the procedure for examination by the time they reach adolescence, they also express similar concerns to their able-bodied peers.

It is possible that a child with a handicapping condition will have no option but to experience an inpatient stay either for observation or for medical/surgical treatment. On these occasions, attention has to be paid in order to ensure that the child does not develop psychological problems. Children and their parents may elect to come into hospital, e.g. to loosen a tendon in order to facilitate more functional motor control. Although the child and family are in more control of the situation, it does not protect them from becoming stressed by being in hospital and by having to adjust to what is happening and why they are having to endure the procedure.

DEPENDENCY

The issue of dependency/independency is a crucial one for all children but for those with a chronic illness the issue has heightened significance. Initially, children with diabetes are dependent upon their parents to give them their injections. However, it is possible to promote independence by ensuring that children take responsibility for knowing about the disorder and for being able to give injections themselves as early as possible. Dependency does not have to be an invariable accompaniment of chronic illness, but is related to the nature of the illness. Other researches found epileptic children were more dependent than diabetic children who were no different to healthy controls.

Children who have mental or physical handicaps also have to negotiate the issue of dependency. Parents have to provide a secure base for much longer and have to provide appropriate learning experiences for their children in order to foster their independence. In certain circumstances, young people will never be able to attain full independence from adults. However, this should not prevent them from gaining some privacy and independence from their parents by living in sheltered accommodation if this is what they and their parents wish.

ILLNESS REMISSION

Illness remission occurs for most children. This may be either a favorable response to treatment or a remission of the illness when the symptoms are in abeyance. Such periods may continue for days, months or years. It is at such times that the illness and related matters may retreat into the background and other age-appropriate activities may take precedence. Frequently, parents report concerns about their child's health and also worry about the recurrence of the illness. At these times, parents require much support in order to foster adjustment.

Returning to normal routines such as school and other pre-illness activities, as soon as treatment permits, contributes to psychological adjustment and self-esteem. In addition, it is important to re-establish the old family routines and appropriate disciplines as, paradoxically, poor adjustment is likely to result where parents maintain a permissive attitude with poor limit-

setting as far as the children's behavior is concerned.

Although children with a handicapping condition do become ill and have these adjustment problems, they do not experience a remission in their condition whether it is cerebral palsy, developmental delay or diabetes. Instead parents have to come to terms with visits to other healthcare professionals, e.g. physiotherapists, occupational therapists, podiatrists, in order to enhance their child's development and quality of life. They will have to confront the issue of mainstream or special needs schooling. Later in adolescence the issue of leaving home becomes more complex depending upon the child's level of dependency.

DISCHARGE

A variety of ambivalent feelings may be produced once the treatment is completed; relief that the discomfort and inconvenience have ended but also concern that the protective element has also finished. Families require support in order to foster their own self-reliance and independence of the medical team. It is important at this time to help the child return to a normal pattern of life. Of particular concern to both the parents and children are the problems associated with losing contact with the peer group, falling behind with school work and the types of restrictions that may be placed on recreation.

Parents of children with a handicap do not experience discharge from the medical team in the same way. Depending upon the area in which they live, once young people have reached 16 to 19 years of age, they have to be transferred to the adult services. Children with a physical or mental handicap will be transferred to the appropriate community team. This transfer may be difficult as families lose contact with a set of professionals that they have come to trust. At the same time the family has to make new decisions about the young person's future.

TERMINAL ILLNESS

This is a major area and owing to space constraints will not be discussed here. There is a large body of literature available on this subject. An article by Pettle-Michael & Lansdown[31] and a book by Barbara Sourkes[32] are recommended for those who wish to explore this topic in greater depth.

CONCLUSION

In focusing on the challenges that families have to confront when they have a child with a chronic illness, it is clear that many families adjust and cope well using their own support networks. However, there are some children and families who require positive help in order to find the appropriate strategies to support themselves and each other. It is at this point that mental health professionals have a major role to play. They have to be sensitive to each family's differing coping styles and such professionals must be able to offer help and support without undermining the family's own strengths in this area. To be able to do this requires training and time with the families to gain an understanding of their individual needs.

REFERENCES

1. Cunningham C, Davis H. Working with parents: framework for collaboration. Milton Keynes: Open University Press;1985.
2. Bridges K, Goldberg D. Psychiatric in-patients with neurological disorders: patients' views on discussion of emotional problems with neurologists. BMJ 1984;289:656–658.
3. Wilkinson G, Borsey D, Leslie P, et al. Psychiatric disorder in patients with diabetes mellitus attending a general hospital clinic. Psychol Med 1987;17:515–517.
4. Rosser J, Maguire G. Dilemmas in general practice: the care of the cancer patient. Soc Sci Med 1982;16:315–326.
5. Maguire P, Rutter D. Training medical students to communicate. In: Bennett A, ed. Communication between doctors and patients. London: Oxford University Press;1976.
6. Hardman A, Maguire P, Crowther D. The recognition of psychiatric morbidity on a medical oncology ward. J Psychosom Res 1989;32:235–240.
7. Macguire P. Communication skills. In: Steptoe A, Matthews A, eds. Healthcare and human behaviour. London: Academic Press;1984.
8. Bradford R, Singer J. Support and information for parents. Paediatr Nurs 1991;May:18–20.
9. Melamed BG, Bush JP. Family factors in children with acute illness. In: Turk DC, Kerns KD, eds. Health illness and families: a life span approach. New York: Wiley;1985.
10. Pinto RP, Hollandsworth JG. Using video tape modelling to prepare children psychologically for surgery: influence of parents and costs versus benefits of providing preparation services. Health Psychol 1989;8:79–95.
11. Melamed BG, Siegel LJ. Reduction of anxiety in children facing hospitalization and surgery by use of filmed modelling. J Consult Clin Psychol 1975;43:511–521.
12. Eiser C. Changes in understanding illness as a child grows up. J Child Psychiatry Psychol 1985;31(1):85–98.
13. Miller SM, Green ML. Coping with stress and frustration: origins, nature and development. In: Lewis M, Saarni C, eds. Origins of behavior. Vol 5. New York: Plenum;1984.
14. Dahlquist LLM, Gil KM, Armstrong FD, et al. Preparing children for medical examinations: the importance of previous medical experience. Health Psychol 1986;5:249–259.
15. Kübler-Ross E. On death and dying. New York: Macmillan;1969.
16. Eiser C. Chronic childhood disease: an introduction to psychological theory and research. Cambridge: Cambridge University Press;1990.
17. Wallander J, Varni J, Babani L et al. Family resources as resistance factors for psychological maladjustment in chronic ill and handicapped children. J Pediatr Psychol 1989;14:157–173.
18. Bradford R. Children, families and chronic disease: psychological models and methods of care. London: Routledge;1997.
19. Leventhal H. A perceptual motor theory of emotion. In: Berkowitz L, ed. Advances in experimental social psychology. New York: Academic Press;1984.
20. Skinner TC, Hampson SE. Social support and personal models of diabetes in relation to self care and well being in adolescents with type 1 diabetes mellitus. J Adolesc 1998;21:703–715.
21. Donovan AM. Family stress and ways of coping with adolescents who have handicaps: maternal perceptions. Am J Ment Defic 1988;92:502–509.
22. Dyson L. Adjustment of siblings of handicapped children. A comparison. J Pediatr Psychol 1989;14(2):215–229.
23. Suelzle M, Keenan V. Changes in family support networks over the life cycle of mentally retarded persons. Am J Ment Defic 1981;83(3):267–274.
24. Bibace R, Walsh H. Development of children's concepts of illness. Pediatrics 1980;66:912–917.
25. Robertson J. Young children in hospital. New York: Basic Books;1958.

26. Bowlby J. Attachment and loss. Volume 1. Attachment. London: Hogarth Press;1969.

27. Bowlby J. Attachment and loss, Volume 2. Separation, anxiety and anger. London: Hogarth Press;1973.

28. Sroufe LA. Infant caregiver attachment and patterns of adaptation in preschool: the roots of maladaptation and competence. In: Perlmutter M, ed. Minnesota symposium in child psychology. vol. 16. 41–83 Hillsdale, NJ: Erlbaum;1983.

29. Ainsworth MDS, Blehar M, Waters E, et al. Patterns of attachment: a psychological study of the strange situation. Hillsdale, NJ: Erlbaum;1978.

30. Main M, Salomon J. Discovery of a new, insecure-disorganised/disorientated attachment pattern. In: Yogman M, Brazelton TB, eds. Affective development in infancy. Norwood NJ: Ablex;1986:95–124.

31. Pettle-Michael SA, Lansdown RG. Adjustment to the death of a sibling. Arch Dis Child 1986;61:278–283.

32. Sourkes B. Armfuls of time: The psychological experience of the child with a life threatening illness. London: Routledge;1995.

2

Growth and development

Linda Lang

INTRODUCTION

In podiatry, the structure and function of the lower limb are of primary interest. Many foot pathologies have their origin in early development. For this reason, the understanding of normal patterns of development is essential in order to recognize and clinically manage these pathologies. This chapter will review the phenomena of human growth and development, with particular reference to the lower limb. The review will focus on the development of the lower limb in early intrauterine life, and continue to the conclusion of physical growth in the second decade after birth. The process of ossification and bone growth, which underpins normal growth, will be looked at in some detail. The development of locomotion will be considered with reference to the standard motor milestones. Infant motor progress proceeds in parallel with neurological development, and those functional and structural links, which underpin clinical evaluation, will be highlighted.

INTRAUTERINE GROWTH AND DEVELOPMENT

Despite many technological advances in medicine, estimating the age of the unborn child is still an inexact science. For clinical purposes, pregnancy is conventionally measured from the first day of the mother's last menstrual period. Therefore, a full-term infant is born at 280 days or 40 weeks (plus or minus 2 weeks) after this date.

In embryology, development is measured from conception, the moment when the female oocyte

17

is fertilized by a male spermatozoon. The time of this event is not precisely known. What is known is that the oocyte is viable up to about 24 hours after its release from the ovary (ovulation). Conception may occur between 8 and 20 days after the onset of menstruation; however, for clinical purposes it is assumed to take place around the 14th day. Thus human gestation from fertilization to birth is estimated to be 266 days or 38 weeks. Gestation is conventionally divided into two main stages: the embryonic and fetal periods. The embryonic period is one of initial tissue and organ differentiation. The fetal period begins from the end of the 8th week and culminates in birth. Measurements of the fetus can be used to assess fetal age. However, the flexed position of the lower limbs makes total length difficult to measure. For this reason, the most commonly used linear measurement is crown-to-rump length. In addition, biparietal width of the skull and linear measurement of the femur, and even the foot, have been used as indicators of fetal age.[1] In the 1950s, Streeter[2] developed a system of developmental stages based on physical features, and this is used in embryology to describe the maturity of an embryo. For clinical purposes, gestation may also be subdivided into three monthly periods or trimesters.[2]

Fertilization of the female's egg or oocyte by one of the male's spermatozoa marks the beginning of life. The fertilized egg or zygote takes approximately 7 days to progress along the fallopian tube to the uterus. During this time, the organism undergoes mitotic cell division from a two-cell structure to one that is multicellular, the morula. As the number of cells increase, a split appears in the cell mass and a fluid-filled cavity forms – this is termed the blastocyst stage. The blastocyst eventually embeds in the endometrium (lining of the wall of the uterus). During this period, the cells of the blastocyst differentiate into two masses. The outer mass, or trophoblast, embeds deeper in the endometrium and culminates in the formation of the placenta. The inner cell mass, or embryoblast, forms the embryo. At the beginning of the 2nd week, the embryoblast differentiates into two layers, the ectoderm or outer layer and the endoderm or

inner layer. By the middle of the second week, a third layer – the mesoderm – develops. All tissue and organs of the body develop from these three germinal layers. The ectoderm gives rise to the nervous system, the epidermis of the skin and its appendages. The gut develops from the endoderm. The cardiovascular, lymphatic and musculoskeletal systems together with the dermis all germinate from mesoderm.

Development of the lower limb

The limb buds first appear at about the 4th week after fertilization. The upper limb bud precedes the lower limb bud by almost a week. The relative advance of the upper limb reflects a general cephalocaudal developmental gradient. In fact, the length of the lower limb does not catch up with the upper limb until the second year after birth. The limb buds are located on the anterolateral aspect of the embryo. The lower limb bud is initially level with the umbilical cord and the lumbosacral spinal segments (L2–S3).

The period between 4 and 8 weeks is critical for the normal development of the lower limb. Rapid cell division and tissue differentiation occur at this time. Clinically, it is the most vulnerable period. Certain drugs such as thalidomide are known to be teratogenic and abnormalities may result when the mother takes such drugs during this critical time in the pregnancy. These abnormalities may vary in severity depending on the timing and magnitude of the event. In the case of the lower extremities, there may be total absence of a limb or limbs (amelia), or a segment of the limb may be absent (phocomelia), or there may be deformity of a segment or part.

Initially, the limb bud consists of loose embryonic mesenchyme covered by a single layer of epithelium, the ectoderm. These two components give rise to the majority of subsequent limb tissues and structures. Surface ectoderm forms the epidermis and its associated structures, hair, nails, sweat and sebaceous glands. Mesenchyme forms the dermis, superficial and deep fascia, muscles, tendons, bones, ligaments, blood and lymphatic vessels.

For ethical reasons, most of our current knowledge of tissue and organogenesis is based on animal models. In the process of tissue differentiation, a critical interplay or 'inducing' effect occurs between adjacent embryonic components. For example, the ectoderm is considered to have an inducing effect on the proliferation and differentiation of the adjacent mesenchyme and vice versa. At an early stage of development, ectoderm at the tip of the limb bud is induced by subadjacent mesoderm to thicken and form the apical ectodermal ridge (AER). The apical ectoderm plays a critical role in establishing the initial orientation of the limb bud along its axis, with a cranial or pre-axial border, and caudal or post-axial border. It is also involved in the separation of digits. It appears to influence accretion of mesenchyme and differentiation into tissues such as cartilage. The AER is also involved in the development of the skeletal and of the vascular patterns of the limb.[3]

Between the 5th and 6th weeks, the limb bud becomes segmented, and constrictions appear marking the location of future joints. The terminal segment, the precursor of the foot, initially has the appearance of a paddle, which then develops radial ridges and clefts. These ridges form the digital rays and the clefts become interdigital webs that will recede as the toes separate (Fig. 2.1). At this stage, the upper and lower limbs have the same orientation, with the thumb and great toe appearing on the side of the limb nearest the head (pre-axial borders) of their respective limbs.

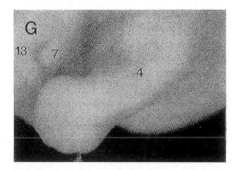

Figure 2.1 Fetus, days 38–40 (reproduced with permission from England M. A colour atlas of life before birth. London:Wolfe;1983).

As these external changes are occurring, internal changes are also taking place. Mesenchyme condenses centrally as a precursor to the development of bone and muscle. Certain bones, e.g. the clavicle, develop directly from this primary tissue by intermembranous ossification. The majority of bones develop by passing through an intermediate stage, where condensed mesenchyme is replaced by cartilage before ossifying (endochondral ossification). Linear growth of all long bones, both pre- and postnatal, is dependent upon viable cartilage cell division. Cartilage cells in the middle of the shaft of long bones begin to hypertrophy then degenerate. The center of the shaft is then invaded by bone-forming cells (osteoblasts) originating from an invading periostial bud. This area is known as the primary center of ossification. Bone is generated progressively outward from these primary centers. Ossification of bones in the lower limb first begins from about the 7th week, with the appearance of a primary center of ossification in the shaft of the femur. By birth, the shafts of all the long bones are ossified. However, their extremities (the epiphyses) are for the most part still cartilaginous.

A number of classical studies, such as those of Straus[4] in 1927 and Gardner et al[5] in 1959, have looked at the development of bones and joints in the foot. Although meticulous, these earlier studies were confined to aborted specimens, which by definition meant that the development of the samples might not have been typical of healthy fetuses. Furthermore, some confusion arises owing to the variety of different methods used to evaluate skeletal development. Nevertheless, these studies provide fascinating and detailed information on the prenatal development of the foot.[4,5]

The skeletal elements of the foot begin to form by condensation of mesenchyme during the 6th week when the embryo is about 0.5 inches (13 mm) crown-to-rump length. Mesenchyme is replaced by cartilage by the end of the embryonic period. The bones of the foot begin to ossify from the 9th week, starting with the lesser metatarsals. By birth, the shafts of all the miniature long bones of the foot (phalanges and metatarsals) are ossified. The short bones of the tarsus ossify by a combination of intramembranous and endochondral processes. Only three tarsal bones begin to ossify before birth. The calcaneus and the talus start to ossify around the 19th and 24th weeks respectively and the center of ossification for the cuboid usually appears, in a full-term pregnancy, at the time of birth. Congenital complete or partial fusion or coalition can occur between any closely adjacent bones such as those of the tarsus, e.g. between the talus and the calcaneus, and between the calcaneus and the navicular.[6]

Postnatal growth of long bones is primarily dependent on an actively dividing cartilage layer located between the shaft and epiphyses, the epiphyseal growth plate. The structure and function of the growth plate are reviewed later in this chapter in the section on postnatal lower limb growth.

Muscle and joint development begin around the same time as bone, i.e. in the 7th week of intrauterine development. The precursor of muscle, condensed mesenchyme, first appears at the root of the limb bud. As the limb bud elongates, mesenchyme progressively condenses along the dorsal and ventral aspects, forming flexor and extensor pre-muscle masses or myotomes. Simultaneously, branches of spinal nerves L2–S3 grow into the limb bud. As these nerves develop, they branch and intermingle to form the plexuses of mixed nerves, which supply the segmental motor myotomes, and sensory dermatomes of the limb. The myotomes in turn segment into different muscles each with their own nerve supply.[7]

Joint formation begins in the undifferentiated areas between the developing cartilage models of the future skeleton, the 'interzonal mesenchyme'. Depending on the type of joint, the interzonal mesenchyme differentiates into different tissue. For example, collagen forms at the sites of future fibrous joints such as the distal tibiofibular joint. In the case of the more complex and functionally important synovial class of joints, the center of the interzone breaks down to form a cavity. Slow generalized movement of the fetus, occurring as early as the 8th week, further promotes this process. The peripheral part of the interzone differentiates into the essential tissues of the joint: synovial membrane which lines the cavity, a surrounding fibrous capsule and associated ligaments. Initially, synovial membrane lines all the internal surfaces of the joint cavity. However, the membrane disappears from the articular surfaces with the onset of motion. Straus suggested that the joints of the foot are defined by at least the 9th week. Joint cavities were reported present as early as the end of the 8th week by Gardner et al in a large study of 184 human embryos and fetuses.[4,5]

The fetal period begins at the end of the 8th week. At about this time, there is a gradual progressive change in orientation of the limbs. Characteristically, the upper and lower limbs rotate in opposite directions. The upper limb twists externally (laterally) and the lower limb twists internally (medially). This twisting or torsion of bone positions the hallux on the pre-axial border medially and the foot moves more toward the midline of the body. At the same time, flexion occurs around major joints. In the lower limb, the hip and knee flex so that the knee points forward and toward the head, while in the upper limb the elbow flexes and points posteriorly and toward the tail. These changes mark the beginning of the fetal period. The twisting of the limbs affects all tissues including the end organs supplied by spinal nerves. An awareness of these early changes is important to understand the complex arrangements of dermatomes and myotomes in the limb and is essential in postnatal clinical assessment of motor function and reflexes. Bony torsion does not end here, but continues to be modified throughout infancy and childhood.

An acceleration in general linear growth characterizes the second trimester, and prenatal growth peaks during the 5th month, at about 20 weeks of gestation. This is a period of particular sensitivity to the developing central nervous system. It should be noted that the human brain continues to develop throughout prenatal life and on into postnatal life. Although reflex movements begin at about the 8th to the 10th week after fertilization, it is not until much later, at approximately the 20th week of pregnancy, that the mother becomes aware of the movements of her unborn child.

Although the number of neurons is already established by the third trimester, the development of the nervous system is far from complete. The spinal cord increases in length and the brain continues to grow in size and complexity. The fetus continues to grow rapidly, but linear growth is now decelerating from peak-velocity in the second trimester. In the latter part of this period, subcutaneous fat is laid down. With a general increase in size of the fetus, there is a corresponding reduction in available space, which in turn restricts movement and increases flexion of the limbs. The lower limbs remain folded in the fetal position with one leg crossing over the other at the level of the ankle (Fig. 2.2). Normally, the feet are still slightly inverted and plantar-flexed. In the early postnatal period, if manually coaxed into a flexed position, the lower limbs will characteristically assume their former fetal position.

Although there is some controversy regarding the natural history of non-neurological congenital foot abnormalities, such deformities are often attributed to intrauterine compression.

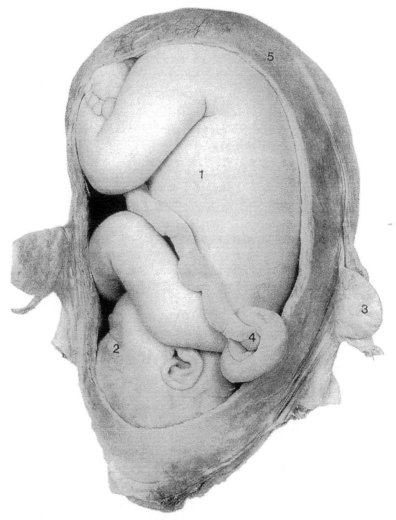

Figure 2.2 Fetus, week 28 (reproduced with permission from England M. A colour atlas of life before birth. London:Wolfe;1983).

Commonly, the foot assumes an extreme of the normal fetal position, e.g. in talipes equinovarus and metatarsus adductus. However, intrauterine molding has also been cited as the probable cause of conditions where the foot is compressed in an atypical fetal position, e.g. in talipes calcanovalgus, where the foot is excessively everted and dorsiflexed. Certain asymmetrical abnormalities are said to be associated with compression of one foot by the other in the folded fetal position.

GROWTH PATTERNS FROM BIRTH TO MATURITY

The posture of the full-term neonate is recumbent with limbs flexed, which reflects the fetal position and intrauterine space restrictions during the weeks leading up to birth. Absence of flexion of the neonatal lower limb is one of the clinical indications of prematurity.[8]

Although birth is a major event and is significant for the onset of certain independent vital functions, it is irrelevant in the continuum of growth. There is a temporary fluctuation in weight in the immediate postnatal period, but linear growth continues uninterrupted. Growth is a defining feature of a healthy childhood. Certain children experience a midchildhood growth spurt, and there is a normal, individual variability in growth patterns. However, overall, the deceleration in growth velocity, which began in the midfetal period, continues until it is reversed by the adolescent growth spurt.

There is considerable individual variability in the age of onset of the adolescent growth spurt, but in general it begins 2 years earlier in girls, at between 8 and 12 years compared to 10 and 14 years in boys. Thus, in early adolescence, girls have a height advantage over boys of the same age. Adolescent growth peaks just prior to the achievement of sexual maturity, which in girls is clearly marked by the onset of menarche. Thereafter, growth rapidly decelerates until it is complete. On average, this occurs between the ages of 16 and 18 years in girls and 18 and 20 years in boys. In boys, the adolescent growth spurt is generally of greater magnitude as well as later than that of girls, enabling them to achieve greater adult stature. Men are on average 5 inches (13 cm) taller than women.

POSTNATAL LONG BONE GROWTH IN THE LOWER LIMB

From birth, secondary centers of ossification begin to appear at the extremities (epiphyses) of long bones. The bony shaft and epiphyses are prevented from uniting by the presence of an intervening cartilage disc, the growth plate. This structure is essential for normal postnatal growth. Cartilage cell division in growth plates is regulated by growth hormone and its mediators and influenced by many intrinsic and extrinsic factors.[9] As long as cell division in the growth plate exceeds the rate of ossification in the shaft and epiphyses, growth will continue. The thigh and leg appear to grow at similar rates after birth. The most active epiphyseal growth plates are those close to the knee, at the distal end of the femur and proximal end of the tibia. Thus, it is bone growth from the distal femoral and proximal tibial epiphyses, which are most important in achieving adult stature.

The growth plate has been described as having layers or zones. Closest to the epiphysis, cartilage cells in zone I form a buffer. Zone II is where maximum cell division occurs and from where cartilage cells are pushed in columns in the direction of the shaft. As they progress into zone III, cartilage cells hypertrophy and die. They then calcify in zone IV and are then invaded by osteoblasts from the shaft and convert to bone in zone V.

As previously stated, while the growth plate is present and active, a long bone can grow. At puberty, growth plates narrow as cartilage production slows and osteoblasts progressively invade. Eventually, the bony shaft and extremity are united and growth ceases. As with the initial appearance of primary and secondary centers of ossification, the closure of growth plates follows a predictable sequence related to the bone age of the child. This is a useful tool in evaluating children with suspected growth disorders. Systems of bone aging based on the tarsal bones of the foot, or more commonly the carpal bones of the hand, are used to determine bone age and predict ultimate stature. The shape of the bone is maintained throughout life by continual remodeling. This remodeling is achieved by hormone control that balances the activity of osteoblasts, and osteoclasts. As osteoblasts lay down new bone, osteoclasts remove excess bone in a constant process of remodeling.

TORSION AND ANGULAR ALIGNMENT OF THE LOWER LIMB

The angular alignment of the thigh and leg changes dramatically during infancy and early childhood. The lower limbs of neonates and young infants are characteristically bowed at the knee (genu varum). This alignment is a continuation of the fetal position and is associated with a wide angle between the neck and shaft of the femur (the angle of declination). By about the age of 3 years, most children have become knock-kneed (genu valgum). These angular changes appear to be associated with the onset of weight-bearing in walking. There is a gradual straightening of the limb during midchildhood. From adolescence onward, there may be a reoccurrence of genu valgum in some girls, which is associated with the width of the female pelvis and is a feature of human sexual dimorphism.

Torsion describes mechanical twisting of a structure about its longitudinal axis. Torsion is seen in the long bones of the lower limb and appears to be unique to human development and has been linked to the development of bipedal gait.[10] It begins with the re-orientation of the limbs at the time of transition from embryo to fetus. The medial or internal twist of the lower limb adducts the feet and brings them together. After birth, torsion of the femur and tibia continues to influence the alignment and angle of the feet in standing and walking. In healthy neonates, the head and neck of the femur are angled forward with reference to the frontal plane. This is referred to as anteversion. In contrast, the tibia at birth exhibits very little torsion. During infancy and childhood, femoral anteversion is gradually reduced so that the adult angle of femoral anteversion is much lower than

that of the neonate – mean angles of 8° to 20° have been reported.[11] During this period, lateral or external torsion, primarily of the tibia, causes the axis of the adult malleoli to be angled externally with reference to the frontal plane. Reported mean malleolar angles range from 10° to over 30° dependent upon the method used. Clinical measurement of this angle in children is even more difficult to achieve and no single measurement method, including computed tomographic imaging, is without error.

Both femoral and tibial torsion contributes to the angle of the feet leaving them slightly abducted in the healthy adult. Intoeing may be associated with delayed or arrested torsion. There appears to be a relationship between the torsion of the thigh and leg bones. For example, in cases where there is insufficient reduction of femoral anteversion, there may be observed greater external tibial torsion. It is important to evaluate the whole limb in clinical decision-making and essential to consider the age and stage of development when treating children with an apparent angular or torsional problems of the lower limb.[10,12]

GROWTH OF THE FOOT

The fetal foot is characteristically triangular in shape with a small narrow heel and wide forefoot. The tarsus accounts for approximately 40% of total foot length. With growth, the foot changes in proportion and shape. The heel grows proportionally longer and broader so that in the adult, the heel projects more and the tarsus accounts for approximately 50% of foot length. This change in proportion is unique to man and is mechanically significant in achieving bipedal stance and walking.[13]

Boys generally have larger feet than girls. In a study of healthy infants, Lang[14] found that from as early as 12 weeks of age, the average foot length in boys appeared to become significantly greater than in girls. Although not conclusive, certain proportional differences in the foot growth were also noted between the sexes. Boys appeared to demonstrate proportionally greater tarsal growth velocity during infancy compared to girls.[14,15]

While the lower extremity lags behind the upper in embryonic development, in adolescence the foot appears to be in the vanguard. The onset of the adolescent growth spurt often occurs first in the foot.[16] During this time, the child's feet rapidly outgrow shoes, and if neglected will be subject to potentially damaging compression. In addition, this acceleration in growth often causes a temporary proportional increase in foot length, which may contribute to the general awkwardness of early adolescence.

It is difficult to measure the human body accurately and all such measurements are prone to error. In children, the interpretation of measurements is further complicated because physiological age does not always correspond exactly to chronological age. Therefore, normal values should only be used as a guideline and never in isolation. Clinical decision-making should involve a consideration of all the evidence.

PROPORTIONAL CHANGES

Substantial proportional changes occur throughout the human growth cycle. The cephalocaudal maturity gradient noted in the embryonic phase gives a vital developmental advantage to the head and upper body, which persists into postnatal life. In the neonate, the head constitutes one-quarter of total length and the lower limbs just over a quarter. During infancy and childhood, the lower limbs generally grow at a higher rate than the trunk, so that they ultimately constitute approximately half of total adult height.[17]

As early as infancy, boys are generally bigger than girls. In a longitudinal study of healthy infants, Lang found that from the 12th week, infant boys in the study sample were on average significantly longer and heavier than the girls were.[14] Surprisingly, no differences were noted in total lower limb length or in the length of the thigh and the leg segments. Few studies have considered growth of the lower limb and foot, and these findings are not conclusive, but they appear to suggest a proportional difference between girls and boys emerging early in infancy.

GENERAL FACTORS INFLUENCING GROWTH IN STATURE

Growth is under genetic control, but gender, race and familial factors will all influence stature, body shape and proportion.[18] The gender differences in growth have already been noted. Generally, tall parents will produce tall children. The average parental height adjusted for gender is used to predict the adult height of offspring.[19] However, illness and disease may confound these genetic influences and prevent the achievement of optimum adult stature.

Certain genetic factors and congenital diseases may cause general growth problems. Dwarfism can be caused by a number of different disorders. Achondroplastic dwarfism is caused by a genetic abnormality that affects cartilage cell growth, most notably in zone II of growth plates. Inadequate cartilage cell division at this site leads to premature closure of growth plates in all long bones. This condition results in disproportionate growth with normal trunk and cranial growth, but short limbs. Pituitary dwarfism is attributed to a failure in growth hormone production, although similar manifestations may be caused by a failure of growth hormone mediators. The result is a general lack of growth leading to overall small stature but with normal proportions. Other hormones, which influence growth, include thyroxin, corticosteroids and adrenosteroids.[20]

Other factors affecting intrauterine growth are maternal disorders such as pre-eclampsia and diabetes. Maternal smoking, drug and alcohol abuse and malnutrition are all known to have adverse affects on growth of the unborn child. Nutrition plays an important part in growth throughout childhood and malnutrition may have a devastating effect on a child's growth and development.[21,22]

Socioeconomic and other environmental factors, which may influence growth, include emotional disturbance and child abuse.[23] Illness, especially chronic diseases, may cause a disruption in growth and a delay or even an arrest of normal growth. However, depending on the nature, intensity and duration of the event, temporary growth disruption is often followed by a period of acceleration known as 'catch-up growth'. This phenomenon brings the child back on, or closer to, the former growth curve.

LOCAL PATHOLOGIES AFFECTING GROWTH IN THE LOWER LIMB

General disturbances in growth of the long bones of the lower limb may affect total stature as seen in achondroplastic dwarfs. However, local disturbance of growth of one limb may result in a consequent limb length discrepancy. The cause may be either congenital or acquired. Genetic research using avian and small mammalian animal models has demonstrated that congenital shortening or ectopic structural formations may be due to failure in the regulation of the expression of specific genes.[24] Those teratogenic agents that disrupt skeletogenesis, particularly when taken during the critical developmental period for the lower limb, may cause growth failure or abnormal morphology. The most devastating effects result from disturbances during the first trimester and in the case of the lower limb between the 5th and 8th weeks. However, less dramatic effects may result from local disruption later in the fetal period. Overgrowth may occur in the presence of an arteriovenous fistula, either posttraumatic or congenital. Disturbance of lymphatic drainage caused by hypoplasia or obstruction of lymphatics may lead to general enlargement of the whole limb.

As previously mentioned, the growth plates above and below the knee are the most active in the body. Factors that may indirectly cause asymmetrical limb length include congenital neuromuscular disorders. Certain disorders such as cerebral palsy produce abnormal position and function of limbs with secondary contractures. Subsequently, this may result in a range of complex motor and cognitive problems where each child has to be assessed individually. Lower motor neuron disorders associated with limb length discrepancies include spina bifida. Spina bifida has a wide spectrum of severity.

Congenital dislocation of the hip (CDH) may result in an apparent limb length discrepancy owing to displacement of the femoral head. CDH ranges in severity and fortunately is usually diagnosed at birth. If neglected, functional consequences related to the severity of the dysplasia will follow. Lack of mechanical forces on the femoral head and on the greater and lesser trochanters has been known to result in underdevelopment of these secondary centers of ossification on the affected side.

Acquired conditions affecting local growth include the development of a local bone tumor. Indirectly, a tumor compressing a spinal nerve may cause limb or foot length discrepancies as well as scoliosis. Poliomyelitis was a common infectious disease prior to the development of successful vaccines in the 1950s. The poliovirus targets the anterior horn cell causing flaccid paralysis. Muscle wasting is a characteristic result of this disease. In young victims, secondary limb length discrepancies often developed owing to asymmetrical paralysis and consequent lack of the mechanical stresses necessary for the promotion of bone development during growth.

Any local disturbance to nerve or blood supply may affect the nutrition of the epiphysis, and result in asymmetrical changes in growth. As the growth plates above and below the knee are the most active in the body, trauma affecting a growth plate, particularly at one of these sites, may result in a segmental limb length discrepancy. A fracture can cause a temporary or permanent cessation of cell division in zone II of a growth plate and may result in premature closure of the plate and/or deformity of the bone. On occasion, a fracture may accelerate local growth because of hyperemia.[25] Hyperemia caused by an arteriovenous fistula may also produce local hyperemia and may stimulate growth on the affected side.

Angular deformities of the lower limb are not necessarily symmetrical and although the actual length of the bones may be equal, any asymmetry in angle may result in a functional limb length discrepancy, e.g. in hyperextension of the knee joint (genu recurvatum) in a child with ligamentous laxity. Bowing of the tibia in Blount's disease may be another underlying cause for a limb length discrepancy and needs timely investigation and treatment. Certain types of trauma may also cause an epiphysis to slip in a growing bone leading to asymmetrical bone deformity. When this occurs, function is usually affected, e.g. a slipped upper femoral epiphysis may limit hip joint motion. However, immediate reduction of the slipped epiphysis will usually resolve the condition without leaving any permanent deformity.

MOTOR DEVELOPMENT

Developmental motor milestones and related factors

Primarily based on the work of Gessell from the 1920s to the 1950s, the sequencing of functional achievements attained from birth through to the age of 6 years has been timetabled into a series of milestones.[26] These cover the development of gross and fine motor skills as well as cognitive and social skills. Such milestones are used to evaluate the child's progress and are directly related to the stages of maturity of the nervous system.[27–29] For this reason, it is important to understand the critical stages of neural development which underpin the child's developmental performance.

The human brain is immature at birth; approximately 85% of brain growth occurs after birth. For example, the cerebral cortex is only one-half of adult thickness and the convolutions, which increase the surface area of the cortex, are not complete. The brain grows from 14 oz (400 g) at birth to 2 lb 3 oz (1000 g) by the end of the first year. Although some of this growth is due to division of glia cells, it is also due to rapid incremental growth of neurons. While axons lengthen, new dendrites sprout and branch in what is termed dendritic arborizations. Through this process, cortical interneuronal connections become increasingly more complex and in turn enable progressive functional development of the infant.

In addition to the growth and development of the neuronal network, progress in postnatal motor development is greatly dependent on myelination of peripheral nerves and spinal tracts. The laying down of this fatty substance around the nerve sheaths enhances nerve conduction. Myelination of regions and tracts in the central nervous system is closely related to the achievement of motor milestones. Myelination of one of the major motor pathways, the pyramidal tract, begins around birth and is largely complete at about 12 to 15 months, the age the average child begins to walk. This is the most intense period of the myelination cycle. However, certain areas of the central nervous system are myelinated before birth and in others this process appears to continue through the second decade.[30] The progress of myelination is more advanced in ascending sensory tracts than in descending motor tracts. This reflects the greater importance of sensory input, both exteroception and proprioception, for effective meaningful movements. It is important to note that neural maturity is related to the child's age from conception and not birth. Thus, in assessing the developmental status of an infant, its maturity at birth, especially if the child was significantly premature, is relevant information.

Reflexes and the development of neurological control mechanisms

At birth, the human infant is unable to perform purposeful movements. Certain primitive reflexes can be elicited at this stage and these reflect the immaturity of the nervous system. In the process of normal development, those reflexes associated with righting and balancing of the body later replace these primitive reflexes, which essentially precede the development of upright posture.

Primitive reflexes are present at birth and are linked to basic survival; they include rooting, sucking, grasping and the startle and Moro reflexes. The startle and Moro reflexes are similar in appearance, but are elicited differently. The startle reflex is a normal response to sudden noise. The Moro reflex may be observed when the infant's head is allowed to drop from a flexed position into extension. In response, the upper limbs of the healthy infant first abduct and extend and then adduct with hands open and the fingers usually curved.

In early infancy, a grasping reflex, similar to that of the hand, may be elicited by stroking the plantar aspect of the foot. The planter response or Babinski is said to be extensor in early infancy, although Illingworth states that an extensor response may be due to poor examination technique and is an abnormal finding even in neonates.[31] Pressure on the heel of the foot will cause a limb extension response. In the first 6 weeks of life, automatic walking and placing are normal features.

Holding an infant vertically over a table so that the plantar aspect of the foot contacts the surface of the tabletop will normally evoke the automatic walking reflex. Holding the infant so that the anterior part of the leg touches the edge of a table will elicit the placing reflex, where the foot is lifted as if to step up onto the table.[31,32]

At this early stage, many similar reflexes can be seen in the upper limb. The infant is incapable of performing righting and saving responses when tilting or falling are simulated during examination. These more complex specialized responses begin to appear in sequence from about the 8th week and precede the onset of independent control.

The labyrinth righting reflexes are linked to the development of purposeful balancing movements. First seen in the head and upper body, these responses lead in turn to the development of purposeful movements. The head-righting reflex usually appears at about 8 weeks and is associated with the infant's ability to lift its head when first lying prone, and later supine. This reflex is the precursor to rolling and sitting. The body-righting reflex appears during the second half of the first year and is critical in achieving upright posture. The landau reflex, in which the head, trunk, hips and knees extend when the child is held in ventral suspension and flex when the head is pushed down, usually appears at about 3 months, but disappears during the early part of the second year. The parachute reaction, in which infants extend their arms in response to a falling motion, may be prompted by holding the child in ventral suspension and performing sudden downward dropping motion. It normally appears just prior to the onset of independent standing and walking, at between 6 and 12 months of age. This is an important saving response which persists throughout life.

Clinical significance of reflex patterns and motor milestones

Absent or abnormal primitive reflexes, or their persistence beyond their normal age span, are considered indicative of a neural pathology. While there is a healthy variability in human development, any delay in the timetable of reflexes and developmental milestones may be indicative of underlying disease, and referral to a pediatrician or a pediatric neurologist is indicated. Congenital neuromuscular conditions such as cerebral palsy may be identified in this way.[33,34] However any serious illnesses and disease in infancy may impact on the child's progress toward maturity. Infants infected with human immunodeficiency virus (HIV), particularly those with a high viral load, are generally observed to be smaller than their non-infected peers. Such children also exhibit comparatively delayed motor and cognitive development.[35] Fortunately, vertical transmission of this disease from mother to baby can now be significantly reduced. The standard of care is for the mother to receive anti-retroviral therapy during pregnancy and labor. At birth, the baby is immediately started on a course of anti-retroviral therapy. This strategy, plus the use of cesarean section to reduce risk of infection during birth, together with bottle- instead of breast-feeding by the mother, has dramatically reduced the incidence of HIV in children in the West. Unfortunately, this prophylactic care is not consistently available to mothers and babies in many developing countries.

The achievement of walking

Milestones that mark the infant's progress measure gross motor development. A number of studies have attempted to chart the achievement of such motor milestones.[17,26–29,31] Surprisingly, there is a marked variation in age at which healthy infants have been reported to achieve

Table 2.1 Variations in reported motor milestone norms

Milestone	Mean age achieved (expressed in weeks)	Age (as originally expressed by authors)	Authors	Year
Rolling	21.0	21 weeks	Lang	1990
	29	7 months	Towen	1971
	12	2.8 months	Frankenberg & Dodds	1969
	30	7 months	Giffiths	1954
	24	24 weeks	Gessell	1952
	29	25–32 weeks	Shirley	1932
Sitting	24.4 weeks	24.4 weeks	Lang	1990
	27	6.18 months	Towen	1971
	24	5.5 months	Frankenberg & Dodds	1969
	30	6–8 months	Giffiths	1954
	30	28–32 weeks	Gessell	1952
	25	20.5–26 weeks	Shirley	1932
Crawling	32.6	32.6 weeks	Lang	1990
		8.5–14.5 months	Towen	1971
	39	9 months	Giffiths	1954
	40	40 weeks	Gessell	1952
	37	32.5–41 weeks	Shirley	1932
Standing supported	38.7	38.7 weeks	Lang	1990
	47	11 months	Towen	1971
	33	7.6 months	Frankenberg & Dodds	1969
	47	11 months	Giffiths	1954
	40	40 weeks	Gessell	1952
	47	47 weeks	Shirley	1932
Walking supported	42.3	42.3 weeks	Lang	1990
	40	9.2 months	Frankenberg & Dodds	1969
	52	12 months	Giffiths	1954
	48	48 weeks	Gessell	1952
	45	40–46 weeks	Shirley	1932
Standing unsupported	50.6	50.6 weeks	Lang	1990
	71	16.4 months	Towen	1971
	42.5	9.8 months	Frankenberg & Dodds	1969
	56	13 months	Giffiths	1954
	56	56 weeks	Gessell	1952
	62	56–66 weeks	Shirley	1932
Walking unsupported	54.6	54.6 weeks	Lang	1990
	78	18 months	Towen	1971
	52.4	52.4 weeks	Frankenberg & Dodds	1969
	61	14 months	Giffiths	1954
	65	15 months	Gessell	1952
	64	59–67 weeks	Shirley	1932

various motor milestones, including walking. While the child's first steps are a landmark event remembered fondly by most parents, the definition of walking used in infant development studies ranges from 7 to 10 consecutive steps and in some studies no definition was stated. Furthermore, certain investigators have relied on parental observation, which may be flawed. Difference in methodology may explain some of the discrepancies between published standards. However, with some exceptions, there does appear to be a trend for more recent studies to report an earlier age for the achievement of walking than studies conducted in the 1940s and

50s. Table 2.1 shows the range of differences from a number of studies, some of which formed the basis of standard clinical evaluation criteria. One of the most recent studies suggests a mean age of just over 12 months for the onset of walking. Racial differences have been noted with children of African origin walking earlier than their Caucasian counterparts. Environment may be influential and greater opportunity for freedom of movement may encourage earlier attempts at independent locomotion. However, there is no known advantage related to early walking and it is not thought to be a reflection of a child's intellectual ability. Furthermore, caution is recommended in the use of early walking aids such as baby-walkers mainly because these devices have been implicated in accidents and related trauma.

SUMMARY

Human development is a dynamic process with its own timetable. There are clearly recognized and defined patterns of normal development which help to guide clinical evaluation. However, when assessing a child, it is important to remember that variability is a characteristic of normal human development. The child's physiological as well as chronological age needs to be considered, together with the birth and the gestational history.

REFERENCES

1. Croft MS, Desai G, Seed PT, et al. Application of obstetric ultrasound to determine the most suitable parameters for the aging of formalin-fixed human fetuses using manual measurements. Clin Anat 1999;12:84–93.
2. Streeter WL. Developmental horizons in human embryos. Age groups XI to XXIII. Embryology 1927 reprint II. Washington DC: Carnegie Institute;1951.
3. Kuhlman J, Niswander L. Limb deformity proteins: role in mesodermal induction of the apical ectodermal ridge. Development 1997;124:133–139.
4. Straus WL. Growth of the human foot and its evolutionary significance and joints of the foot. Embrydogy 1927;19:93–134.
5. Gardner E, Gray DJ, O'Rahilly R. The prenatal development of the skeleton and joints of the foot. J Bone Joint Surg 41A(5):847–875.
6. Antonetti C. Order of appearance of the ossification centers in the foot during the period of intrauterine life in human material. Invest Clin 1997;38(3):127–138.
7. Yamamoto M, Gotch Y, Tamura K, et al. Coordinated expression of Hoxa-11 and Hoxa-13 during limb muscle patterning. Development 1998;125(7):1325–1335.
8. Dubowitz LMS, Dubowitz V, Goldberg BA. Clinical assessment of gestational age in the newborn infant. J Pediatr 1970;77:1–10.
9. Spagnoli A, Rosenfield R. The mechanisms by which growth hormone brings about growth. Growth and Growth Disorders 1996;25:615–628.
10. Lang LMG, Volpe R. Measurement of tibial torsion. J Am Podiatr Med Assoc 1998;88:160–165.
11. Upadhyay SS, Burwell RG, Moulton A, et al. Femoral anteversion in healthy children: application of a new method using ultrasound. J Anat 1990;69:49–61.
12. Fabry G, Cheng LX, Molenaers G. Normal and abnormal torsional development in children. Clin Orthop 1994;302:22–26.
13. Wood-Jones F. The foot. London: Baillière Tindall and Cox;1944.
14. Lang LMG. A longitudinal study of general and lower limb growth in infants. PhD thesis. London: Council for National Academic Awards;1990.
15. Gould N, Moreland M, Trevino S, et al. Foot growth in children aged one to five years. Foot Ankle 1990;10:211–213.
16. Cameron N, Tanner J, Whitehouse R. A longitudinal analysis of the growth of the limb segments in adolescence. Ann Hum Biol 1982;11:211–220.
17. Sun H, Jensen R. Body segment growth during infancy. J Biomech 1994;27:265–275.
18. Ramen S, Tech T, Nagaraj S. Growth patterns of the humeral and femur length in a multiethnic population. International J Gynecol 1996;54:143–147.
19. Tanner JM. Fetus into man. Cambridge, Mass: Harvard University Press;1990.
20. Grant DB. Growth in early treated congenital hypothyroidism. Arch Dis Child 1994;70:464–468.
21. World Health Organization Working Group on Infant Growth. An evaluation of infant growth: the use and interpretation of anthropometry in infants. Bull World Health Organ 1995;73:165–174.
22. Rosenfield RL. Essentials of growth diagnosis. Growth and Growth Disorders 1996;25:743–758.
23. Montgomery SM. Family-conflict and slow growth. Arch Dis Child 1997;77:326–330.
24. Merino R, Macias D, Ganan Y, et al. Expression and function of Gdf-5 during digital skeletogenesis. Dev Biol 1999;206:33–45.
25. Reichard KW, Reyes HM. Vascular trauma and reconstructive approaches. Semin Pediatr Surg 1994;3(2):124–132.
26. Gessell A. The mental growth of the preschool child, a psychological outline of normal development from birth to the sixth year including a system of developmental diagnosis. New York: Macmillan;1925.
27. Shirley MM. The first two years: a study of twenty-five babies. Vol 1: Posture and locomotor development. Minneapolis: University Press of Minneapolis;1931.

28. Griffiths R. Abilities of babies. London: University Press of London;1954.
29. Towen BCL. A study of the development of some motor phenomena in infancy. Dev Med Child Neurol 1971;13:435.
30. Adams RD, Victor M, Ropper AH. Principles of neurology. 6th ed. New York: McGraw-Hill;1996.
31. Illingworth RS. Development of the infant and young child: normal and abnormal. Edinburgh: Churchill Livingstone;1987.
33. Towen BCL. Neurological development in infancy. Clinics in developmental medicine, no 58. London: Spastics International Medical Publications;1976.

33. Darrah J, Redfern L, Maquire TO, et al. Intra-individual stability of rate of gross motor development in full term infants. Early Hum Dev 1998;52(2):169–179.
34. Allen MC, Alexander GR. Using motor milestones as a multistep process to screen preterm infants for cerebral palsy. Dev Med Child Neurol 1997;39(1):169–179.
35. Drotar D, Olness K, Wiznitzer M, et al. Neurodevelopmental outcomes of Ugandan infants with HIV infection: an application of growth curve analysis. Health Psychol 1999;18(2):114–121.

BIBLIOGRAPHY

Adams RD, Victor M, Ropper AH. Principles of neurology. 6th ed. New York: McGraw-Hill;1996.

Larsen WJ. Human embryology. 2nd ed. New York: Churchill Livingstone;1997.

3

History-taking and the physical examination

Peter Thomson

The means by which a history is taken is age-dependent; the younger the child, the more the clinician has to rely on the carer for information. However, even very young children may be able to offer clues. Such clues may be given directly, e.g. in the manner and degree by which the child responds to palpation of a tender area or indirectly as in the case of the child who intoes, by observing the child's posture when sitting or playing.

This chapter will demonstrate the importance of obtaining a comprehensive and cohesive history and carrying out a physical examination before embarking on any management plan for the patient.

GENERAL CONSIDERATIONS

Prior to the first encounter with the patient, consideration should be given to certain intangible factors that may nevertheless help shape the outcome of this and of subsequent visits.

Time

In most cases, the podiatrist has a very short time in which to build a relationship with the patient. This task is made especially difficult when the child is frightened or apprehensive. It should be remembered that for the child, previous visits to clinics may have involved pain or discomfort. Therefore, the child may have preconceived ideas concerning the reasons and likely outcome of the visit. In very young children, it may be helpful not to rush into the consultation. A little time spent getting to know the child and trying to allay any fears will pay dividends later on. It must never be seen as time wasted.

FIRST IMPRESSIONS

Body language sends strong messages to even young children. Watching, listening and adopting an 'open' posture, i.e. sitting with legs uncrossed, arms and hands open, leaning forward and getting close, all convey the impression of warmth and acceptance and that the clinician cares and is interested in the problem.[1]

The clinician should make an introduction to both the parent and the child. The offer of a hand to shake or a reassuring hand on a young shoulder gives the impression of friendliness.[1]

Trust may be created between the clinician and young children by acknowledging their presence early on in the consultation and by having eye contact with them at their level. It is important that the child knows that the purpose of this meeting is for the child.

It has been said that, 'One of the most obvious facts about grown-ups to a child is that they have forgotten what it is like to be a child'.[2] Empathy is an essential personal attribute that the clinician should nurture. Empathy means only that the clinician recognizes and understands the feelings the child is experiencing. If the child can detect that the clinician can appreciate how the child is feeling, then the child is more likely to place trust in the clinician.[3]

The creation of a non-threatening environment is also to be recommended with only essential equipment on show. In addition, paying attention to detail such as the use of color on walls and having available child-size furniture and toys appropriate to the child's age may help to lessen the impact of a clinic visit to an apprehensive young patient.[3] Such measures are also useful in occupying the attention of attending brothers and sisters. However, as most consultations take place in general, non-dedicated clinics, it may not be possible to achieve this objective.

PSYCHOLOGICAL DEVELOPMENT

Up to the age of 6 months, babies are comfortable with strangers and will generally allow you to approach them and to touch them, especially when in close contact with their carer. However, from approximately 6 months to 3 years all children suffer from 'stranger anxiety'. Such children cling strongly to their parents and will become very distressed if any attempt is made to separate them from their carer. With time, the child will venture further away from base and become more adventurous. In the meantime, examinations may be conducted with the child sitting on a parent's lap.[4]

Slightly older children, although wary of strangers and of unfamiliar surroundings, tend to be more cooperative, especially when encouraged to do so by their parents.

Adolescents may be more cooperative but may be less communicative. Young people at this age may also be embarrassed about the changes that are happening to them physically. Therefore, great sensitivity may be required when requesting that articles of clothing need to be removed for the examination.

BEHAVIOR

Inappropriate behavior may be the result of fear. The child may also be expressing more deep-seated worries about family issues such as divorce, terminal illness or a recent death in the family (see Ch. 1).

THE CONSULTATION

The purpose of the consultation is to gather enough information for a management plan to be devised in order that the patient may be relieved of a problem. In a study by Hampton et al[5] in 1975 it was shown that out of 80 patients attending an outpatient department, doctors could make an accurate initial diagnosis in 60 from the medical history alone. However, for the information to be of value, a carefully structured plan of investigation needs to be formulated. Although the questioning needs to be structured, its form should not be too rigid in order to allow patients or parents to express themselves fully.[3]

Suggested essential information would include the following:

Personal details

- Name (including the name by which the child prefers to be known)
- Address
- Contact telephone number
- Date of birth.

Referral details

- Who referred the child?
- Reason for referral?

It is important that this information is read by the clinician before the consultation. To begin the consultation by demonstrating that it is known who referred the child and for what reason signifies to the parents the importance of the current consultation. It also allows the parents to build on previous consultations and to express dissatisfaction about what has gone before and to expand on issues that in their opinion were insufficiently covered.[6] It also shows that the clinician is concerned enough to have taken the time to read the referral sheet and to become familiar with the case. However, it is wise to request that the parents confirm the details of the referral.

Chief complaint

When considering a diagnosis, the following information should be noted:

- Date of onset and pattern
- Duration
- Progression
- Symmetry
- Pain on rest or with activity
- Weakness or limp
- Family history
- Previous treatments.

Date of onset and pattern

It is important to record when the problem was first noted and by whom. Certain gait problems appear worse at times of rapid growth when there may be temporary imbalance between certain muscle groups. Other conditions may be present from birth or first noticed only when the child began to walk.

Duration

For how long has this latest episode been noticed?

Progression

Is the problem static or is it progressively getting worse? In neurological cases, the prognosis may be less favorable when the condition is progressive in nature, e.g. Charcot–Marie–Tooth disease or Duchenne muscular dystrophy

Symmetry

Is the condition one-sided? In intoe, there is almost a 2:1 bias on the left side being affected.[7,8]

Pain on rest or with activity

When considering conditions where pain is a feature, it should be noted whether or not this is aggravated by activity. Systemic conditions, e.g. juvenile chronic arthritis, would involve pain whether the child was at rest or not, as would infection. Sever's disease would typically cause discomfort at heel-strike and be relieved with rest.

It should be recorded at what time in the day the child experiences the pain, i.e. whether on rising from bed in the morning or only as the day proceeds. It is also important to note not only the type of pain but attempts should also be made to quantify the pain. This can be done even with quite young children with visual analogue scales, where the child is asked to mark on a line drawn between two faces – one sad, one happy – where the child considers the pain would lie (Fig. 3.1).

Weakness or limp

A child who presents with a limp should be treated with some urgency. In particular, checks should be made of the hips and referral on to another

Figure 3.1 Visual analogue scale. This simple version is used to quantify pain in young children. They are asked to mark on the black line where they feel their pain would lie.

specialist if appropriate. Weakness in muscle groups, e.g. difficulty in climbing stairs, getting out of chairs or in getting up from the floor, particularly in boys, will have a neurological basis.

Family history

Certain conditions may appear in other family members. It is important that this information is available as it may give clues to the likely outcome if the condition is treated or not and of what secondary problems, if any, have arisen in these people. Such information may also indicate what treatments are likely to be successful.

Previous treatments

It is desirable to be aware of what has gone before in the form of previous treatments by other healthcare professionals and whether or not these treatments are still ongoing. Every effort should be made to obtain copies of treatment records. However, unless clear written notes or prescriptions are available, it may not be unwise to start again and to monitor any progress. Conversely, when such records are available, it cannot be justified to waste any more time repeating unsuccessful treatment plans. However, a new plan of action that concurs with a previous unsuccessful treatment plan is an opportunity for the clinician to consider a differential diagnosis for the complaint.

FULL MEDICAL HISTORY

In order to assess a child thoroughly, a complete past medical history is essential. Since there are

several stages in early life when the child is particularly vulnerable, this history must start with the pregnancy and with details of the mother's health at that time. It should include information about the birth and the delivery, i.e. was it a spontaneous vaginal delivery or was the child delivered by cesarean section? On first impression it may be thought that a child born by section would be less likely to suffer any of the trauma involved by being delivered by the vaginal route. However, cesarean sections are normally carried out for a reason, e.g. fetal distress. Was the child breech? Breech delivery increases the incidence of limb damage, including dislocated hip.

Was the child premature, or did the child go past term? What was the status of the infant at delivery? Was the child cyanosed? Was oxygen required? Did the infant suffer from any convulsions? Was any time spent in the special care unit? How heavy was the child? Was the child's weight appropriate for the gestational age?

In addition to the above, information should be sought about other family members with similar conditions. The logical sequence of investigation should be as follows:

a. Prenatal
b. Birth
c. Immunizations
d. Previous illness or surgery
e. Family history.

Prenatal

Pregnant women are well advised on the risks that certain substances or infectious agents may have on their unborn children. In the early stages of pregnancy, the woman must guard against anything that has the potential to cross the placental membranes and thus exert potentially harmful effects on the embryo. Damage to the child in utero may have adverse effects on neural development and hence on motor control and on locomotion.

Pregnancy

The embryonic period is the period of organogenesis, where systems and organs are being developed. Any insult, no matter how minor, may have catastrophic effects on the developing child at this stage. The fetal period is a period of growth and maturation and is a time when the child is less likely to be damaged by environmental factors. However, because of an increase in size, the fetus may be more at risk from compressional forces.

Human teratogens

A teratogen may be defined as any substance that may by its action cause birth defects.

Drugs and chemicals

Thalidomide. Thalidomide was first patented for use in Germany in 1954. It was prescribed as a sedative and was found to be safe, non-dependent and non-toxic in its clinical dose.[9,10] However, soon after its introduction many children were being born with deformities that in nature were rare occurrences such as amelia and phocomelia. Researchers found that the common denominator in all these cases was the use of thalidomide by mothers in the early stages of their pregnancies. Thalidomide was withdrawn in 1961.[11] However, thalidomide is now being re-introduced into clinical practice as a successful therapy for certain forms of cancer, human immunodeficiency virus (HIV) infections, erythema nodosum leprosum and cutaneous lupus erythematosis.[11–15]

Anticonvulsant drugs. Phenobarbitone and phenytoin have been shown to cause conditions such as talipes equino varus (TEV), polydactyly, metatarsus varus, hypoplasia of the distal phalanges and mental disorders.[16–18]

Sodium valproate and carbamazepine may give rise to an increase in neural tube defects.[18] However, it is reported that 90% of mothers prescribed anticonvulsants can expect a favorable outcome.[19]

Alcohol (ethanol). Chronic alcoholism affects 1–2% of women of childbearing age.[20] The effects on the child of the maternal consumption of alcohol during pregnancy may range from spontaneous abortion to intrauterine growth retardation (IUGR) through to full fetal alcohol syndrome where the child is affected intellectually and will also suffer from craniofacial dysplasia.[17,20–24] There may be no safe threshold of consumption.

Cocaine. Cocaine is a powerful vasoconstrictor and because of this action on the fetal vessels may result in IUGR. Children born to mothers who were cocaine users during their pregnancy also show signs of central nervous system deficit.[17,25,26]

Marijuana (cannabis). Marijuana is a natural substance and pregnant women, with reported incidences of between 3 and 16%, commonly use it. Effects on the fetus include IUGR, congenital anomalies, e.g. syndactyly, TEV and neurobehavioral problems in the newborn, including exaggerated startle reflexes and tremors.[17]

Vitamin A. It has been reported that the high intake of vitamin A in the form of vitamin supplements in the early stages of pregnancy may be associated with an increased risk of malformation.[17] Synthetic retinoids (isotretinoin, etretinate) are strictly contraindicated in pregnancy.[27]

Tobacco. Maternal smoking is a well-established cause of retarded fetal growth.[28] In a heavy smoker (over 20 cigarettes per day), premature delivery is twice as frequent compared with mothers who do not smoke and also their infants weigh less than normal. In active smokers, this results in an average 7 oz (200 g) decrease in birthweight.[29] These women also run the risk of a higher than normal incidence of stillbirth. Nicotine causes a decrease in uterine blood flow thereby lowering the supply of oxygen.[30] The resultant deficit impairs cell growth and may also have an adverse effect on mental development and small but significant differences in balance and fine control.[31] Research has found that passive smoking may also be significant in the health of the fetus and studies are now centered on these effects.[29,32–34] It is reported that a non-smoker living with someone who smokes 20 cigarettes per day will be exposed to at least 1% of that smoker's nicotine levels.[29]

Miscellaneous. In the 1950s, several cases of cerebral palsy were notified along the shores of

Minimata Bay in Kumamoto, Japan. These were traced to the eating of fish contaminated with alkyl mercury compounds, which had been discharged from a factory into the sea.[35]

Infectious agents

Cytomegalovirus. Infection may bring about abortion, growth failure, retinopathy, microcephaly, epilepsy or hearing loss. Cytomegalovirus infection in adults causes mild symptoms.

Rubella. In addition to causing poor fetal growth, infection may also cause malformations of the eye, the inner ear and the heart. The prevalence of infections has decreased in North America and in the UK owing to successful triple vaccination programs for measles, mumps and rubella.

Toxoplasmosis. This is caused by a protazoan parasite (*Toxoplasma gondii*) found in cat excrement. Infection may also be contracted by eating undercooked meat. Toxoplasmosis may affect developing brain tissue.

Herpes simplex type II. Infection may occur during delivery. The virus may affect the child's eyes, central nervous system and liver.

Human immunodeficiency virus. Infection in utero may cause microcephaly and growth failure.

Other factors causing deformity

During periods of rapid bone growth, any abnormal or excessive load applied to that bone may result in its permanent deformity. The fragile embryo is well cushioned against any deforming pressures by being suspended in amniotic fluid, which reaches a peak volume of approximately 1 L at 37 weeks (Fig. 3.2). However, as the child matures, the amount of amniotic fluid decreases. When the pregnancy continues past term, the volume may be as low as 0.5 L at 42 weeks. Fortunately, the fetus becomes increasingly able to resist deformation because of its slowing growth rate and from being less plastic owing to an increase in ossification (see Ch. 2).

Oligohydramnios. Oligohydramnios is a condition where the total amount of amniotic fluid is less and the peak volume reached earlier. Infants born to such women have been recorded as

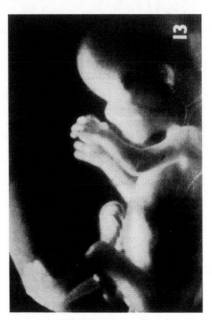

Figure 3.2 Fetus in utero suspended in amniotic fluid. Note also position of feet and legs.

having an increased incidence of postural birth deformity, e.g. oligohydramnios owing to fetal renal agenesis in Potter syndrome causes severe compression on the fetus resulting in TEV, multiple joint contractures, plagiocephaly, torticollis and developmental dysplasia of the hip.

Position of the feet and legs. The normal foot/leg position is knee–chest with the feet dorsiflexed at the ankle (Fig. 3.2). Such a position is a strong kicking position; one that will enable the fetus to stretch and to deflect abnormal external forces away. The legs and feet of a child who adopts a breech position are at a distinct mechanical disadvantage when trying to redirect such forces (Fig. 3.3). A breech position may also lead to an increased incidence of dysplasia of the hip.

Malformation. The limbs may already be flail because of spinal muscular atrophy or dystrophia myotonica or from neural tube defects such as spina bifida. In such cases, the legs and feet may be held in such an abnormal position throughout the pregnancy as to cause great deformity.

Multiple pregnancy. The more infants there are, the less space any individual will have to move around (Fig. 3.4).

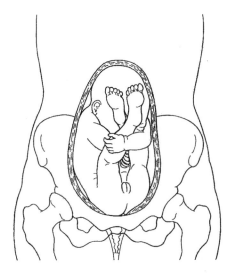

Figure 3.3 Breech position.

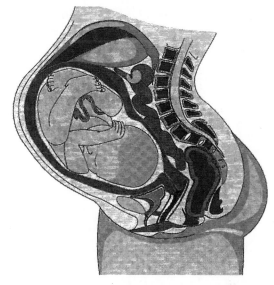

Figure 3.5 Prima gravida: fetus tight against maternal spine

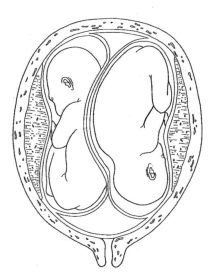

Figure 3.4 Multiple pregnancy.

Prima gravida. Dunn[36] reported that there was a higher incidence of postural deformity in the firstborn than in subsequent births (54% : 35%). He attributed this finding to well-toned abdominals in the young mother keeping the fetus tight against the immovable maternal spine, hence lessening the space in which the child had to move and grow (Fig. 3.5).

Birth

Examples of neonatal injury:

- *Dislocation* of the hips from breech presentation.
- *Palsies* of arms and legs from breech presentation.
- *Edema* of skull.
- *Hematoma* (cephalhematoma) which may take several weeks to subside.
- *Intraventricular hemorrhage* may be found in premature babies because of the friable cerebral vasculature of these infants. This type of bleeding may result in cerebral palsy.
- *Subarachnoid hemorrhage* is commonly due to a compressional head injury after a prolonged and difficult labor, e.g. from a baby that is very large for its gestational age. This type of bleeding has serious implications. Frequently, babies damaged in this way appear quite normal for some time but then they may become hypotonic and their reflex actions diminish. Muscle tone is a very good indicator of brain-damaged infants as their legs can be seen to be held in marked extension. Gradually, such children become very irritable, do not like to be handled and may fit.

- *Asphyxia* damages brain cells and interferes with brain function by compromising the patency of the blood vessels.

Stimuli to breathe

Temperature change. The infant leaves a steady environment of 37° to one of only 25°. As the head appears, it is cooled, and peripheral thermoreceptors on the skin stimulate the hypothalamus to initiate respiration.

Passage through the birth canal. As the infant's chest is squeezed through the birth canal, fluid is forced from the lungs; the arms are released and, as a result of a recoil action, air is sucked in.

Cord clamping. The effect of clamping the umbilical cord is to raise the blood pressure, reduce arterial oxygen (Po_2) and increase arterial carbon dioxide (Pco_2). Respiratory chemoreceptors in the carotid bodies monitor changes in these blood gases and also in blood pH and they respond to both low levels of Po_2 and to high levels of Pco_2 by initiating a reflex action in the lungs in order to maintain homeostasis.

Catheter insertion. If there is still no response from the child, a catheter is inserted into the airway in order to stimulate and to aid in respiration. The insertion of the catheter may be a sufficient irritant to provoke the child to breathe.

Apgar scoring system. Babies are assessed 1 minute after delivery and again at 5 minutes by a system devised in the early 1950s by Dr Virginia Apgar.[37] Her scoring system highlighted those children who would need resuscitation at birth and who would therefore run the risk of suffering some handicap (Fig. 3.6).

- The child who scores between 0 and 3 requires vigorous resuscitation.
- The child who scores between 4 and 6 requires some assistance.
- The child who scores between 7 and 10 needs no intervention.

It is likely that children who score low, especially at 5 minutes, will end up with some degree of handicap.

Postnatal influences

Prior to skeletal maturity, the child is not a static structure. The child grows not only in a linear fashion, but the bones of the lower limb also unwind and derotate. It is possible to use such information to advantage, e.g. in serial casting or when using splints. However, the same principles that help bring about correction may also be the cause of many of the gait problems for which parents consult.

After birth, many children commonly adopt 'positions of comfort'. This may be observed at its most obvious in the prone newborn who sleeps in a knee–chest position with the feet

POINTS	2	1	0
COLOUR	Completely pink	Pink with blue extremities	Blue or white
HEART RATE	> 100 bpm	< 100 bpm	Absent
RESPIRATION	Crying lustily	Shallow and irregular	Absent
MUSCLE	Active movement	Some flexion of extremities	Flaccid
REFLEX IRRITABILITY	Cough	Grimace	Nil

Figure 3.6 Apgar scoring system.

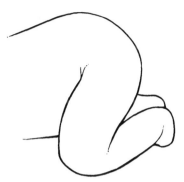

Figure 3.7 Typical newborn knee–chest position.

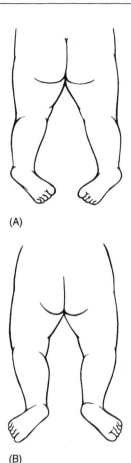

(A)

(B)

Figure 3.8 Typical sleeping positions giving rise to gait problems. (A) Hips extended, internal rotation, ankle equinus. (B) Hips extended and in external rotation with abduction of feet.

crossed at the ankles, the position the child had been molded into in utero (Fig. 3.7). Unfortunately, such a position encourages low tibial position, equinus at the ankle and metatarsus adductus. A similar foot and leg type may be seen in children who prefer to kneel. Hutter & Scott[38] observed that a low tibial torsion and adducted foot type was common in the Japanese population because of their propensity to kneel.

Sleeping positions may also give rise to undesirable leg and foot positions. For example, internal tibial torsion, ankle equinus and adduction at the forefoot encourage an intoe gait and/or toe-walking which may be the result of allowing the child to sleep prone with the hips in extension and the feet internally rotated. Conversely, an abducted gait can be encouraged when the child lies prone with the hips in extension and the feet externally rotated. Such a position forces the hips into external rotation with lateral torsion on the tibiae and a valgus attitude to the feet (Fig. 3.8A, B).

Children who exhibit marked ligamentous laxity may also show a preference to sit in a particular position of comfort, i.e. the reversed tailor or 'W' position (Fig. 3.9). Sommerville[39] described how the normal unwinding of the femoral neck takes place as a result of the torsion exerted on it by the normally tight hip capsule during that time when the infant's leg position changes from the early knee–chest to one that is in extension. When ligaments are lax, this torsion does not take place and the fetal internal femoral torsion persists. In such children, it is not only comfortable, but it is natural to sit this way. However, by doing so, these children prevent, or at the very least delay, the unwinding of this segment. In addition to persistent internal femoral torsion, an excessive external force is directed to the distal tibial epiphyses.

Immunizations

Immunization is one of the single most important developments in the promotion of child health. For example, since the introduction of immunization, smallpox has been eradicated and cases of polio have dropped from reported highs

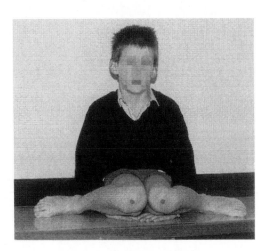

Figure 3.9   Reversed tailor or 'W' position.

of 8000 in 1 year in the late 1940s and early 1950s in England and Wales to only 25 in the 10 years from 1980–1989. Similarly, in the USA, notifications of outbreaks of measles (vide supra) have dropped from nearly 800 000 in 1958 to only 138 confirmed cases in 1997.[40] Therefore, immunization uptake should be encouraged and noted.

Previous illness or surgery

A concise history of previous illness or surgery may give insight to the present wellbeing of the child. At this stage of the consultation, details of any systemic or endocrine disorders such as diabetes mellitus should be noted and any bone disorders such as osteogenesis imperfecta identified. Children who suffer from osteogenesis imperfecta may be of short stature and may already have a considerable history of multiple fractures of the lower limbs, some of which may have involved the epiphyses of the long bones.

Notes should also be made of any adverse reactions to drugs or of any other known allergies.

Family history

In order to assess the child fully, an account should be made of the family history. This is important for three main reasons:

1. It highlights other family members with the same complaint and it may instigate the screening of other siblings.
2. It assists in assessing the value of particular treatment methods for that condition from what has gone before.
3. It also acts as an indicator of possible secondary effects as a result of unsuccessful treatments or of neglect.

PHYSICAL EXAMINATION

The physical examination takes place before the child enters the consulting room. Ideally, the clinician should try to observe the child unawares, e.g. while still in the waiting area and the clinician should pay particular attention to the child's posture and general demeanor while the child is in a relaxed state. Where possible, the clinician should then escort the parent and the child to the room where the examination will take place. If the child is walking, it is during this period that the first assessment of the child's gait will take place. Once again, the child should be unaware that such an observation is being made.

Review of systems

Every opportunity should be made at the first consultation to conduct a review of major systems. Examinations should be quick and efficient. Enough clothing should be removed in order to allow effective visualization of the part in question. Children should be requested to undress themselves with or without the assistance of a parent. Even young children will feel uncomfortable with a stranger removing their clothes. Young children will also feel very nervous about lying flat. Therefore, that part of the examination which requires the child to be supine should be left until last. Simple explanations should be given to the child of what is about to take place.

Dermatological review

The most readily available structure to examine is the child's skin. Observations should be made of the color and integrity. Notes should be made of any bacterial, fungal or viral infections. Similarly, any eruptions or frank disease such as psoriasis or eczema should be mapped and recorded, as should any medication, systemic or topical, that has been prescribed. It should be remembered that severe eczema of the flexure creases of the knee may inhibit full stretch of the knee in the swing phase of gait. This will naturally contribute to an abnormal gait pattern. Likewise, any stretching program given for tight hamstrings in such a child will be doomed to failure.

As a general rule, the younger the child, the more clothing that needs to be removed for the examination. Advantage should be taken of this to examine as much of the child as possible, including the lower back. Any dimples or sinuses or hairy tufts in the lower back should alert the clinician to spina bifida occulta. A description of the more common skin afflictions can be found in Chapter 8.

Vascular examination

A quick assessment of the vascular supply is readily done by noting digital color, capillary filling time and by running the backs of the hands down both the child's legs to the toes. Notes should be made of any differences in temperature between one leg and the other. Vasospastic disorders such as chilblains or Raynaud's, which is more common in females, should also be recorded. Enquiries should be made of adolescents suffering from such disorders as to whether or not they smoke. Discretion is advised since it is not only unlikely that any underaged patients will voluntarily offer such information in the presence of a parent but they may view being put in this position as a breach of trust. However, it is essential that the facts are established in order that the appropriate health education message is delivered, especially as to the effects of nicotine on the peripheral circulation.

Pedal pulses are also readily detected in children recording, when necessary, rate, rhythm and volume. Below 1 year a child's pulse rate is between 110 and 160 beats per minute (bpm). Between 2 and 5 years, it is between 95 and 140 bpm and from 5 to 12 years, it is between 80 and 120 bpm. These figures will be increased by fever or stress.[41]

Neurological examination

A comprehensive account of pediatric neurology may be found in Chapter 7. However, what follows is the type of routine examination that may be carried out in all infants, as part of a first assessment. Initially, the child's motor development may be assessed in one of two ways: (1) developmental reflexes and (2) developmental milestones.

A child is born with certain reflexes such as rooting, coughing and yawning. Other reflexes are dependent upon myelinization of the corticospinal tracts, e.g. Babinski (see also Ch. 7). Noting the timing and the quality of certain milestones and reflexes may assist in assessing normal development. The spectrum of normal in respect of a child walking unsupported is great. Parents may report that their child walked as early as 11 months or as late as 15 months. However, if a parent presents with a child who is unable or unwilling to walk at 18 months (two standard deviations from the mean), investigation directed at the child's hips plus a full neurological workout are indicated. In addition, further enquiry regarding the achievement of other milestones may also be useful, e.g. sitting unsupported. The child should be sitting unsupported by 10 months at the latest. However, it may be that all milestones were reached late.

Milestones should therefore be viewed with caution. For instance, it does not follow that a child who does not crawl is not eventually going to walk. Hence, any milestone should be considered as a 'snapshot' of the child's development at that time only and should be weighted against other information. For example, primitive reflexes are spinal reflexes and give no indication of damage to higher centers whereas irritability, hypotonia or hypertonia, a high-pitched cry or convulsions are more likely to be associated with cerebral injury.[18]

Developmental reflexes.

Cortical thumb position. When born, the child will hold the hand in a fist, with the thumb enclosed by the fingers. It is an abnormal finding to have continual, tight fist-clenching or when the above thumb position continues past 4 months (Fig. 3.10).

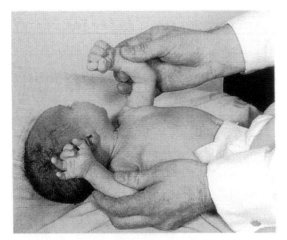

Figure 3.10 Cortical thumb position.

Moro reflex. While holding the child securely and in a position facing the examiner, the Moro reflex may be induced by suddenly dropping the child's head backwards 2 to 3 inches (5 to 7.6 cm). The examiner should look for symmetry of movement from the arms as they are flung into extension and abduction. At the same time, the hands should open and the legs should extend. The same symmetry should be seen as the legs and arms are drawn back into flexion at the end of the test (Fig. 3.11). Because of the nature of this test, it is likely the child will cry. Therefore, testing for the Moro reflex is best done at the end of the assessment. The Moro response is normally not observed past 5 months of age by which time it is considered to be abnormal.

Asymmetrical tonic neck reflex. With the child lying supine, the head is first placed in the midline, then turned to one side. On doing this, it may be seen that the arm the head is turned towards extends, while the other arm flexes, i.e. the 'en garde' position (Fig. 3.12). This reflex

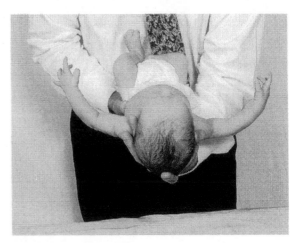

Figure 3.11 Moro reflex.

should not be present beyond 6 months. After this time, the reflex is always abnormal.

Plantar grasp. The plantar grasp is similar to the palmar grasp whereby placing an object (examiner's finger) in the palm of the child's hand elicits strong flexion of the fingers around the object. The toes will flex in a similar fashion when the same stimulus is given to the area around the webbing of the toes, on the plantar aspect of the foot. This response disappears between 9 and 12 months; the palmar grasp at around 8 months.

Plantar response. The classic, positive, Babinski response may be difficult to isolate from a withdrawal response to the stimulus, therefore the value of this test in the newborn is in doubt by many clinicians. In addition, certain authors[42]

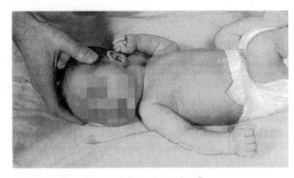

Figure 3.12 Asymmetric tonic neck reflex.

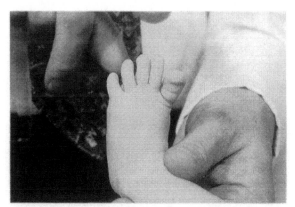

Figure 3.13   Plantar response – positive Babinski or poor technique?

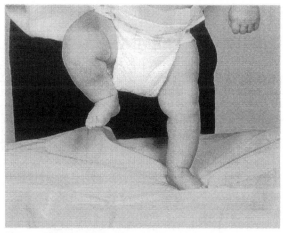

Figure 3.14   Stepping reflex.

believe that until 6 months a positive sign, i.e. the hallux in extension, is normal in infancy whereas others consider a true positive to be abnormal at any age[43,44] (Fig. 3.13).

The stepping response. The child is held over a table top or other firm surface. On making contact with the surface with the soles of the feet, the child will extend one leg while simultaneously making a stepping movement with the other. When this leg comes back down onto the table, the supporting leg will then make the same movement. This reflex is lost at approximately 8 weeks (Fig. 3.14).

Tendon jerks. Patellar and ankle jerks are both present at birth.

Myelinization. Myelinization proceeds in a cephalic to caudal direction. As this process matures and power is developed in muscle so

---

Significant developmental milestones (see also Appendix VI, p 359)

Birth
- When the child lies prone, the head is turned to one side and there is flexion of the hips and knees.
- Head control is absent.

6 weeks–2 months (Fig. 3.15A, B)
- Hips are now much less flexed.
- When lying supine, the heels can reach the supporting surface.
- The child can sit with assistance but is very unstable.

4 months
- The child can raise the head when lying prone.

5 months
- The child can extend the upper limbs when lying prone.

6 months
- The child can self-support with the hands when lying prone.
- The child can roll from prone to supine.

7 months (Fig. 3.16A, B)
- The child is able to sit unassisted.
- The child can reach the mouth with the toes.
- The child can roll back into prone.

9 months
- The child begins to crawl and can stand momentarily.

11 months
- The child can walk upright with double support.

12 months
- The child can walk with single support.

13 months
- Using a wide base for support, the child can squat in order to pick up a toy (Fig. 3.17).

15 months
- The child can walk, kneel and stand up unaided (Fig. 3.18).

2 years
- The child can climb stairs without help, two feet per step.
- The child can run and jump.

3 years
- The child can now run and hop.

4 years
- The child can walk downstairs one foot per step.

5 years
- The child is able to skip.

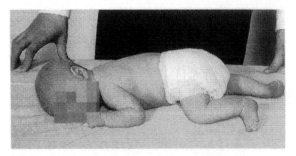

(A)

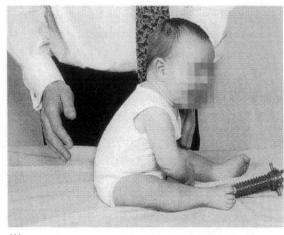

(A)

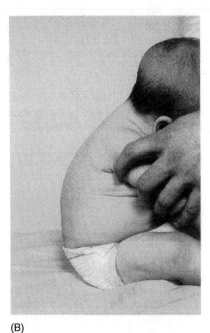

(B)

Figure 3.15 (A) Baby aged 6 weeks. Hips much less flexed than in the newborn. (B) Baby aged 6 weeks. The baby can sit with assistance but is very unstable. Note lack of back contour.

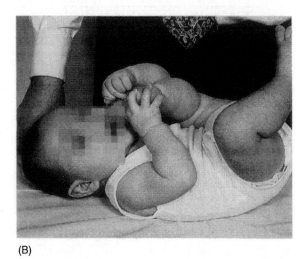

(B)

Figure 3.16 (A) Baby aged 7 months. The baby can sit unassisted. (B) Baby aged 7 months. The baby can reach the mouth with the toes.

the ability to resist gravity is greater. This process may most easily be seen with head lag. (Fig. 3.19A, B, C). In certain children, e.g. with cerebral palsy, this head lag may persist for much longer than that indicated or it may never be lost.

Orthopedic examination

If the child is walking, it is important to assess the child's footwear and to try to analyze the wear pattern on the shoes. For example, exces-sive wear on the posterior heel is suggestive of a calcaneal gait; wear on the medial heel, of a foot that is hyperpronating. Wear at the tip of the sole may indicate a child with a neurological problem, i.e. a spastic gait with weak evertors/dorsiflexors or it may simply demonstrate a shoe that is too small. This in itself may contribute to an abnormal gait especially of intoe.

Wear from a lateral heel to a medial sole is normal. However, when this pattern is excessive, together with distortion of the uppers, it demon-

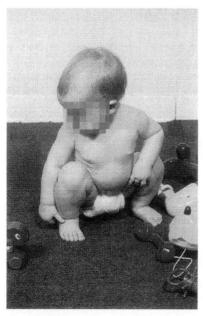

Figure 3.17   At 13 months, the infant is confident enough to squat to pick up a toy.

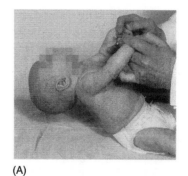

(A)

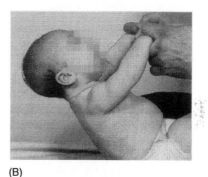

(B)

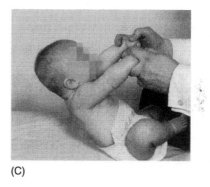

(C)

Figure 3.19   Head lag. (A) Newborn. (B) Aged 6 weeks. (C) Aged 6 months.

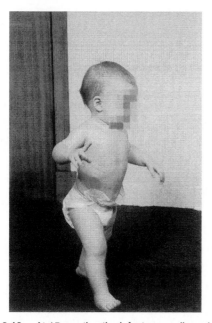

Figure 3.18   At 15 months, the infant can walk unaided

strates a foot that is not recovering after mid-stance and therefore one that is pronating throughout the stance phase. Clinical examina-tion may typically show a child with excessive tibial torsion. It is not uncommon to find in such cases measurements in excess of 40° external rotation at the malleoli.

Lateral wear on the heel and sole is of a foot that is supinating throughout the gait cycle, com-monly as the result of an uncompensated hind-foot varus. In such children, there may be a history of lateral ankle injury.

Finally, judgment must be passed on the shoe's suitability and the importance of appropriate footwear must be relayed to the parents and to the child.

A full account of developmental biomechanics may be found elsewhere in the book. However, all clinicians involved in podopediatrics should familiarize themselves with assessing the infant hip. Such is the dire consequence of a missed hip dysplasia that every opportunity should be taken to test for range and quality of motion at the hip. Further discussion may be found in Chapter 11.

MANAGEMENT PLAN

Children should be involved in the discussion of their treatment at a level appropriate to their comprehension. The problem should be explained in jargon-free language that the child (and the parents) can understand and realistic, achievable goals then set. This should include an outline of what is realistic for the podiatrist to achieve and equally important what is expected of the child in order for these goals to be met.

REFERENCES

1. Kent G, Dalgleish M. Psychology and medical care. 3rd ed. Saunders, London;1996.
2. Jarrell R. Third book of criticism. New York: Farrer, Strauss and Giroux;1965.
3. Myerscough DR. Talking with patients–a basic clinical skill. Oxford: Oxford Medical;1989.
4. Levene M. In: Levene M. ed. Jolly's diseases of children. 6th ed. London: Blackwell Scientific;1991.
5. Hampton JR, Harrison MJG, Mitchell JRA, et al. Relative contributions of history taking, physical examination and laboratory investigations to diagnosis and management of medical outpatients. BMJ 1975;ii:486–489.
6. Newell R. Interviewing skills for nurses and other health care professionals. London: Routledge;1994.
7. Dunn P. Congenital postural deformities: further perinatal associations. Proc R Soc Med 1974;67:1174–1178.
8. Tax H. Podopediatrics. 2nd Ed. Baltimore: Williams and Wilkins;1985.
9. Taussig H. A study of the German outbreak of phocomelia: the thalidomide syndrome. JAMA 1962;180:1106–1114.
10. Lenz W. A short history of thalidomide embryopathy. Teratology 1988;38:203–215.
11. Miller MT, Strömland K. Teratogen update: thalidomide: A review, with a focus on ocular findings and new potential uses. Teratology 1999;60:306–321.
12. Benchikhi H, Bodemer C, Fraitag S, et al. Treatment of cutaneous lymphoid hyperplasia with thalidomide: report of two cases. Am Acad Dermatol 1999;40(6P+1):1005–1007.
13. Duong DJ, Spigel GT, Moxley RT 3rd, et al. American experience with low dose thalidomide therapy for severe cutaneous lupus erythematosis. Arch Dermatol 1999;135(19):1079–1087.
14. Larkin M. Low dose thalidomide seems to be effective in multiple myeloma (news). Lancet 1999;354(9182):925.
15. Ollivier S, Bonnet J, Lemann M, et al. Idiopathic giant oesophageal ulcer in an immunocompetent patient. The efficacy of thalidomide treatment. Gut 1999;45(3):463–464.
16. Loughnan PM, Gold H, Vance JC. Phenytoin teratogenicity in man. Lancet 1973;i:70–72.
17. Briggs GG, Freeman RK, Yaffe S. Drugs in pregnancy and lactation: a reference guide to fetal and neonatal risk. 5th ed. Baltimore: Williams and Wilkins; 1998.
18. Johnston PGB. The newborn child. 8th ed. Edinburgh: Churchill Livingstone;1998.
19. Malone FD, D'Alton ME. Drugs in pregnancy: anticonvulsants. Semin Perinatol 1997;21(2):114–123.
20. McKnight A, Merrett D. Alcohol consumption in pregnancy: a health education problem. J R Coll Gen Pract 1987;37(295):73–76.
21. Wright JT, Barrison I. Alcohol and the fetus. Br J Hosp Med 1983;March:260–266.
22. Jones KL, Smith DW, Ullebrand CN, et al. Patterns of malformation in offspring of chronic alcoholic women. Lancet 1973;i:1267–1271.
23. Johnson VP, Swayze VW II, Sato Y, et al. Fetal alcohol syndrome: craniofacial and central nervous system manifestations. Am J Med Genet 1996;61(4):329–339.
24. Bagheri MM, Burd L, Martsolf JT, et al. Fetal alcohol syndrome: maternal and neonatal characteristics. J Perinat Med 1998;26(4):263–269.
25. Plessinger MA, Woods JR Jr. Cocaine in pregnancy. Recent data on maternal and fetal risks. Obstet Gynecol Clin North Am 1998;25(11):99–118.
26. Richardson GA, Hamel SC, Goldschmidt L, et al. Growth of infants prenatally exposed to cocaine/crack: comparison of a prenatal care and no prenatal care sample. Pediatrics 1999;104(2):18.
27. Monga M. Vitamin A and its congeners. Semin Perinatol 1997;21(2):135–142.
28. Butler NP, Goldstein H, Ross EM. Cigarette smoking in pregnancy: its influence on birthweight and perinatal mortality. BMJ 1972;ii:127–130.
29. Law MR, Hackshaw AK. Environmental tobacco smoke. Br Med Bull 1996;52(1):22–34.
30. Economides D, Braithwaite J. Smoking, pregnancy and the fetus. J R Soc Health 1994;114(4):198–201.
31. Trasti N, Vik T, Jacobsen G, Bakketeig LS. Smoking in pregnancy and children's mental and motor

development at age 1 and 5 years. Early Hum Dev 1999;55(2):137–147.

32. Roquer JM, Figueras J, Botet F, et al. Influence on fetal growth of exposure to tobacco smoke during pregnancy. Acta Pediatr 1995;84(2):118–121.

33. Fortier I, Marcoux S, Brisson J. Passive smoking during pregnancy and the risk of delivering a small for gestational age infant. Am J Epidemiol 1994;139(3):294–301.

34. Jauniaux E, Gulbis B, Acharya G, et al. Maternal tobacco exposure and nicotine levels in fetal fluids in the first half of pregnancy. Obstet Gynecol 1999;93(1):25–29.

35. Matsumoto H, Koya G, Takeuchi T. Fetal minimata disease: a neuropathological study of two cases of intrauterine intoxication by methyl mercury compound. J Neuropathol Exp Neurol 1965;24:563.

36. Dunn P. Congenital postural deformities. Proc R Soc Med 1972;65:735–738.

37. Apgar V. Proposal for a new method of evaluation of newborn infants. Anesth Analg 1953;32:260–267.

38. Hutter CJ Jr, Scott W. Tibial torsion. J Bone Joint Surg 1949;31A:511–518.

39. Sommerville EW. Persistent foetal alignment of the hip. J Bone Joint Surg 1957;39B:106–113.

40. Morbidity and Mortality Weekly Report. Measles – United States 1997. MMWR 1998;47(14):261–273.

41. Curtis N, Klein N. In: Lissauer T, Clayden G, eds. Illustrated textbook of paediatrics. London: Mosby;1996.

42. Gingold M, Jaynes M, Bodensteiner J, et al. The rise and fall of the plantar response in infancy. J Pediatr 1998;33(4):568–570.

43. Forfar J, Arneil G. Textbook of paediatrics, vol I. 3rd ed. Edinburgh: Churchill Livingstone;1985.

44. Illingworth RS. Development of the infant and young child: normal and abnormal. Edinburgh: Churchill Livingstone;1987.

4

Pediatric gait

Russell G. Volpe

The typical clinician is more comfortable observing the gait of adults than that of children. After all, a reference model for 'normal' gait exists for the adult, enabling easy comparison of any patient to that standard. Clinician discomfort associated with watching children walk and trying to make meaningful assessments stems from difficulties identifying what is normal and at what age. The development of mature, adult-like gait in a growing child is an ongoing process tied closely to maturation of the nervous system and growth of the lower extremity. The clinician needs to be familiar with the intricacies of this ongoing process in order to identify the child with variations in gait that, at particular ages, may be associated with pathology. Furthermore, the child is not a 'mini-adult' and it is important to know the many differences in normal gait between these two groups.

Pediatric patients with lower extremity concerns may be classified into two groups:

1. The infant under 1 year of age who does not bear weight and, consequently, most of the problems seen are congenital in nature.
2. The toddler, who at about 1 year of age, starts to walk and it is around this time that the family may show concerns about how the child walks. Anxieties may run high with reference to 'normal' gait as the journey to mature, adult ambulation begins. Parents see a wide-base, significant bow, and noticeable out-toe. They are often concerned that these are abnormalities that may impair the child's growth, development and normal function.

The first step in identifying when a pathological or abnormal gait event may be present in a child is to understand the development of gait over the early years of walking.

GAIT OF THE 1-YEAR-OLD

The gait of the earliest walker, at approximately 1 year of age, is typically abrupt and choppy. To assist with balance and support, the base of gait is wide during double limb support. This has been described as a low pelvic-span:ankle-spread ratio.[1] This relationship may also be defined as the base of gait and is about 70% of the pelvic width at the age of 1 year.

Single support is 32% of the gait cycle in the 1-year-old as compared to 38% in the average adult.[1] This is sometimes referred to as a high stance to swing ratio. Immaturity of the motor control system contributes to a lower percentage of single support in the gait of an early walker. The step length is also short in the new walker (average 7.8 inches (20 cm)). A lack of stability in the support limb may be the reason for the short step length. The lack of balance, weakness of the ankle plantar flexors or lack of control of muscles creates instability of the support limb. This lag or lack of muscle control may play the greatest role in creating instability in the new walker. The pattern of myelinization in the developing human is known to be cephalocaudad.[2,3] This places the lower extremity behind the trunk and upper body in maturation of the nervous system which may lead to this early instability found in the new walker. The short single support phase may also correlate with the instability in the immature walker with a short step length.[4]

As a consequence of this lack of neuromotor stability, the cadence is increased (average 180 steps per minute) and the walking velocity is slow (average 66 yards (60 meters) per second).[4] The upper extremities are held stiffly, with elbow extension and abduction. Reciprocal arm swing with contralateral footstep, a hallmark of gait maturation, is notably absent in the earliest walker.

Swing phase

In the sagittal plane during the swing phase, there is reduced dorsiflexion of the ankle resulting in a relative mild foot drop. Normally, flexion of the knee in swing is slightly reduced in the 1-year-old. As a result, the ankle is in slight plantarflexion at the end of swing, leading to a flatfoot-strike. This may be accompanied by pelvic tilt, pelvic rotation, hip abduction, hip joint rotation and knee joint rotation. Burnett & Johnson[5] in their study of 28 children found that pelvic tilt was present at an average age of 13.4 months and pelvic rotation was present at an average age of 13.8 months. Pelvic tilt appears close to the onset of independent ambulation (average 3 weeks after independent ambulation) with onset of pelvic rotation (average 4 weeks after independent ambulation) close behind.

Stance phase

There is exaggerated dorsiflexion of the weight-bearing foot on the ankle during stance phase. There may be an earlier onset to knee-flexion after foot-strike with minimal knee-extension during late stance.[4] Sutherland attributes this reduced knee-extension in the early walker to inadequate strength of contraction of the posterior ankle muscles. Knee-extension is a result of deceleration of the forward movement of the tibia from action of the posterior ankle muscles coupled with other extrinsic factors.[1] Reduced activity of the quadriceps muscles does not appear to be the cause since the quadriceps show prolonged stance phase activity at this age.

In the transverse plane, the hip joint remains externally rotated throughout the gait cycle. This leads to circumduction to aid in ground clearance during swing. This finding, which may be indicative of pathology in an older individual, is normal in the early walker and should not be cause for suspicion (Fig. 4.1).

GAIT OF THE 2-YEAR-OLD

The gait of the 2-year-old has matured to include reciprocal arm swing of the opposite side in 75%

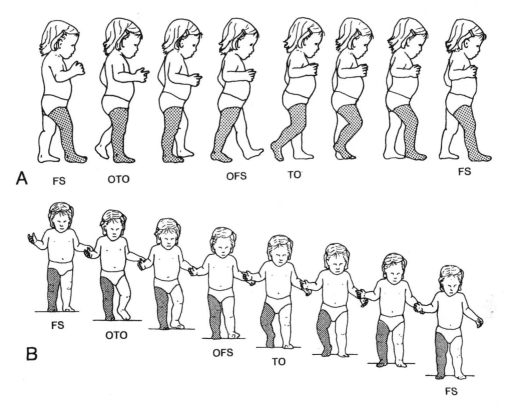

Figure 4.1 (A) Sagittal view of the gait of a 1-year-old girl. Tracings from individual move frames throughout one full gait cycle. The individual frames coincide with significant gait events. Gait cycle begins with right foot-strike (shaded) and ends with foot-strike of the same foot. (B) Frontal view. (FS, foot-strike; T, opposite toe-off; OFS, opposite foot-strike; TO, toe-off.) (Reproduced with permission from Sutherland DH. Gait disorders in childhood and adolescence. Baltimore: Williams and Wilkins; 1984.)

of individuals.[6] Burnett & Johnson[5] reported an average age of onset of 18 months for synchronized arm movements. There is an increase in single support time to 35% of the gait cycle. In the sagittal plane, swing phase ankle dorsiflexion increases eliminating the mild dropfoot that was seen in the 1-year old and facilitating greater ankle dorsiflexion at contact.

This is the earliest age to exhibit a heel-strike contact pattern. After contact, the knee goes into greater flexion and then extends before toe-off to at or near the original knee-flexion angle. Burnett & Johnson[5] reported an average age of onset of 19.5 months (27 weeks after onset of ambulation) for the mature foot and knee mechanism referred to as 'double-knee lock'. They stated that the development of the mature foot and knee mech-

anism depends on the development of a greater knee-flexion in midstance at an average age of 16.3 months (15 weeks after onset of ambulation) and a heel-strike contact pattern at an average age of 18.5 months (22½ weeks after onset of ambulation). There continues to be greater dorsiflexion of the ankle during stance phase than was seen in the 1-year-old. The shift from dorsiflexion to plantarflexion of the ankle occurs at 40% of the cycle in mature 7-year-olds. In the 2-year-old, this shift is delayed until 50% of the cycle (Fig. 4.2).

The amount of pelvic tilt, abduction and external hip rotation is also reducing at this age. At age 2, progressive neuromuscular maturation leads to increasing step length and decreasing cadence with some narrowing of the base of

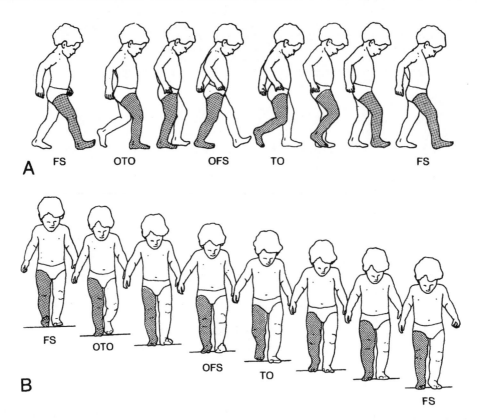

Figure 4.2 (A) Normal male gait pattern in a 2-year-old boy demonstrates presence of heel-strike at the time of foot contact, reciprocal arm swing and greatly increased step length. (B) Frontal view. (See Fig. 4.1 for abbreviations.) (Reproduced with permission from Sutherland DH. Gait disorders in childhood and adolescence. Baltimore: Williams and Wilkins; 1984.)

support. The step factor, defined as step length divided by limb length, has been shown to increase between the ages of 1 and 4 years, with the greatest change occurring before the age of 3 years.[7] Sutherland[4] reported step-length increases in a linear manner with increasing limb length. This linear relationship may be useful in evaluating children with suspected delay in neuromuscular maturation. The child who is developing normally will show corresponding increases in step length with growth in limb length. Lack of correlation between limb length and step length in a child may support the possibility of such delays.

GAIT OF THE 3-YEAR-OLD

The gait of the 3-year-old approaches that of a mature gait, but relative high cadence and

low walking velocity are still present. Immature ankle muscles limit length owing to persistent increased stance phase ankle dorsiflexion. A well-developed heel-strike, mature hip rotations, narrowing of the base of gait and smooth movements make the gait of the 3-year-old nearly indistinguishable from the gait of the adult. Sutherland[4] reported that by age 3½ years all children had a reciprocal arm swing. The base of gait is reduced to 45% of pelvic width by age 3½. This has also been described as a pelvic-span:ankle ratio of 0.45 (Fig. 4.3).

GAIT OF THE 7-YEAR-OLD

In 7-year-olds, cadence remains higher than it is in adults (although it is greatly reduced from what it was in the early ambulator), walking

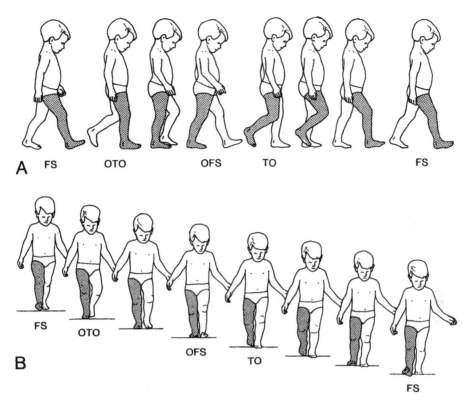

Figure 4.3   (A) Normal male gait pattern in a 3-year-old boy shows vigorous gait, reciprocal arm swing, well-developed heel-strike and smooth movements which differ only slightly from an adult. (B) Frontal view. (See Fig. 4.1 for abbreviations.) (Reproduced with permission from Sutherland DH. Gait disorders in childhood and adolescence. Baltimore: Williams and Wilkins; 1984.)

velocity is lower and pelvic rotation and hip joint rotation are slightly increased. Cadence reduces to 140 steps/minute by age 7 with an average velocity of 3.74 ft/s (1.14 m/s). The typical adult values for velocity are 4.78 ft/s (1.46 m/s) for males and 4.26 ft/s (1.30 m/s) for females.[4] Hip abduction during swing phase is also slightly greater. The step length increases as the limb is lengthening which correlates with the reductions in cadence seen with development.

In order of importance, walking velocity, pelvic span divided by ankle spread, duration of single support and cadence are the major variables in discriminating between the gait of a child under age 2½ and the gait of a child age 3 years or older[4] (Fig. 4.4).

MUSCLE FUNCTION IN DEVELOPING GAIT

Sutherland et al studied the phasic activity of muscles in children using surface electrode electromyography (EMG). Seven muscles were studied in the lower extremity of cooperative children for a total of 369 studies. Generally, the muscle phasic activity in children is similar to adults with only a few muscle groups demonstrating noteworthy differences.

Tibialis anterior muscle activity demonstrates prolonged stance phase activity with delayed onset of swing phase activity. This is consistent with the mild foot drop in swing and absence of heel-strike seen in the earliest walker. By age 2, EMG analysis demonstrates mature anterior

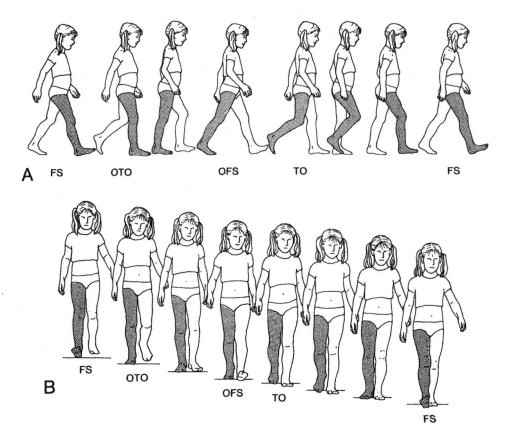

Figure 4.4 (A) Normal female gait pattern in a 7-year-old girl. (B) Frontal view. (See Fig. 4.1 for abbreviations.) (Reproduced with permission from Sutherland DH. Gait disorders in childhood and adolescence. Baltimore: Williams and Wilkins; 1984.)

tibial activity just prior to toe-off and continuing until approximately 40% of stance phase.[1]

Gastrocsoleus activity in swing phase is usually absent in adults. Activity of the gastrocsoleus in late swing phase and premature stance phase activity have been reported in children age 1 and 1½.[3] In a related report, Sutherland et al[1] reported 66% of 1-year-olds and 25% of 2- to 7-year-olds demonstrated gastrocsoleus activity from midswing to opposite side heel-strike.

Studies have also shown that on EMG analysis of 1- and 1½-year-olds, phasic activity began prematurely in swing phase in the vastus medialis as well as the gastrocsoleus. Stance phase prolongation was found in the gluteus maximus, vastus medialis and lateral and medial hamstring and tibialis anterior. Immaturity in the development of muscle control may lead to the characteristic phasic alterations in the gait of the earliest walkers. This immaturity in the development of muscle control is most likely a result of delay in myelinization. These phasic alterations have been shown to reduce as the child matures.[4]

MATURATION OF GAIT

The first milestone in normal neuromuscular development of the child is the ability to roll over from prone to supine by age 6 months. Sitting begins concurrently, with crawling by age 9 months and walking unassisted at 1 year.[4] Burnett & Johnson[5] reported an average age for unsupported sitting of 6¼ months (range 4½ to 9½ months). Crawling was seen at an average age of 7 months, creeping 8½ months, cruising 10 months and walking by 12⅓ months (range

9 months to 17 months). Boys were found to walk on average 2 weeks earlier than girls. The 28 children studied attempted to run between 10 and 24 weeks after independent ambulation. Also, with few exceptions, heel-strike, flexion at midstance, mature foot and knee mechanism were seen within 40 weeks after initiation of independent gait.[5]

There are two components of development that must be considered in order to understand why humans take a longer time to ambulate independently when compared to other quadripeds. The first component is that walking is a complex task that requires learning over a period of time. This was studied by Scott[8] who looked at congenitally blind children and found that they never attempted to stand on their own and had to be taught to walk. This supports the theory that walking is at least in part a learned activity. The second component is that onset of ambulation is dependent upon reaching a maturational threshold around the first year of life. That the nervous system undergoes growth and maturation in the postnatal period is known. All neurons are present by the 8th month of gestation but myelinization does appear to correlate with increase in size and neuromuscular control in children.[1,9] There is a differential pattern of myelinization at various levels of the nervous system that may help us to understand the gradual maturation of the control system. We know the importance of myelin in ambulation from our understanding of the effect demyelinating diseases have on motor function.[10] Development of mature gait is most likely a result of a combination of learning and of maturation of the nervous system. The child learns a complex task while neuromotor maturation occurs. Undoubtedly, a safe, supportive environment will help infants to learn a new, complex task. However, concurrent maturation of the nervous tissue appears essential to reaching the goal of walking independently.[11]

VERTICAL FORCE AND TORQUE IN DEVELOPING GAIT

Gait maturation of vertical force distribution is evidenced by the development of a secondary peak after heel-lift and increased drop in these forces corresponding to midstance. Increases in single support duration, stride length and walking most likely contribute to the more sinusoidal nature of the vertical force distribution with maturing gait.[1] The mean loading peaks reported by Sutherland et al[1] were approximately 110% of body weight for all age groups from 1 to 7. This is up to 20% lower than the average loads in adults reported by Cunningham.[6]

A beginning walker demonstrates an internal torque with internal rotation. This is present throughout the gait cycle. By age 2½ to 3, external torque emerges in late stance phase, resulting in establishing the sinusoidal internal/external torque cycle found with mature gait.

DETERMINANTS OF MATURE GAIT

Sutherland et al[4] have described five factors as predictive of gait maturation. Increase in single support is from 32% of the gait cycle in the 1-year-olds to 38% in the 7-year-olds. Walking velocity increases from 24 inches/s (60 cm/s) at 1 year to 47 inches/s (120 cm/s) at 7 years which results from increases in step length as the limb lengthens and neuromotor maturity occurs. Step length is a function of age, walking velocity and internal rotation of the pelvis at foot-strike. The most rapid increase is until age 2½ and then increase proceeds at a slower rate. The increasing velocity and step length lead to a decrease in cadence. The rate of decrease in cadence is greatest from age 1 to 3.

The base of gait narrows with age which has been described as a decrease in the ankle spread relative to pelvic width.[4] This is described as a rapid rise in the ratio of pelvic span to ankle spread until the age of 2½ and increases more slowly until the age of 3½, after which it remains about the same until the age of 7.

The findings of two major studies on the development of mature gait in children are consistent. Burnett & Johnson[5] reported that heel-strike and synchronous arm movements were present at an average age of 18.5 months for heel-strike and 18 months for synchronous arm movements.

Sutherland et al[4] found that heel-strike and reciprocal arm swing were usually established by age 1½. They found that heel-strike, knee-flexion wave, reciprocal arm swing and an adult pattern of joint angles throughout the walking cycle are acquired at an early age. These events precede the development of mature cadence, step length and walking velocity. Joint motions during gait of normal children are not age-dependent. They differ only slightly from those of adults. Deviations in joint-angle measurements from normal values do not suggest immaturity but rather indicate disease or dysfunction.

ANALYZING PEDIATRIC GAIT

There are several methods available to the clinician to analyze the gait of children. They range from the simple, such as observing the gait for detectable deviations from the norm, to the complex such as measurement of three-dimensional joint kinematics and kinetics. In a typical clinical setting where sophisticated technology for quantitative gait analysis is often not available, observational gait analysis is most often used.[12] Simple observation may prove adequate, particularly in children with non-neurological causes for their gait disturbance. Even in those situations where the level of involvement would make the use of systems to objectively analyze the gait ideal, the observation of gait is an appropriate starting point. Observation will draw the observer's attention to gross deviations and set the stage for further testing.

The observation of gait may provide insight into stability and balance, velocity and control, symmetry and movement of the upper and lower extremity and trunk, weight transfer, foot placement, positional foot deformities, and the changes occurring with the use of assistive devices.[13]

The observer is able to see the child function unencumbered by technology with a gait that is closest to how the child ordinarily walks. Computerized gait analysis, which usually involves the placement of sensors or attachments to other tethering devices, may produce an altered gait that does not represent the child in normal function.

The use of a form to document observations made during gait analysis will assist the observer in maintaining consistency and in remaining thorough from patient to patient and from day to day. Video recording of children walking is a useful adjunct to observational gait analysis. It enables the observer to review the recorded material after the patient has left, avoiding the problems of patient fatigue and hasty analysis when observation is done in real time.

Krebs et al[12] found in a study of the reliability of observational gait analysis that it is only moderately reliable for investigating kinematic gait deviations. Their study, which created near-ideal conditions for the observation of gait, found raters achieved an average of less than 7 agreements out of 10 observations. These limitations were found when the same raters repeated their assessment and between different raters. Therefore, caution should be exercised in making precise conclusions from observational gait analysis.

In spite of these limitations, the benefits of simple or video observation of gait, which include ease of execution and close approximation of normal walking conditions, make it a useful tool in pediatric assessment.

TECHNIQUES FOR THE OBSERVATION OF GAIT

The child should be observed standing before beginning to walk. Observe the posture of the child and the base of gait. A wide base may suggest an effort to remain stable in the child with ataxia or an angular deformity such as genu valgum (knock-knees). Asking the child to bring the feet together at the heels and the toes may bring out instability in stance with a narrow base of gait. This may suggest a cerebellar ataxia. The child may then be asked to close the eyes to remove visual input for balance. Instability present only with the eyes closed may suggest a sensory ataxia or unilateral vestibular disease. Children without pathology should be able to maintain these positions for 30 seconds without falling.[14]

The child's gait should be seen with the shoes on as well as barefoot. Certain gait components may be affected by the wearing of shoes. For example, children with an abnormally pronated gait often will appear normal in supportive shoes that mask the deformity. Conversely, intoe gait will appear worse in shoes, particularly heavier shoes that weigh inward the relatively lightweight limb of the child during swing phase.

If the child walks with braces or other assistive devices, attempts should be made to observe the gait with and without these aids. When practical, the child's gait should be observed on the way to the consultation room from the waiting room since the gait will be more natural when the child is unaware of formal observation. The area for gait analysis should be not less than 15 ft (4.6 m) in length to minimize turning frequency and to allow acclimation the child should be allowed to walk back and forth several times before commencing the formal analysis.

Basic components of observational analysis might include head and shoulder position, arm position and swing, pelvic height in stance, symmetry and length of step and the relationship of foot and leg segments to each other. In swing phase, the quality and length of leg swing and the flexion/extension positions of the hip, knee and ankle should be noted.

In those cases of neuromuscular disease where a subtle abnormality is suspected and may not be evident during simple walking, the child may be asked to perform certain activities that stress the gait. The first of these is to ask the child to walk away from you on toes, then return to you on heels. The observer should look for differences in the distance the forefoot or rearfoot is raised from the ground in either heel-walking or toe-walking. Subtle asymmetries in the ability to toe- or heel-walk may point to a weakness or hemiparesis that was not evident earlier. An arm weakness or alteration of arm position may also emerge under these conditions.

The child with cerebellar disease will have difficulty walking tandem with a heel-to-toe gait. It is not useful to test for tandem-walking before age 6 or 7 as in normal children the ability to walk tandem may not be fully realized until this age. The child below this age threshold may be asked to execute quick turns to stress the balance

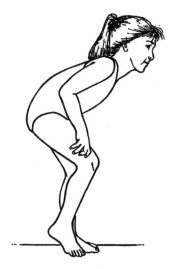

Figure 4.5   The Gower maneuver. Note the need to prop up the trunk with the hand on the thigh for children to right or erect themselves from the floor. (Reproduced with permission from Valmassay RL, ed. Clinical biomechanics of the lower extremities. St Louis: Mosby–Year Book; 1996.)

mechanism. The base of gait will widen during these turns in the child with midline cerebellar disease.

The child suspected of having proximal muscle weakness may be asked to perform the Gower maneuver as part of the gait assessment. The child is asked to rise to a standing position from a seated starting point without the use of a supporting surface for assistance. Children with normal strength to the muscles around the pelvis will be able to erect themselves without placing their hands on the thighs or floor for push or assistance to right themselves (Fig. 4.5).

Attempts to stress or challenge the child's gait may reveal subtle abnormalities even in children where specific neuromotor problems are not suspected. Simply asking the child to run or climb stairs may bring out subtle abnormalities. These activities require a higher level of motor and muscle function and will reveal deviations that were not apparent in normal ambulation.

TIME–DISTANCE VARIABLES

Quantification in gait analysis begins with the measurement of time–distance variables. These

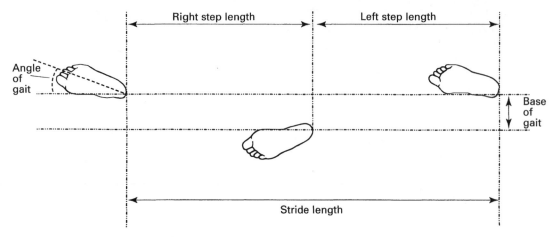

Figure 4.6 Subdivision of stride length, step length, angle and base of gait. (Reproduced with permission from Valmassay RL, ed. Clinical biomechanics of the lower extremities. St Louis: Mosby–Year Book; 1996.)

may include step length, stride length, cadence, cycle time and walking velocity. Simple tools such as a marked walkway, a stopwatch and powder on the subject's feet on a dark surface make measurement of these variables possible. Step length is defined as the distance from initial contact point of one leg to the initial contact point of the *other* leg. Stride length is defined as the distance from the initial contact point of one leg to the next contact point of the *same* leg (Fig. 4.6). Cadence is the number of steps per unit of time.

Information about the symmetry, stability and function of the child may be obtained from assessment of these variables. Care must be taken to recognize that these parameters are the result of the interaction of numerous component activities and do not, in themselves, determine the cause of the alteration in function. In addition, step and stride lengths as well as walking velocity are variables related to height.[1] Serial changes in these variables over time may be a result of growth and not improvements in function and therefore efforts should be made to consider the effects of growth before conclusions are reached.

Comparison of step and stride length and stance/swing phase ratios from left to right may assess symmetry. Stability may be assessed with analysis of time spent in the stance phase versus time spent in the swing phase. Instability in gait may lead to an increase in stance-phase duration

and efforts to improve stability over time will show a corresponding decrease in stance-phase duration. Overall function may be assessed with a look at walking velocity and cadence. A high cadence, particularly with a decrease in step length, may point to increased instability and reduced function.

ELECTROMYOGRAPHY

The most useful method to determine the phasic activities of muscles is with EMG. EMG measures the electrical signal which occurs with muscular contraction.[15] Data from EMG analysis help the user to determine whether a particular muscle is normal, out of phase, continuous or clonic. This may be useful in identifying the specific cause of a movement abnormality and may aid in planning surgical interventions such as tendon transfers.[16] An EMG, which indicates out-of-phase or prolonged activity of a particular muscle, may not, in itself, suggest pathology. The EMG finding may have resulted from the position of the joint upon which that muscle is acting as well as the demands placed on the muscle as a result of positioning. Therefore, many factors should be analyzed before conclusions are reached about muscle activity based on EMG findings. Interpretation of abnormal EMG data is best done after careful review of kinematic, kinetic and clinical data.[13] (Fig. 4.7).

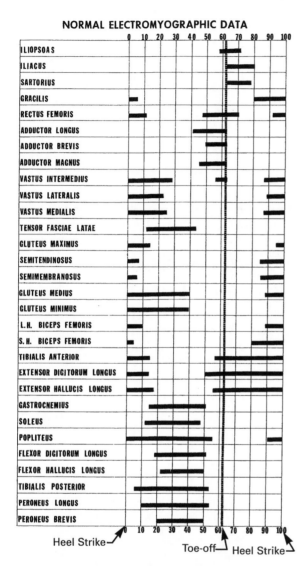

NORMAL ELECTROMYOGRAPHIC DATA

Heel Strike — Toe-off — Heel Strike

Figure 4.7 Adult muscle phasic activity chart used at Shriner's Hospital, San Francisco.

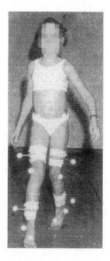

Figure 4.8 Gait laboratory patient with body markers. (Reproduced with permission from Bronstein AM, Brandt T, Woolacott MH. Clinical disorders of posture and gait. New York: Arnold/OUP; 1996.)

KINEMATICS

Kinematics is the study of the angular displacement of joints. It measures joint motions but does not identify the cause of the movement. Systems for the assessment of kinematics use a reference system such as markers that are placed on specific anatomical landmarks. The markers are used to define the relationship of segments that are used by the systems to determine the joint angles. Typical systems include active or passive

markers in order to identify the landmarks for a camera. Active markers emit light for detection by a camera and require direct connection to a power source. This may be cumbersome for the subject and may alter the gait. Passive markers are illuminated for the camera by a separate light source, do not require direct connection to a power source and therefore tend to be less intrusive to the patient (Fig. 4.8). There are numerous commercially available systems to measure kinematics using either active or passive sensors. The use of computer-automated tracking, a feature of most of the currently available systems, has significantly decreased the time for data processing to a useful clinical form.

Kinematics may be done in two- or three-dimensional analysis. In a two-dimensional analysis, out-of-plane measurement is not accounted for and may introduce error in the sagittal plane measurements.[17] Three-dimensional analysis attempts to eliminate this problem by presenting motion data in three dimensions. Motion at each joint is represented in the frontal, sagittal and transverse planes.

Kinematic data in children with pathology may be compared to data in a control group to document joint ranges during function.[1,18] Care should be taken to ensure that data from two populations are comparable.

KINETICS

Kinetics refers to those factors that cause or control movement. Kinetics requires more complex computation to be determined and therefore is more difficult to understand than joint kinematic patterns. A joint moment represents the body's internal response to an external load. The net joint moment determines which muscle group is dominant at a specific joint. Sagittal plane moments are the greatest in the lower extremity in gait followed by those in the frontal plane. Transverse plane kinetics may not have any clinical significance.[15] There are two commonly used methods for determining the joint moment in kinetics. The first involves the use of the ground reaction force and the second involves inverse dynamics. Specifics of the two methods are beyond the scope of this chapter.

The use of kinetics in clinical medicine may be in assessing the ability of muscles to generate power during gait. When a particular muscle is found to be generating much of the power in gait, it would be useful to preserve that muscle in any treatment that might be rendered. This information would be valuable to have in a preoperative assessment of function in a child with a complex movement disorder. Kinetic information is also useful in refining data obtained in kinematic analysis. For example, a hyperextended knee detected in kinematics may have an exaggerated net flexor moment. This could suggest to the clinician what protective measures for other soft-tissue structures affected by this flexor moment may be indicated. Joint kinetics are also useful in determining the effectiveness of various braces and orthoses.[13]

ENERGY EXPENDITURE

Assessment of energy expenditure is useful to the clinician as a method of determining whether or not a given treatment or procedure has been of benefit to the patient. Reduction in energy expenditure after a procedure would suggest functional improvement as a result of the treatment. One of the methods used to do this is to determine the mechanical work for walking using kinetics or kinematic data with joint measurements.[19] A second method for determining energy expenditure is through measures of oxygen consumption. This method is useful in determining overall expenditure as it measures a total end product of energy used. Studies have shown an increase in oxygen consumption in subjects with pathology as compared with subjects without pathology.[19,20]

ABNORMALITIES OF GAIT

NON-NEUROLOGICAL
Rotational gait assessment

Rotational gait assessment begins with the angle of gait. The angular deviation from the line of progression is noted and an estimate in degrees of the amount of any turning is recorded. The normal early walker will be markedly external (10° to 20°) decreasing to 7° to 10° external by the age of 6. Next, the position of the patella is marked and noted. An inward pointing or

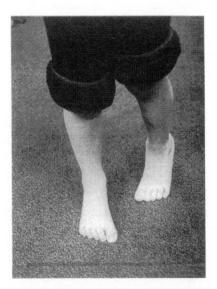

Figure 4.9 Intoe gait with 'squinting' patella. Note the femur, knee and lower leg appear inwardly rotated as a unit. This is suggestive of proximal (hip, femur) etiology of the intoe.

'squinting' patella may be found in the child with an internal or reduced-for-age external angle of gait. Such a finding suggests that one component of the rotational disorder is at the level of the hip/femur (Fig. 4.9). Finally, the angle made between the patellar position and the angle of gait at the foot level is measured. An internal angle of gait greater than the patellar position suggests additional intoe at the foot or leg level.

When a reduced or internal angle of gait is observed and the patella position is external, then rotational deformity at the foot and/or lower leg should be suspected. This may be from internal tibial torsion or rotation, talipes equino varus or metatarsus adductus (Fig. 4.10A, B). The dorsal and plantar surfaces of the foot, particularly on weightbearing, are checked in order to rule out metatarsus adductus. In metatarsus adductus, adduction is apparent between the forefoot and the midfoot. Other than this abnormality, the foot appears normal. If talipes equino varus is suspected, inward deviation of the foot will be noted more proximally, at the level of the midtarsal joint. The gait will exhibit equinus in the sagittal plane, frequently in an uncompensated form with absence of heel contact. A high arch and varus or inverted position of the foot will be evident throughout the stance phase. If the foot and ankle complex appear normal in the intoed child with externally pointed patellae, then internal tibial torsion or rotation should be suspected. Examination of malleolar position with the knee in the frontal plane will help confirm this diagnosis. Rotational disorders are often combined deformities at multiple levels, and it is not unusual to find the aforementioned causes for intoe present simultaneously (Table 4.1).

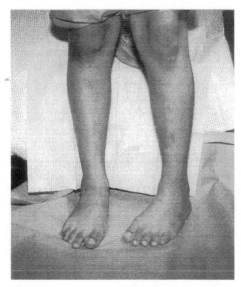

A

B

Figure 4.10 A & B   Intoe gait with an external patella and a markedly internal position to the tibia and foot. This is suggestive of distal (knee, fibia, foot) etiology of the intoe.

Table 4.1   Rotational deformities by level

Level	Causes
Patella (knee) pointing inward Angle of gait inward	Internal femoral torsion Soft tissue at hip
Patella rectus or outward Angle of gait inward No foot deformity	Internal tibial torsion or position
Patella rectus or outward Angle of gait inward Foot deformity	Clubfoot Metatarsus adductus
Patella (knee) outward Foot outward	External femoral torsion External hip contracture
Patella rectus Foot outward	Acquired valgus foot Congenital calcaneovalgus

Angular gait assessment

Frontal plane deviations at the hip, knee and tibia are readily apparent watching the child walking to and from the examiner. Complaints of bow-legs (genu varum) and knock-knees are among the most common gait-related problems in the pediatric population. Many of these children have normal frontal plane angulations appropriate for their age at different stages of development. For example, it is normal for the infant to be bow-legged until the age of 2. From the age of 4 until the age of 6, genu valgum is a normal developmental stage (Box 4.1).

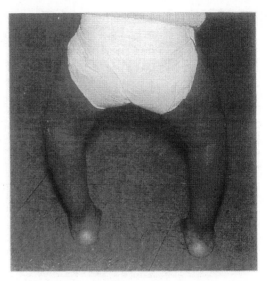

Figure 4.11   Significant tibial varum left > right.

Box 4.1 Normal values for frontal plane knee position by age.	
<2 years:	genu varum
2–4 years:	straight
4–7 years:	genu valgum
7–12 years:	straight
13–18 years	genu valgum
Adult:	straight
Geriatric	genu varum

Pathological bowing in the toddler usually has the apex of the deformity in the shaft of the tibia (Table 4.2). The bow will be a sharp, angular one as opposed to the gentle one seen with physiological tibial varum – a developmental norm. The newborn has up to 10° of normal tibial varum that reduces to 2° by age 6. Significant bowing should be monitored for progression over time. This can be done with measurements of the intercondylar distance between the knees. The length of the leg should also be measured to determine the significance of serial change. A measurement of leg length over subsequent visits will enable the clinician to judge the significance of changes in the distance between the knees. Among the causes for severe, progressive bowing in this age group are Blount's disease (an osteochondrosis of the medial capital tibial epiphysis) and rickets (caused by a disturbance in calcium metabolism that leads to weakening at the epiphyseal plate and may present with bow-legs or knock-knees).

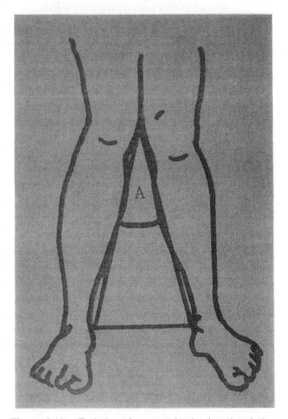

Figure 4.12   Technique for assessing leg length to judge significance of changes over time in knee or ankle spread in genu varum or valgum.

Medical treatment often leads to at least partial correction of these deformities (Fig. 4.11).

Genu valgum will be evident in gait with the knees in contact with each other and a wide intermalleolar distance at the ankles. This is apparent in the anterior–posterior view and will vary in significance with the age of the child. When genu valgum is particularly severe or when it occurs before or after the physiological age for this position, the child should be further evaluated. Rickets or bone dysplasia are possible causes for this condition. Measurement of ankle distance may be performed to assess progress with a technique similar to that described earlier for bowing (Fig. 4.12).

Children with genu valgum should be observed during gait for excessive out-of-phase pronation. This may be a result of medial displacement of body weight over the foot caused by the genu valgum creating a moment arm medial to the center of body mass which encourages pronation. Genu valgum may also be the result of excessive out-of-phase pronation in an individual compensating for intrinsic or extrinsic biomechanical faults. The mechanics of closed-chain pronation may include knee-flexion and internal leg rotation with resultant increased genu valgum (Fig. 4.13).

In a study of physiological knock-knee in 305 preschool children,[21] gait analysis revealed a

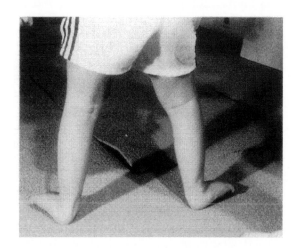

Figure 4.13 Increased closed chain subtalar joint pronation with genu valgum and a wide base of gait.

Table 4.2 Angular deformities by level

Level	Causes
Bowing	
Apex at the knee	Genu varum (physiological)
Apex in the tibia	Physiological tibia vara True tibia vara (Blount's disease) Rickets
Knocking	
Apex at the knee	Genu valgum (physiological) Rickets Excessive pronation
	Lateral epiphyseal Disruption (femur/tibia)

shorter stride length and a slower walking speed than in those in a control group. In the control group (n=163), the stride length was 33.5 inches (85.3 cm) and the velocity was 39.2 inches/s (99.7 cm/s). In the group with physiological genu valgum (n=142), the stride length was 32.7 inches (83.1 cm) and the velocity was 37.9 inches/s (96.4 cm/s).

In the child with a propulsive gait, usually present by the age of 3, the rearfoot position at heel contact and throughout the stance phase should be assessed. Normal gait requires pronation at contact to dampen shock followed by resupination throughout the remainder of stance. The child lacking pronation at contact may have a rigid foot type, possibly caused by a talipes equino varus, convex pes plano valgus (vertical talus) or tarsal coalition. In the last two conditions, the foot may appear pronated, but little or no motion at the subtalar joint will be evident after heel contact. Failure to resupinate in midstance in preparation for propulsion may indicate excessive, out-of-phase pronation. This may be a result of compensations for conditions such as equinus, persistent internal limb rotations, and frontal plane imbalances. The quality of propulsion as evidenced by the direction of weight passing throughout the foot should be assessed. In the child with severe medial roll of body weight in propulsion, resupination has not occurred, setting the stage for possible forefoot deformities such as juvenile hallux valgus and digital deformities.

Limps

Antalgic gait

Pain or inflammation in the leg or hip causes an antalgic gait. The causes of the pain are numerous and the presence of an antalgic gait signals to the clinician that a thorough work-up to identify an etiology is indicated. The affected side is favored and a limp results. A short stance phase and increased swing phase is noted on the affected side as the child is anxious not to weight-bear on the painful side. Physical examination will usually reveal normal muscle strength and tone, but deep tendon reflexes may be diminished as a result of guarding in the painful extremity.

Abductory lurch

In both abductory lurch and the antalgic gait, an attempt to get off or unload an involved extremity is present. This causes a shortening of the stance phase with increase in swing phase. The abductory lurch is usually a faster, less-hampered gait than the antalgic gait which is often slowed by pain or discomfort. The abductory lurch includes lateral movement of the head and may demonstrate trunk shift toward the affected hip.

Short leg gait

The limp of the child with a structurally short limb differs from that found with an antalgic gait or an abductory lurch. The observer will note sagittal plane movement of the head in the child with a limb length discrepancy. This appears as up and down or 'bobbing' movement of the head when the child is walking. This gait pattern has been described as a step up in stance onto the longer side and a step down in swing onto the shorter side.

The sideward head-leaning and trunk-shifting described for the abductory lurch are not present in the short leg limp. As pain is generally not a component of a limb length discrepancy, the observer should not expect to see the salient features of an antalgic gait such as marked shortening of the stance phase on the affected side.

A recent study[22] examined the effect of limb-length discrepancy on the gait of 35 neurologically normal children, average age 13 years (age range 8 to 17 years). They had a shortening of one limb that ranged from 0.8 to 15.8% of the length of the long extremity (0.23–4.4 inches (0.6–11.1 cm)). This study found that discrepancies of less than 3% of the length of the long extremity were not associated with compensatory strategies. In those subjects with discrepancies of greater than 5.5%, there was a greater displacement of the center of body mass with toe-walking as the principal compensatory strategy. However, in this group toe-walking alone could not equalize the work performed by the two extremities. This difference in mechanical work occurred at the hip and knee. Those children with discrepancies between 3 and 5.5% used a variety of compensatory strategies in combination to minimize the deleterious effect on energy expenditure.

In contrast to previous reports of significant pelvic obliquity in patients with limb-length discrepancy, Song et al[22] found that pelvic obliquity is not a common finding and that most individuals develop compensatory mechanisms to maintain a level pelvis.[23,24] The compensatory strategies included toe-walking, flexion on the long limb, vaulting over the long limb and circumduction of the long limb. Of these, only toe-walking and flexion of the long limb could be defined with objective descriptions of the movements. Vaulting and circumduction could not be defined with objective criteria. This may be because these are complex movements that are used in combination with other movements making it difficult to document them objectively.

The clinician should approach the child with a limp in a systematic way. The age of the child and the nature of the limp are clues that can focus on a differential diagnosis. For example, in the 2-year-old presenting with a limp, the differential diagnosis might include a developmental dislocated hip, septic hip, toxic synovitis, juvenile rheumatoid arthritis and diskitis. The child with the dislocated hip usually does not have pain and would be expected to have a short-leg or abductory lurch limp but would not have an antalgic limp. The other conditions listed are usually associated with pain and would be more likely to present with an antalgic limp in gait. It should also be considered that those conditions associated with pain might also lead to a child who refuses to walk or avoids walking.

In an older child, such as a 5- to 7-year-old, the possible causes of a limp vary. The likelihood of an undiagnosed dislocated hip and the incidence of a septic hip are reduced. Legg–Calvé–Perthes disease would be more likely as this condition is found in this age group. If the presenting limp was in a 12-year-old, the differential diagnosis would now include slipped capital femoral epiphysis as well as a septic hip and Legg–Calvé–Perthes disease. Dislocated hip, generally detected in the early years of walking, would now be extremely unlikely in this age group.

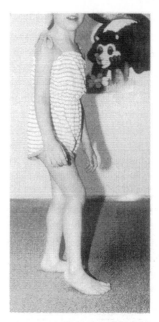

Figure 4.14   Child with right hemiplegia. Note internal leg rotation and forefoot contact with ankle equinus of the right side. The left or 'normal' side exhibits compensatory pes valgus.

NEUROLOGICAL

Hemiplegia

Hemiplegic gait is found in a child with a contralateral lesion of the corticospinal tract above the level of the medulla of the brain. The involved side will show stiffness in swing phase with reduced knee-flexion and a raised pelvis or hip. Equinus of the foot with dragging during swing phase is often evident. Reciprocal arm swing may be absent and the arm on the involved side may be held stiffly with excessive elbow-flexion. Stress activities such as heel-walking may show reduced height to the forefoot on the involved side. In the child with hemiplegic gait, the clinician should evaluate the contralateral limb as well. This other leg, although essentially normal, is often subject to increased stresses from the hemiplegia and may compensate as a result (Fig. 4.14).

Spastic gait

Spastic gait results from bilateral lesions of the corticospinal tracts that may be caused by a variety of conditions. These may include

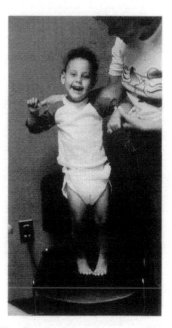

Figure 4.15   Spastic diplegia in a pre-walking child. Note internal limb position and ankle equinus and upper limb posture for balance.

hypoxic–ischemic injuries and encephalitis. Increased tone leads to out-of-phase or prolonged phasic activity of muscles. This may manifest as toe-walking from overactive gastrocsoleus muscles or as scissoring from increased adductor tone (Fig. 4.15). The ankle equinus may lead to a toe-drag in swing and adductor tone may lead to the thighs brushing together in gait. Tight flexors may lead to a crouching gait with flexion of the hips and knees and tilting of the pelvis. The feet are often in an equinovarus or equinovalgus position. Laxity of ligaments in the foot facilitating compensation for the equinus at the midtarsal joint is among the factors leading to an equinovalgus position of the foot in some spastic children (Fig. 4.16).

Ankle–foot orthoses (AFOs) are frequently used as an aid for children with spastic gait. Solid and hinged or articulated AFOs are commonly used. AFOs are best used in patients who do not have a tendency to crouch which appears to correlate with poor knee-extensor strength.[25] In Rethlefsen et al's study,[25] AFOs did not appear to contribute to a crouch gait in those individuals not predisposed to this position by extensor weakness. AFOs may be appropriate for patients with calf spasticity of varying amounts as long as passive range of motion to neutral or a 90° angle of the foot to the leg is available at the ankle (Fig. 4.17).

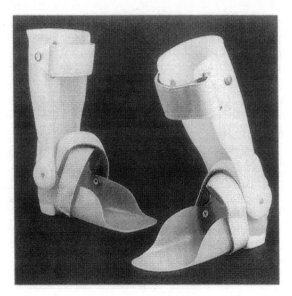

Figure 4.17 Hinged or articulated ankle–foot orthoses (courtesy of Langer Biomechanics Group).

Greater dorsiflexion of the ankle was found at initial contact with both solid and articulated AFOs as compared with subjects wearing shoes alone. Dorsiflexion at terminal stance was greatest in articulated AFOs. It was also reported that plantarflexor power generation at preswing was preserved in articulated AFOs.[25]

Cerebellar ataxia

Causes of cerebellar ataxia may be grouped based on the onset of the gait change. If the child has shown signs of ataxia from earliest walking, the cause may be from dysplasia of the cerebellum or injury or other lesion affecting this part of the brain. When the history points to a gradual onset to the gait change, a disorder marked by deterioration should be considered. Such an example would be Friedreich's ataxia. An acute onset to the ataxia would point to a toxic ingestion or a viral or postviral inflammation. Ataxia associated with toxic ingestion may involve other changes such as increased muscle tone, slurred speech and changes in mental status.

The gait in the child with cerebellar ataxia will have a wide base and reveal difficulty with tandem-walking. The child may diverge from

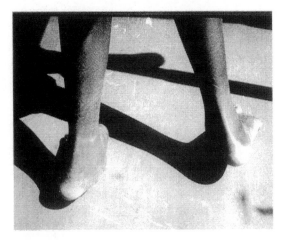

Figure 4.16 Equinovalgus foot deformity with spastic diplegia. Note the absence of heel contact with prominence of the talus with breakdown of the midtarsal joint.

the line of progression in a lurching movement. This gait pattern resembles the characteristic gait of the individual with alcohol intoxication. Stressing the gait with activities such as running or rapid turning may bring out instability not evident during walking.

Sensory ataxia

Sensory ataxia shares the principal characteristics of cerebellar ataxia, including instability and a wide base. Disorders that affect the posterior columns of the spinal cord will produce gait changes associated with sensory ataxia. In children, these include Friedreich's ataxia, demyelinating disease and polyneuritis.

This gait pattern is caused by decreased sensory input from the feet. This failure of sensory input from the feet causes the child to raise the leg high in swing phase with a heel-first strike pattern and a tendency to fix the eyes on the ground out of concern for stability.

Steppage gait

Steppage gait is caused by disorders of the anterior horn cells or peripheral nerves. Spinal muscle atrophy, Charcot–Marie–Tooth disease and Guillain–Barré syndrome are among the more likely causes.

This gait pattern is associated with weakness of the dorsiflexors leading to a dropfoot. To aid in ground clearance in the presence of the dropfoot, the child will increase flexion of the hip or knee. A bilateral steppage gait can resemble a sensory ataxic gait, but in steppage gait the forefoot usually contacts first.

The child with a steppage gait will have difficulty walking on the heels because of weakness in ankle dorsiflexors. The combination of increased hip- and knee-flexion with forefoot contact can give this gait the appearance of a prancing horse. A variation occasionally observed is a dropfoot with a toe–heel gait and no compensatory hip- and knee-flexion. In the absence of proximal sagittal plane compensation, foot dragging may occur in order to help clear the ground.

Waddling gait

Disorders that lead to weakening of the pelvic musculature produce a waddling gait. These include primary myopathies, muscular dystrophies, polymyositis, anterior horn cell disease and myelodysplasia. A variation of this gait pattern, either unilaterally or bilaterally, may be seen in the toddler with a developmental dislocated hip.

Waddling gait is easy to picture as it matches a mental image of a creature that waddles. The base of gait is wide for stability and there is a drop of the pelvis on the swing-phase side caused by a weakness in the hip abductors and extensors on the stance-phase side. The Trendelenburg test where the child would be asked to stand on one leg and drop of the pelvis is noted on the unloaded side suggests the presence of proximal muscle weakness. In the child with bilateral involvement, this drop of the pelvis on the swing side leads to the characteristic waddling appearance (Fig. 4.18). In order to help stabilize the trunk, the child may develop a lumbar lordosis that is characteristically seen on lateral observation. Children with a waddling gait may demonstrate the Gower maneuver, as described earlier in this chapter, when they are asked to rise from a seated position.

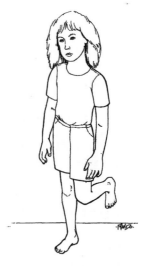

Figure 4.18 Trendelenburg test. Child is standing on one leg and drop of the pelvis is noted on the raised side. (Reproduced with permission from Valmassay RL, ed. Clinical biomechanics of the lower extremities. St Louis: Mosby–Year Book; 1996.)

OTHER LESS COMMON GAIT ABNORMALITIES

Short swing gait

This gait pattern is associated with tight hamstrings. The tight hamstrings limit the extension of the knees and the full excursion of the swing limb leading to an early contact of the heel and premature onset of stance.

Pelvic hike

A pelvic hike characterizes this gait pattern in swing phase in the presence of a dropfoot. It is most often used as a means of creating ground clearance during swing when stiffness in the hip or knee limits flexion of these joints.

Circumduction gait

This is a variation on the pelvic hike gait. The inability to flex the knee with stiffness places a demand on the swing limb to shorten. The normal motion at the hip facilitates the circumduction of the limb in swing phase.

Recurvatum or back-knee gait

This gait pattern is seen as a means of compensation for a gastrocsoleus equinus. Hyperextension of the knee joint is a compensatory mechanism in order to help the trunk pass over the planted foot in the sagittal plane during stance phase.

Flexed knee in stance gait

Tight or overactive hamstring muscles or weakness in the gastrocsoleus muscles usually cause this gait pattern. This hyperactivity of knee flexors or weakness of knee extensors leads to a prolongation of knee-flexion during stance phase.

Calcaneus gait

This is the opposite of a toe-walking or an equinus gait. The child may appear to heel-walk or may demonstrate lifting of the heel and toe at the same time. Weakness of the gastrocsoleus muscles as might be seen in a low myelodysplasia is a likely cause of this gait pattern.

THE EMERGENT GAIT ABNORMALITY

A 1985 study[26] of the cause of gait disturbance in children looked at 425 pediatric patients who sought medical attention for painful or painless alteration of gait. Traumatic causes of abnormal gait were excluded in this study. Singer[26] reported that of total hospital admissions over a 1-year period, 3.71% were related to altered gait. He also looked at total visits to the emergency department and reported 0.46% of all emergency visits were related to altered gait. These findings establish the frequency with which pediatric patients seek medical care for non-traumatic altered gait. It should be remembered that trauma to the lower extremities is the principal cause of altered gait in early childhood.[27]

In the study of pediatric patients whose gait disturbance led to a hospital admission, a wide variety of etiologies for the gait change were found with a significant percentage from infectious diseases (Table 4.3). Clinicians and emergency departments must recognize those conditions that require immediate hospitalization and intervention because of their potential to 'create deformity, functional disability or death'.[26] These should be distinguished from self-limiting conditions which require less urgent attention. Singer proposed a list of 10 disease states associated with gait changes that require urgent attention (Table 4.4). Even in those cases where the gait disturbance does not seem to require urgent attention, efforts should be made to identify the specific pathological process involved so as to plan management based on a specific diagnosis.

CONCLUSION

An overview of the emergence and development of gait in children has been presented. It is useful for the clinician to understand the development of normal walking. This understanding will enable the reader to consider pathology as the

Table 4.3 Etiology of gait disturbance in 425 patients (reproduced with permission from Singer JI. The cause of gait disturbance in 425 pediatric patients. Ped Emer Care 1985;1:7–10)

	No. of inpatients	No. of outpatients
Unknown	57	84
Osseous		
Osteomyelitis	21	
Sickle cell thrombotic	17	2
Legg–Calvé–Perthes	12	
Bone tumor	7	
Lymphoblastic leukemia	5	
Occult fracture	4	
Osgood–Schlatter	2	6
Sacroiliac infection	1	
Intervertebral disc infection	1	
Articular		
Transient synovitis	13	7
Pyarthrosis	13	
Juvenile rheumatoid arthritis	9	
Acute rheumatic fever	6	
Henoch–Schönlein purpura	5	1
Slipped capital epiphysis	5	
Systemic lupus erythematosus	1	
Dermatomyositis	1	
Inflammatory bowel disease	1	
Serum sickness	1	
Popliteal cyst		2
Soft tissue		
Cellulitis	42	3
Myositis	5	6
Diphtheria–pertussis–tetanus reaction		5
Prepatellar bursitis	2	
Perirectal abscess	2	
Muscular dystrophy	1	
Erythema nodosum	1	
Thrombophlebitis	1	
Sexual assault		1
Vaginitis	1	1
Central nervous system		
Drug intoxication	13	1
Acute cerebellar ataxia	6	2
Brain tumor	6	
Malingering	5	
Meningitis	4	
Cerebral vascular accident	3	
Acute infantile hemiplegia	1	
Hemiplegic migraine	1	
Encephalitis	1	
Febrile seizure	1	
Pseudotumor cerebri	1	
Arteriovenous malformation		1
Peripheral nervous system		
Guillain–Barré	3	
Multiple sclerosis	1	
Reflex sympathetic dystrophy	1	
Lead intoxication	1	
Hypokalemia	1	
Intra-abdominal		
Appendicitis	10	
Iliac adenitis	4	
Mesenteric adenitis	2	
Retroperitoneal abscess	1	
Total	303	122

Table 4.4 Disease states associated with altered gait that demand immediate recognition (reproduced with permission from Singer JI. The cause of gait disturbance in 425 pediatric patients. Ped Emer Care 1985;1:7–10)

Osteomyelitis
Paraspinal abscess
Cord tumor
Pyarthrosis
Guillain–Barré
Tick paralysis
Cerebral abscess
Meningitis
Encephalitis
Appendicitis

underlying cause of a presenting gait change when that change is not consistent with normal gait for a child of that age.

In order to enhance the reader's ability to analyze gait, the various methods for gait assessment have been reviewed. These range from simple observation to sophisticated analyses requiring elaborate technology. The clinician should review these options and determine the level of analysis appropriate for each individual child.

Finally, a review of the key characteristics of typical gait abnormalities seen in children has been presented. Care has been taken to describe these gait patterns in a clear and concise manner. However, it is difficult to create a complete picture of the changes associated with a gait abnormality on the printed page. The reader should be reminded that gait is a three-dimensional event and that complete understanding of its many facets requires dynamic observation of individuals in function.

REFERENCES

1. Sutherland DH, Olshen RA, Biden EN, et al. The development of mature walking. London: MacKeith Press;1988.
2. Inman VT, Ralston H, Todd F. Human walking. Baltimore: Williams and Wilkins;1981.
3. Morell P, Norton WT. Myelin. Sci Am 1980;242(5):88–117.
4. Sutherland DH, Olsen R, Cooper L, et al. The development of mature gait. J Bone Joint Surg Am 1980;62:354–363.
5. Burnett CN, Johnson EW. Development of gait in childhood II. Dev Med Child Neurol 1971;13(2):207–215.
6. Cunningham DM. Components of floor reactions during walking. Prosthetics Devices Research Project, Institute of Engineering Research, University of California, Berkeley, Series II;1950;Issue 14:Nov.
7. Scrutton DR. Footprint sequences of normal children under five years old. Dev Med Child Neurol 1969;11:44–53.
8. Scott E. Surgery of the foot and ankle. In: Mann R, ed. Biomechanics of the foot. St Louis: Mosby;1989.
9. Rabinowicz T. Cerebral cortex of the premature infant of the 8th month. Prog Brain Res 1964;4:39–92.
10. Rafalowska J. Some problems of the development and aging of the nervous system. II. Myelination of the spinal roots in the second half of life and in early infancy. Neuropatol Pol 1979;3:407–420.
11. Sutherland DH, Valencia F. Pediatric gait. Normal and abnormal development. In: Drennan JC, ed. The child's foot and ankle. New York: Raven Press;1992:19–35.
12. Krebs DE, Edelstein JE, Fishman S. Reliability of observational kinematic gait analysis. Phys Ther 1985;65:1027–1033.
13. Rose SA, Ounpuu S, DeLuca PA. Strategies for the assessment of pediatric gait in the clinical setting. Phys Ther 1991;71:961–980.
14. Crumrine PK. Gait disorders in children. Em Med 1998;7:18–36.
15. Winter DA. Biomechanics and motor control of normal human movement. 2nd ed. New York: Wiley;1990.
16. Perry J, Hoffer MM. Preoperative and postoperative dynamic electromyography as an aid in planning tendon transfers in children with cerebral palsy. J Bone Joint Surg Am 1977;56:531–537.
17. Davis RB, Ounpuu S, Tyburski DJ, et al. A comparison of 2D and 3D techniques for the determination of joint rotation angles. Proceedings of the internal symposium on 3D analysis of human movement. Montreal, Quebec, Canada;1991.
18. Ounpuu S, Gage JR, Davis RB. Three-dimensional lower extremity joint kinetics in normal pediatric gait. J Pediatr Orthop 1991;11:341–349.
19. Olney SJ, MacPhail HEA, Hedden DM, et al. Work and power in hemiplegic cerebral palsy gait. Phys Ther 1990;70:431–438.
20. Rose JR, Gamble JG, Medeiros J, et al. Energy cost of walking in normal children and those with cerebral palsy: comparison of heart rate and oxygen uptake. J Pediatr Orthop 1989;9:276–279.
21. Lin CJ, Lin SC, Huang W, et al. Physiologic knock-knee in preschool children: prevalence, correlating factors, gait analysis and clinical significance. J Pediatr Orthop 1999;19:650–654.
22. Song KM, Halliday S, Little D. The effect of limb length discrepancy on gait. J Bone Joint Surg Am 1997;79:1690–1698.

23. Morscher E. Etiology and pathophysiology of leg length discrepancies. In: Hungerford DS, ed. Progress in orthopedic surgery. Vol 1. Leg length discrepancy. The injured knee. New York: Springer;1977:9–19.

24. Phelps JA, Novachek TA, Dahl MT. Consequences of leg length inequality in young children. Read at the Annual East Coast Clinical Gait Laboratory Conference, Rochester, Minnesota;1993:May 3.

25. Rethlefsen S, Kay R, Dennis S, et al. The effects of fixed and articulated ankle–foot orthoses on gait patterns in subjects with cerebral palsy. J Pediatr Orthop 1999;19:470–474.

26. Singer JI. The cause of gait disturbance in 425 pediatric patients. Ped Emer Care 1985;1:7–10.

27. Singer JI, Towbin R. Occult fractures in the production of gait disturbance in childhood. Pediatrics 1979;64:192–196.

SECTION CONTENTS

5

General medicine and diabetes

Christopher Steer, Kathryn Noyes and Christopher Kelnar

GENERAL MEDICINE

Christopher Steer

The pattern of childhood disease identified in a particular community is influenced by climate, geography, socioeconomic status and notably by the prevalence of malnutrition and reservoirs of disease, particularly diarrheal and respiratory infection. In the past few decades, many countries have witnessed dramatic reductions in childhood mortality and morbidity achieved by improved standards of nutrition and hygiene and by the introduction of immunization and antibiotics. This has allowed greater input and attention to the early diagnosis and management of less common disorders, e.g. congenital malformations, epilepsy, cerebral palsy, mental handicap, and diseases of the endocrine, lymphoreticular and immune systems. Improved understanding of genetic mechanisms and the pathophysiology of disease has also led to the wider application of preventive and screening techniques, e.g. antenatal diagnosis in pregnancy utilizing chorionic villus biopsy or amniocentesis (for alpha-fetoprotein assay to detect spina bifida, and chromosome analysis) and neonatal Guthrie testing (for phenylketonuria, galactosemia, hypothyroidism). 'Gene probe' techniques using methods which cleave DNA have also identified specific gene loci, e.g. for muscular dystrophy and cystic fibrosis. These methods allow early and specific diagnosis in fetal and postnatal life and may yield important clues to the underlying mechanisms operating in some diseases. Although vast resources are being invested to assist in some of these developments, this should not obscure the fact that, in global terms, malnutrition and infection remain the most significant contributors to childhood disease. In podiatric practice, a large number of children will be seen with abnormalities of the feet determined by intrauterine and genetic influences. These disorders will be considered first, followed by discussion of systemic disorders, e.g. those involving the immune and hematological systems, which may influence management of the foot.

CONGENITAL ANOMALIES

Congenital anomalies may be classified as *malformations* (defective formation of tissue and organs), *deformations* (defects caused by unusual forces acting on otherwise normal tissue), and *disruptions* (defects caused by breakdown of previously normal tissue).

Malformations

Such defects in morphogenesis may be single, affecting one structure in an otherwise completely normal child, or multiple where several structural abnormalities are present because of the same underlying cause. A *syndrome* is said to occur when a recognizable pattern of malformation is identified usually with multiple features and again with a single presumed specific cause.

Major malformations affecting, e.g., major organ systems such as brain, heart, kidney or viscera are identified in approximately 2% of children at birth although this figure reaches 5% when allowance is made for diagnosis in later childhood.

Minor malformations are identified in approximately 4% of children at birth and by definition such malformations rarely require treatment and mostly affect the skin and appendages, e.g. sacral dimples, simian creases, clinodactyly of fifth fingers, syndactyly of second and third toes, extra nipples and pre-auricular sinuses.

Table 5.1 Recognized etiology of congenital defects in newborn infants (Nelson & Holmes, 1989)[1] (*n* =1549 from 69 227 births)

Chromosome abnormalities	10.1%
Single mutant gene disorders	3.1%
Familial disorders	14.5%
Multifactorial disorders	23.0%
Teratogens	3.2%
Uterine factors	2.5%
Twinning	0.4%
Unknown	43.2%

The underlying mechanism in malformation syndromes may involve defective tissue and organ formation owing to abnormal cell shape, inappropriate cell matrix (collagen), vascular insufficiency or defective programming of cell regression and death during development.

The etiology of various congenital defects is outlined in Table 5.1. Genetic mechanisms and examples are described more fully in the following pages. 'Teratogens', agents thought to mediate abnormality by direct action during pregnancy, are listed in Appendix II. In general, teratogens have more harmful effects when they influence fetal development in the early stages of pregnancy. Harmful pregnancy influences are easiest to blame for fetal and neonatal abnormality but it should be remembered that in many instances these are difficult to prove unequivocally against a background where the causes of approximately 40% of fetal abnormality are at present not known.

Deformations

Deformations are caused by abnormal mechanical forces acting on normal tissue. The majority involve the musculoskeletal system and are secondary to intrauterine molding. This may be due to 'crowding' caused by such conditions as oligohydramnios (lack of liquor amnii), congenital uterine abnormality (e.g. bicornuate uterus), chronic leak of liquor, persistent breech presentation, twins or uterine tumors. Neuromuscular imbalance or paresis caused by spina bifida cystica, spinal muscular atrophy or dystrophia myotonica may also impair fetal movement and normal joint and muscle development. Intrauterine 'positional deformity' of variable severity secondary to the above may cause relatively simple anomalies, e.g. talipes (equinovarus or calcaneovalgus), congenital dislocation of the hip or scoliosis. However, multiple severe anomalies may occur as in 'Potter's syndrome', usually secondary to oligohydramnios caused by renal agenesis in the fetus; in such cases, the fetus is subjected to severe compression causing marked talipes, multiple joint contractures, plagiocephaly (asymmetry of the skull), torticollis and hip dislocation.

Disruptions

Disruptions represent rare sporadic events where previously normally formed or forming tissues 'break down', e.g. as a result of 'entanglement' in aberrant uterine amniotic bands. This results in uterine reduction deformity or 'amputation', most often involving the extremities but, in rarer cases, the head or thorax (Fig. 5.1).

GENETIC CONSIDERATIONS

Defects in morphogenesis and many other disorders are mediated by interactions between pre- and postnatal environment and genetic endowment. Such effects may be obvious at birth and may manifest as a congenital abnormality or may only become evident with time as a consequence of growth or environmental factors. The three principal genetic mechanisms in operation are single major gene disorders, chromosomal abnormalities and polygenic (multifactorial) inheritance.

Single gene inheritance

Genes located on the X chromosome are known as X-linked genes and those on the autosomes as autosomally linked genes. Chromosomes are arranged in pairs, one of each pair being derived from each parent, with comparable gene determinants located at the same position. The pairs of genes are known as 'alleles' and normally function together. Gene mutation is said to occur when changes in gene structure arise and produce an abnormal characteristic. When a mutant gene produces an abnormality despite the presence of a normal 'allelic' partner, this is regarded as a *dominant* pattern. A mutant gene which only produces an abnormality when mediated by a 'double dose' (i.e. one from each partner) represents a *recessive* pattern. In *X-linked recessive* disorders, the abnormal gene is situated on the X chromosome. In the female, the presence of the normal allele on the other X chromosome protects her from the disease but she is a carrier. However, in affected males, the abnormal gene on the X chromosome is not balanced by the appropriate allele on the Y chromosome, and he manifests the disease state. In *X-linked dominant* disorders, the above mechanism also applies but the female carrier also shows manifestations of disease albeit less severe than in the male. In addition, certain disorders are found almost exclusively in females and apparently are lethal early on in utero in affected males (e.g. Rett's syndrome – a progressive motor disorder with seizures and autism – and Aicardi syndrome – agenesis of the corpus callosum with developmental retardation and seizures). It is not yet clear whether these are X-linked dominant or autosomal dominant disorders although the former is suspected.

Autosomal dominant disorders

More than 1000 disorders result from this mode of inheritance. As noted above, the abnormal gene responsible for disease is carried on one of the autosomes only. Each offspring has a one in

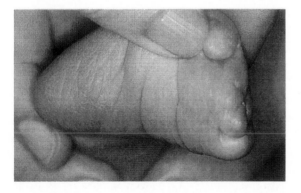

Figure 5.1 Toe 'amputation' secondary to intrauterine bands.

two chance of inheriting the gene and manifesting the disease. The degree of severity of 'expression' of disease may vary considerably from one affected individual to another. In certain examples of dominantly inherited disorders, 'new' cases arise from spontaneous gene mutation within the ovum or sperm (e.g. up to 80% of individuals with achondroplasia, an autosomal dominant disorder, have normal parents). The risk of a similar mutation affecting subsequent offspring is low but the individual arising from the new mutation will still pass the disorder on to 50% of their offspring. A selection of examples of more than 1000 conditions mediated by autosomal dominant inheritance, many of which affect the extremities, are listed in Appendix III.

Autosomal recessive disorders

Whereas autosomal dominant disorders tend to cause gross structural defects and clinically obvious abnormalities, recessively inherited disorders are in addition commonly implicated in biochemical disorders. In recessive inheritance, neither parent shows any sign of the disease but the risk of offspring being affected is 1:4 while the risk of a child being a carrier is 1:2. Many individuals carry abnormal genes but the risk of a spouse carrying similar genes is usually small unless there is consanguinity as, for example, in first cousin marriages. Relevant examples from the 700 or so known autosomal recessive mediated disorders are listed in Appendix IV.

X-linked disorders

As noted, these disorders are carried by the female on the X chromosome and therefore manifest in 50% of male offspring while 50% of daughters perpetuate the carrier state. A selection from the 100 or so recognized X-linked disorders is listed in Appendix V with special emphasis on disorders of the extremities.

Major structural chromosomal abnormalities

Modern cytogenetic techniques permit direct visualization of human chromosomes including

Table 5.2 Incidence of chromosome abnormalities

Down syndrome (21 trisomy)	1 in 600–800 overall
Edwards' syndrome (18 trisomy)	1 in 8000
Patau's syndrome (13 trisomy)	1 in 20 000
Turner's syndrome (XO)	1 in 10 000
Klinefelter's syndrome (XXY)	1 in 1000
Poly-X syndrome (XXX etc.)	1 in 1000
XYY syndrome	1 in 1000
Balanced structural re-arrangements	1 in 520
Unbalanced structural re-arrangements	1 in 1700
Fragile X males	1 in 2000
Fragile X females	1 in 1000

the identification of heterochromic 'bands' alternating with lighter non-staining areas. These bands are ascribed special numbers in order to facilitate the detection of loss (deletion) of even a small part of a chromosome or the addition of extra genetic material. Such changes occur during sperm and ovum formation (gametogenesis) during meiosis.

Disorders caused by chromosomal abnormalities result from changes in the total number of autosomes or sex chromosomes or from alterations in chromosome structure resulting from deletion or interchange of chromosome material from one chromosome to another – *translocation*.

Approximately one in 150 newborn infants has a chromosome abnormality, distributed as in Table 5.2.

The more common disorders will be outlined here. For more detailed description, the reader should refer to detailed illustrated texts[2,3] such as *Smith's Recognizable Patterns of Human Deformation*.

Chromosome abnormalities affecting the autosomes

Trisomy syndromes. Down syndrome is mediated by an extra no. 21 chromosome and is the best recognized and most common chromosomal abnormality. A high correlation exists between increasing maternal age and the non-disjunction during meiosis resulting in an extra chromosome in the conceptus. Approximately 5% of cases are due to translocation, i.e. centric fusion between chromosome 21 and chromosomes 13, 14 or 15. Important features of Down syndrome are sum-

Table 5.3   Trisomy syndromes

	21 trisomy (Down)	18 trisomy (Edwards')	13 trisomy (Patau's)	8 trisomy	9 trisomy
General	Mental retardation Hypotonia	Severe mental retardation Low birthweight	Severe mental retardation Apnea Seizures	Mental retardation Short stature	Mental retardation
Head and face	Brachycephaly Mongolian slant of eyes Prominent epicanthic folds Brushfield's spots (speckled iris) Prominent malformed ears Flat nasal bridge Short broad neck	Micrognathia Low set malformed ears Prominent occiput	Microcephaly Midline scalp defects Cleft lip and palate Microphthalmia	Prominent brow Low set ears High-arched palate Micrognathia	Microcephaly Deep set eyes Prominent ears 'Fish mouth' Micrognathia
Extremities	Simian crease Short broad hands Hypoplastic mid phalanx of fifth finger Widely spaced great toes Abnormal dermatoglyphics	Flexion deformity of fingers Short dorsiflexed big toes 'Rockerbottom' feet or talipes equinovarus Abnormal dermatoglyphics	Polydactyly Hypoplastic or hyperconvex finger nails Simian crease Flexion deformities of fingers Abnormal dermatoglyphics Retroflexible thumb	Deep flexion creases on palms and soles	Clinodactyly Digital and nail hypoplasia Syndactyly Simian crease Abnormal dermatoglyphics
Some other features	Congenital heart disorders Intestinal atresia Hypothyroidism Conductive deafness	Congenital heart disorders Cleft lip and palate Tracheo-oesophageal fistula	Congenital heart disorders Polycystic kidneys Omphalocele	Congenital heart disorders Limited joint mobility Patella dysplasia	Congenital heart disorders Congenital dislocation of the hip Urinary tract anomalies

marized in Table 5.3 along with the principal abnormalities noted in the less common trisomic syndromes. In contrast to Down syndrome, most infants with trisomy 13 and 18 die in early infancy and usually within the first few months although longer survivors are occasionally reported. Long-term management includes early diagnosis and sympathetic counseling.

Autosomal deletions. Chromosomal deletions are associated with a number of clinical syndromes and have been described affecting the short (p) arms of chromosomes 4, 5, 11, 18 and the long arm (q) of chromosomes 9, 13, 18, 21 and 22. Mental retardation is invariable, mostly in association with facial dysmorphism. A variety of abnormalities of the hands and feet occur and include syndactyly, clinodactyly, short metacarpals and metatarsals and dysplastic nails. The commonest deletional disorder affecting the short arm of 5 (5p-) has been dubbed the 'cri du chat' syndrome on account of the high-pitched mewing cry noted in the newborn period. Other features include microcephaly, hypertelorism, micrognathia, prominent epicanthic folds, antimongolian palpebral fissures and occasional congenital heart disease. Such individuals are frequently happy with an engaging outgoing personality.

Table 5.4 Abnormalities of the sex chromosomes

	Turner's syndrome 45 XO and Mosaics	Klinefelter's syndrome 47 XXY	Poly-X Female 47 XXX etc.	Fragile X sites	Y Polysomy 47 XYY etc.
Incidence	1/10 000 females	1/1000 males	1/1000 females	1/1000 females 1/2000 males	1/1000 males
Features include:	Short stature Primary amenorrhea and infertility owing to ovarian dysgenesis Webbing of neck and shield chest Down-turned mouth Micrognathia Downward slanting of palpebral fissures Increased incidence of cardiac defects Congenital lymphedema Short metacarpals or metatarsals Hypoplastic/ hyperconvex nails	Long limbs with low upper to lower segment ratio Impaired spermatogenesis Eunuchoidism Gynecomastia Increased incidence of mental retardation Ulceration of skin over anterior lower legs	Mental deficiency Variable short stature and facies within syndromes Clinodactyly Overriding toes and multiple joint dislocation in 'Penta X' syndrome	Mental deficiency Hypotonia Lax joints Mild cutis laxa Large ears Macro-orchidism	Tall stature Aberrant often anti-social behaviour Increased skeletal length versus breadth in skull vault, hands and feet

Abnormalities affecting the sex chromosomes

Abnormalities of the sex chromosomes constitute approximately half of all chromosomal abnormalities detected in the newborn period. The physical abnormalities encountered vary considerably but nearly all affect gonadal function in some form. Features of the commoner syndromes are summarized in Table 5.4.

Polygenic (multifactorial) inheritance

'Polygenic' inheritance refers to genetic defects which are thought to be caused by the cumulative action of a number of genes. Whether a given polygenic disorder manifests or not is also influenced by environmental factors and whether a given 'threshold' for expression of a disorder is reached. This has led to use of the term 'multifactorial' inheritance. When a particular family member is affected, the risk of first-degree relatives (sons and daughters) also being affected is increased. The commoner disorders currently thought to be multifactorial are listed in Table 5.5.

Several reference atlases (e.g. *Smith's Recognizable Patterns of Human Malformations* and *Recognizable Patterns of Human Deformation*[2,3]) are available for perusal in cases where children are encountered and where a congenital disorder is suggested but not immediately recognized by the clinician. Computerized databases are also

Table 5.5 Polygenic (multifactorial) disorders

Ankylosing spondylitis	Hirschsprung's
Atopy	disease
Congenital cardiac defects	Perthes disease
Isolated cleft lip and palate	Psoriasis
Isolated club foot	Pyloric stenosis
(talipes equinovarus)	Schizophrenia
Congenital dislocation of hip	Spina bifida complex
Diabetes mellitus	and anencephaly

becoming available where a given selection of physical abnormalities may be entered and where a number of differential diagnoses are generated from the program (e.g. the London Dysmorphology Database[4]). These approaches considerably enhance the ability to make an early diagnosis and to arrange appropriate counseling and treatment.

Molecular genetics

Remarkable technical advances have led to improved understanding of basic genetic mechanisms over recent years. As noted earlier, 'gene probe' methodology has allowed for the first time analysis of individual DNA sequences with high degrees of accuracy. Single-stranded DNA 'probes' can 'find' their complementary sequences within human DNA, utilizing labeling techniques such as in situ hybridization or Southern blotting.[5] In situations where very little DNA is available, techniques such as the polymerase chain reaction can be used to amplify and increase the amount of material available for subsequent analysis. Wide application of these and similar methods continues to have a profound impact on genetic research and medical practice.

The 'Human Genome Project', for example, represents a unique international collaborative study which will determine the entire human DNA sequence; this will be completed within the next 3 to 5 years. Recent research has also shown more clearly the basic biochemical mechanisms underlying many inherited diseases. Inherited variations in DNA sequencing have been found to result from change (substitution) in a single base pair of DNA, loss of DNA (deletion) and addition (insertion, expansion and duplication). 'Repetition' (i.e. trinucleotide repeats) has been associated with specific disorders such as fragile X syndrome (cytosine guanine guanine), dystrophia myotonica (cytosine thymine guanine) and Huntington's disease (cytosine adenine guanine). It has also been clearly shown that significant variation occurs in regions of the DNA sequences which have no apparent impact on gene function. Such genetic 'polymorphism' can however be utilized in gene probe assays,

particularly when adjacent to a gene site, whose particular sequence has yet to be accurately characterized.

In an increasing number of disorders, the deficient specific protein normally 'coded' by an identified DNA sequence in a healthy individual has been identified, allowing for the first time the prospect of gene replacement or specific treatment targeting the basic biological fault in a particular disease, e.g. the chloride channel/transporter protein in cystic fibrosis and the muscle protein 'dystrophin' in Duchenne muscular dystrophy. The pace of genetic research shows no sign of slowing; for a regularly updated authoritative source of information, the reader is referred to OMIM (the Online Mendelian Inheritance in Man[6]). Table 5.6 gives some examples of identified genes along with their chromosomal locus.

GROWTH AND GROWTH DISORDERS

Normal growth is mediated by increases in cell number and size, defined as hyperplasia and hypertrophy. While early embryonic growth results mostly from cellular hyperplasia, subsequently the balance between hyperplasia and hypertrophy varies considerably. Postnatal growth is influenced by a given child's genetic endowment, adequate nutrition and normal hormonal

Table 5.6 Examples of identified gene abnormalities responsible for genetic disorders and their chromosomal locus

Disorder	Gene alteration (deletion or point mutation) and chromosomal site
Gaucher's disease	1q
Osteogenesis imperfecta	7q
Sickle cell anemia	11p
Phenylketonuria	12q
Von Willebrand's disease	12p
Factor X deficiency	13q
Alpha-thalassemia	16p
Severe combined immuno-deficiency owing to adenosine deaminase deficiency	20q
Hemophilia A and B	Xq
Duchenne muscular dystrophy	Xp

function. In order to define and to identify disorders of growth in an individual, access is required to appropriate population standards. Such standards are presented in the form of 'growth charts' prepared from longitudinal and cross-sectional data in appropriate populations.

The 97th and 3rd centiles are conventionally taken as the upper and lower limits of normality representing plus or minus two standard deviations from the population mean. There is an increased likelihood of identifying significant pathological causes of short stature in children whose dimensions plot below the third centile. When serial measurement identifies an individual whose measurements are crossing centile lines, or in whom growth velocity is persistently low, active further investigation is indicated.

It is important to ascertain the pattern of growth over time in order to identify and to categorize growth disorders in children. For example, infants and children with a congenital growth disorder show persistent deviation from the normal curve from early on, while those with an acquired disorder progressively decline from a normal point on the growth curve.

In certain situations, it may be useful to determine bodily proportions, e.g. the relationship of trunk length to leg length. The former may be determined by measuring sitting height and leg length (subischial) by subtracting this value from total height. Patients with variants of short limb dwarfism, e.g. achondroplasia, may have normal sitting height but markedly reduced subischial leg length, whereas patients with pubertal delay frequently demonstrate a disproportionately long leg length compared to sitting height.

Factors affecting growth: the role of hormones

Normal growth is sustained by an adequate nutritional intake, adequate sensory stimulation (psychogenesis), satisfactory general health, by genetic endowment and by hormonal influences. Hormones producing significant effects on growth are growth hormone, insulin and insulin-like growth factors (somatomedins), thyroxine, parathyroid hormone, calcitonin, cortisol and the sex steroid group. Hormonal effects are closely interrelated and apart from important effects on growth, they are also vital in maintaining the internal milieu, for withstanding stress, i.e. trauma, infection, starvation and psychological stress, and for normal reproductive function.

Growth hormone itself has a peripheral lipolytic and anti-insulin effect while promoting skeletal growth, protein synthesis and cell proliferation via the intermediary effects of insulin-like growth factors.

Causes of growth failure

The causes of growth failure and short stature are summarized in Table 5.7 and discussed further below.

1. Children with genetically determined short stature are small from the outset and grow parallel to but below the third centile. Growth velocity is normal and a normally timed pubertal growth spurt occurs with ultimately the attainment of a short adult height similar to their parents. Bone age is always appropriate for chronological age and on examination there is no evidence of malabsorption or of any particular 'syndrome' and there is no biochemical abnormality detectable on investigation. At present, the role of growth hormone therapy is being assessed in this group of children even though they are not known to be growth hormone deficient ('small normal'). It is not yet clear whether final attained height will be increased with such treatment.

2. Several chromosome disorders are described more fully in an earlier part of this chapter and it is worthy of note that many are associated with short stature and growth failure.

Table 5.7 Causes of growth failure

1. Genetically determined short stature
2. Chromosome disorders
3. Intrauterine growth retardation
4. Skeletal dysplasia
5. Constitutional delay in growth and puberty
6. Malnutrition and psychosocial deprivation
7. Chronic system disorders, e.g. gut, renal and cardiovascular systems
8. Endocrine disorders, e.g. hypothyroidism and growth hormone deficiency

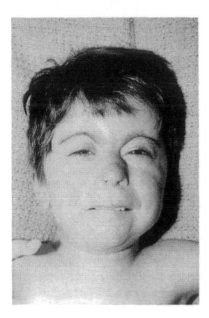

Figure 5.2   Typical facial appearance of Amsterdam (de Lange) dwarf.

3. Intrauterine growth retardation (IUGR) may result from several factors, notably maternal smoking, excessive intake of alcohol during pregnancy (producing the fetal alcohol syndrome) and placental insufficiency, particularly when it is associated with chronic pre-eclampsia and hypertension. Intrauterine infections (see above) and chronic antepartum bleeding may also be implicated. Frequently, neonates with multiple congenital abnormalities show evidence of poor intrauterine growth and there are a small number of low birthweight dwarf syndromes, e.g. de Lange 'Amsterdam' dwarfism (Fig. 5.2), Seckel's 'bird-headed' dwarfism and the Russell–Silver syndrome, in which there is symmetrical, long-standing IUGR.

Although such cases show 'catch-up' growth, often in quite dramatic fashion over the first 2 months of life, this is difficult to predict with certainty and is less likely to occur with long-standing IUGR and does not occur at all in the low birthweight dwarf syndromes.

4. Skeletal dysplasias represent a group of disorders in which development of cartilage and bone is defective, resulting in disproportionate 'short-limbed' short stature with abnormalities in the size and shape of limbs, skull, pelvis and spine. The most widely known is the dominantly inherited condition achondroplasia in which severe limb shortening makes the diagnosis obvious at birth. In certain of the rarer dysplasias (osteochondro-dysplasias), now numbering more than 40,[3] diagnosis may be more difficult and may be aided considerably by detailed radiological examination.

No specific treatment is available to correct the underlying osteochondroplastic disorder although orthopaedic and orthotic support may be necessary, e.g. in order to treat kyphoscoliosis and to stabilize valgus feet.

5. In children who exhibit signs of constitutional delay in growth and puberty, short stature is secondary to a slower than normal rate of maturation. Height *and* bone age are usually delayed by 18 months to 4 years and pubertal onset is delayed until the bone age is appropriate. The exact cause of this condition is unclear although a family history of a similar growth pattern is often obtainable. Final adult stature is eventually reached in the late teens and is appropriate for the target 'midparent' height. The development of secondary sexual characteristics occurs normally. Growth velocity is normal for bone age in such individuals and only occasionally is treatment indicated for amelioration of psychosocial difficulty caused by peer group pressures. In this situation, anabolic steroids are sometimes prescribed.

6. Malnutrition is the most important cause of growth failure on a global scale with, at current estimates, 60% or so of the world's children being undernourished.

7. Chronic disorders of any major organ system are well-recognized causes of growth failure. In long-standing severe congenital heart disease, tissue hypoxia, chronic cyanosis and cardiac strain frequently accompany growth failure. Catch-up growth following successful cardiac surgery is not invariable. Chronic gastro-intestinal, pulmonary, and cyanotic heart disease may all produce the phenomenon of 'clubbing' affecting the fingers and toes. Bulbous swellings of the terminal phalanges are associated with loss of nail angulation and fluctuation of the nail base; occasionally, this is encountered as a benign familial (dominant) disorder (Fig. 5.3).

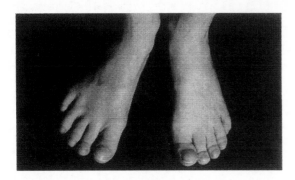

Figure 5.3 Toe clubbing caused by pulmonary disease (cystic fibrosis). Note nail angulation.

8. *Endocrine (hormonal) mechanisms.* Ovarian dysgenesis in Turner's syndrome and severe psychosocial deprivation mediate their effects on growth via these mechanisms. The remaining endocrine disorders which significantly affect growth are growth hormone deficiency, hypothyroidism and excessive cortisol production.

The principal causes of growth hormone deficiency are summarized in Table 5.8.

Estimates of the prevalence of growth hormone deficiency vary considerably and many authors consider this to be an underdiagnosed condition. A figure of 1:3000–4000 would seem to be appropriate at present.

Steroid excess as a result of medical treatment or of increased endogenous secretion of cortisol or adrenocorticotropic hormone, e.g. owing to tumors, causes growth failure by inhibiting growth at tissue level.

Table 5.8 Causes of growth hormone deficiency

Congenital	Other
Autosomal recessive type	Neoplasm of
Autosomal dominant type	hypothalamus or pituitary
Idiopathic type	e.g. craniopharyngioma
Associated with pituitary	Irradiation
hypoplasia/aplasia	Meningitis
Associated with midline	Encephalitis
defects, e.g. cleft palate,	Histiocytosis
septo-optic dysplasia,	Birth asphyxia
holoprosencephaly	Skull trauma
	Hypothyroidism
	Hemochromatosis
	Severe psychosocial
	deprivation

DISORDERS OF THE IMMUNE SYSTEM

Intact and properly functioning skin and mucous membrane and the action of cilia form the primary barriers to invasion by infectious agents. Subsequent defense is mediated by the immune system whose main functional components are listed in Table 5.9. Disorders of different parts of the immune system tend to present with different and distinct clinical syndromes.

Lymphocyte populations

Stem cells of the lymphoreticular system differentiate into two major cell lines known as 'T' (thymus-derived) cells and 'B' ('bursa' or bone marrow-derived) cells. One of the most import-

Table 5.9 Components of the immune system

Lymphocytes	T cells: 'Helper', 'suppressor' and 'killer' subtypes B cells: Immunoglobulin synthesis (IgG, IgM, IgA, IgE)
Lymphokines Complement system Phagocytes	Polymorphonuclear leucocytes Macrophages Mononuclear cells

Table 5.10 B- and T-cell function

Properties of B cells
Major immunoglobulin synthesis (e.g. protection against common major bacteria)
Viral neutralization on initial exposure
Local mucosal protection in gut and respiratory tract
Initiate macrophage killing
Initiate vasoactive amine (e.g. histamine) release from mast cells and basophils

Properties of T cells
T-helper function
T-suppressor function (modulation of immune response)
T-killer function (initiation of cytotoxic processes)
Containment of infection with agents such as mycobacteria, Herpes group viruses, Epstein–Barr virus, fungal and protozoal infection
Allograft rejection
Graft versus host disease

ant differences between B and T cells is the ability of the former to synthesize various classes of immunoglobulin. The major functions of these different lymphocyte populations are summarized in Table 5.10.

Close cooperation between T and B cells is necessary for mounting an immune response – to include neutralization with specific immuno-globulin and the initiation of further processes such as phagocytosis by macrophages and poly-morphs. Such cooperation is augmented by a cascade of complement protein factors in the case of B cells and for T cells by recently discovered proteins known as 'lymphokines', the best known of which are migration inhibition factors and the interleukins.

B-cell secretory products (immunoglobulins) are divided into five main classes each of which is synthesized by a specific cell line. Immuno-globulins are active against staphylococci, strep-tococci, pneumococci and *Haemophilus influenzae* and may initiate adequate initial protection against some viral diseases such as varicella and hepatitis although they are less efective in con-taining established viral disorders. B cells also mediate immediate hypersensitivity reactions such as those seen in allergic rhinitis and asthma. The main subtypes of immunoglobulin are summarized in Table 5.11.

Immune deficiency diseases are summarized in Table 5.12.

Disorders affecting the T-cell system carry a poor prognosis compared with disorders of the B-cell system while 'combined' deficiency states are the most difficult to treat and have the poorest outcome.

Table 5.12 Disorders of the immune system

Panhypogammaglobulinemia (Bruton type)
Selective specific IgA or IgM deficiency
Common variable immunodeficiency

DiGeorge syndrome
Nezelof syndrome

Severe combined immunodeficiency
Ataxia telangiectasia
Chronic mucocutaneous candidiasis
Wiskott–Aldrich syndrome

Complement deficiencies
Chronic granulomatous disease
Myeloperoxidase deficiency
Chèdiak–Higashi syndrome
Leucocyte motility and cidal effects (glucose-6-phosphate dehydrogenase deficiency, glutathione synthetase deficiency, Kartagener's syndrome, Shwachman's syndrome, hyperimmunoglobulin E syndrome)

Secondary immunodeficiency states
Adenosine deaminase and nucleoside phosphorylase deficiency
Nephrosis
Protein losing enteropathy
Protein/calorie malnutrition
Steroid therapy
Other immunosuppressant therapy
Viral infections including HIV virus and acquired immune deficiency syndrome

Disorders of the complement system

Approximately 10% of the globulin fraction of serum is made up of heat-labile protein components known as 'complement' and 'com-plement control proteins'. These proteins act as the principal mediators of the inflammatory response and are important in defense against infection. The 'classical' complement pathway consists of 11 separate proteins; there is a further

Table 5.11 Immunoglobulin subtypes

Class	Molecular weight	Main biological role
IgG	140 000	Complement fixation and neutralizing antibody
Serum IgA	160 000	Polymer formation
Secretory IgA	370 000	Mucosal surface protection and polymer formation
IgM	900 000	Complement fixation and polymer formation. Agglutination; opsonic activity
IgD	160 000	?Biological role
IgE	197 000	Skin and mast cell fixation; elimination of parasites Anaphylaxis

alternative system with constituents designated as B, D and P. Complement C3 is a component of both pathways. The cumulative effect of an activated complement system, triggered by antigen antibody combination, includes viral neutralization, opsonization, induction of granulocytosis, leukocyte chemotaxis, endotoxic inactivation and microbial lysis.

Congenital deficiencies of all the components of the classical complement system and deficiency of factor D of the alternative pathway have been described but are rare.

Disorders of the phagocytic system

The phagocytic system consists of polymorphonuclear leukocytes and monocytes. When monocytes leave the circulation, they develop into macrophages within many organ systems or migrate into areas of inflammation. Polymorphs are usually marginated in the circulation or stored in bone marrow in order to be rapidly released in response to infection and acute inflammation. At sites of inflammation, neutrophils adhere to capillary walls and migrate into surrounding tissues by diapedesis. Bacteria are prepared for phagocytosis by a process of opsonization which involves complement and the action of specific immunoglobulin antibody to neutralize surface virulence factors on a given microorganism.

Disordered phagocytic function is the main abnormality in *chronic granulomatous disease of childhood*. In this disorder, there is defective oxidative metabolism within leukocytes which severely impairs normal function resulting in recurrent severe pyogenic infection in early infancy. Early aggressive and appropriate antibiotic therapy is important; occasionally, granulocyte transfusions may be indicated in resistant cases and surgical drainage procedures are often necessary.

Chèdiak–Higashi syndrome (autosomal recessive) presents in early infancy with oculocutaneous albinism, recurrent infections and neurological problems such as mental retardation, pyramidal and cerebellar dysfunction and peripheral neuropathy. Abnormal granules are demonstrated in leukocytes and all other marrow-derived cells. Polymorph function is significantly impaired although the exact mechanism responsible is not fully understood. This disorder progresses to cause anemia, leukopenia and thrombocytopenia with death from infection or malignancy before the teenage years.

Viral infections, e.g. intrauterine infection with rubella or cytomegalovirus, may influence the differentiation and normal function of B and T cells as may Epstein–Barr virus infection in postnatal life. However, the most important disorder to be considered is the profound disturbance in T-cell function resulting from infection with human T-cell lymphotrophic virus (HTLV3) now known as human immunodeficiency virus (HIV). Infection with this agent results in the acquired immune deficiency syndrome (AIDS).

Childhood AIDS was first described in 1982, and by 1990 more than 1300 cases were reported to the Centers for Disease Control in the USA with more than 500 cases reported in Europe alone and more than 2000 cases worldwide. It has been estimated that on a global scale pediatric AIDS cases may number several million. Approximately 80% of children contract AIDS following transplacental infection with a falling proportion becoming infected via contaminated blood or blood products. Recent studies suggest a seropositive rate of between 0.01 and 0.02% in European women, with maternofetal transmission rates estimated to be 10–30%.[6] Passively acquired maternal antibody is thought to be cleared from the infant's circulation by approximately 18 months of age thus limiting the usefulness of antibody screening in this age group. Definitive diagnosis depends upon the detection of viral antigen; typical immune dysfunction includes elevated levels of IgG, IgM and IgA (polyclonal hypergammaglobulinemia), thrombocytopenia, anemia and a reversal of the normal greater-than-one ratio of helper to suppressor T cells. As the disease progresses, further T-cell dysfunction manifests as a lymphopenia of CD4 lymphocyte subsets, abnormal responses to mitogens and decreased production of interferon and interleukin-2.

The mean age of diagnosis of AIDS in children is at present about 6 months although the trend is for increasing numbers of older children with milder disease to be reported. Early symptoms include recurrent respiratory infections, failure to thrive with persistent diarrhea, candidiasis, pyrexia of unknown origin and generalized lymphadenopathy. Opportunistic infection with *Pneumocystis carinii* presents with fever, cough and tachypnea associated with significant hypoxia. Another troublesome respiratory disorder is lymphocytic interstitial pneumonitis which is usually accompanied by parotid gland enlargement, finger clubbing, hepatosplenomegaly and generalized lymphadenopathy.

Progressively severe candidiasis involving the mouth, pharynx and esophagus compounds the nutritional difficulties in AIDS children who often develop terminal wasting disorder accompanied by enteropathic bowel changes and further opportunistic infection with *Cryptosporidium*, *Salmonella* and atypical *Mycobacteria*. A significant proportion of children also show signs of nervous system involvement manifested by regression in milestones and by signs of pyramidal tract dysfunction. Other signs of multisystem involvement include cardiomyopathy, hepatitis and nephropathy.

At present, AIDS is an irreversible disorder and management is supportive with the emphasis on family management since the mother may already be dead or ill from AIDS herself. Such treatment includes optimizing nutritional status, treatment of recurrent bacterial infection (with monitoring of respiratory flora), and treatment of anemia and thrombocytopenia and regular gammaglobulin infusions. Pneumocytis pneumonia is treated with co-trimoxazole or pentamidine and oxygen therapy and some centers practice regular prophylaxis with inhaled pentamidine to head off infection. Invasive or severe candidal infection is treated with amphotericin B, ketoconazole or fluconazole. Acyclovir is indicated for the management of herpes virus group infections. New 'combined' (reverse transcriptase inhibitors with protease inhibitors) antiviral drug regimens are showing promising results in slowing the progression of HIV infection with careful clinical trials on-going.[7]

Until a specific cure or immunization techniques become available, the emphasis is on prevention by thorough screening of blood donors and blood products and by appropriate counseling with respect to intravenous drug abuse and 'safe sex' whatever the gender of the participants. Maternal/fetal transmission of HIV can also be reduced by administration of antiviral therapy in the third trimester of pregnancy. There are very few cases of proven HIV infection following needle stick injury from an infected patient although a single case report has documented HIV infection in a dental patient thought to have been infected by her dentist. Clearly professionals involved in managing infected patients should take all necessary precautions to avoid self-contamination with virus-laden blood. Other general measures include the washing of potentially infected linen at 95°C for 10 minutes; designated infected waste to be disposed of separately and incinerated. Disposable equipment should be used whenever possible and where reusable equipment is employed, this should be heat-sterilized by autoclaving or where appropriate by gas sterilization using ethylene oxide. Although HIV seroconversion following needle stick injury is very uncommon, guidelines for staff should include the following:

1. Staff with infections such as herpes simplex or eczema should not care for AIDS patients.
2. Cuts and abrasions should be covered with waterproof dressings, and disposable plastic aprons and latex gloves should be worn when exposed to blood and saliva. Eye protection should be worn if splashing into the conjunctiva is possible.
3. Safe handling and disposal of sharps should be undertaken to avoid needle stick injury. Resheathing of needles after use should be avoided in order to reduce the risk of finger needle stick.

A sharps container conforming to Department of Health standards, e.g. 'CIN BIN', should be used and subsequently incinerated. All specimen containers and request cards should be appropriately labeled as 'biohazard' and spillages of blood or blood-stained secretions should be mopped up with 1% sodium hypochlorite (10% bleach diluted 1:10) and the area in question should be left covered in disinfectant for 30 minutes before wiping clean using disposable gloves. Any inoculation incidents should be 'milked' to encourage bleeding and then washed immediately with soap and water. Splashes of blood into the eye should be irrigated with copious amounts of water or saline (see also Miller et al[7]).

DISORDERS OF THE BLOOD AND LYMPHATIC SYSTEM

Disorders of hemostasis

Hemostasis is normally maintained by a complex mechanism involving local reactions of blood vessels, altered platelet activity and the interactions of protein 'coagulation factors' circulating in the blood. After vascular injury, there is active vasoconstriction followed by mobilization of platelets and clotting factors as shown schematically in Figure 5.4.

In the first phase of normal coagulation, thromboplastin is formed by the interaction of plasma, platelets and extracellular fluid; this facilitates conversion of prothrombin to thrombin in the presence of calcium ions. Thrombin then converts soluble fibrinogen into a stable fibrin clot (polymer) which interacts with platelets to form a firm plug. Factors 8, 9, 11 and 12 act through a so-called 'intrinsic' system to activate factor 10 whereas in the 'extrinsic' system this factor is directly activated by factor 7 (proconvertin). Fibrin lysis is mediated by a

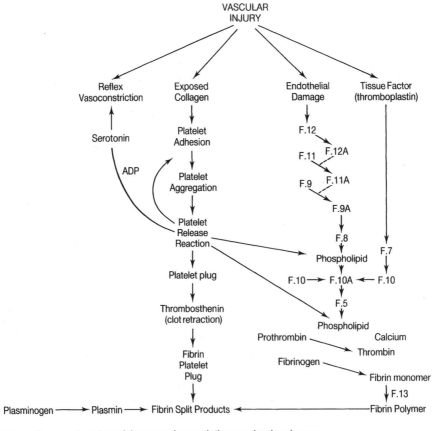

Figure 5.4 Schematic representation of the normal coagulation mechanism in man.

substance known as plasmin which is derived from its serum precursor, plasminogen.

Assessment of coagulation disorders is aided considerably by utilizing several diagnostic tests outlined in Table 5.13. These tests are complementary to history and physical examination; a careful family history is also important since several coagulation disorders have a genetic basis.

The principal disorders manifesting with increased bleeding tendency are listed in Table 5.14. Only the commoner disorders are now discussed.

The hemophilias are X-linked recessive disorders and represent the commonest and most troublesome coagulation disorders. Types A and B are clinically indistinguishable and are secondary to factor 8 and 9 deficiency respectively. Clinical severity depends upon the degree of factor depletion, which becomes clinically progressively severe at levels below 5% although signs are not necessarily apparent in the newborn period. Certain neonates with these disorders do present with, for example, pro-

longed bleeding times from the umbilical cord or circumcision sites. With increased activity, hematomas develop in response to minor trauma, affecting joints and muscles. Multiple painful hemarthroses are followed by progressive joint deformity. Other complications include prolonged bleeding from trivial lacerations, hematuria and intracranial hemorrhage. Diagnosis may be expected from the family history and will certainly be confirmed by demonstrating a prolonged partial thromboplastin time and low factor levels. Management is by minimizing trauma in early infancy, avoiding exposure to aspirin and expeditious specific factor replacement using specially formulated concentrate. Other local measures to reduce bleeding include the application of cold compresses and careful pressure. Initial immobilization should be followed by gentle remobilization in the event of hemarthroses in order to reduce the risk of ankylosis. Careful genetic counseling is mandatory in this disease; antenatal diagnostic techniques are now available utilizing chorionic villus biopsy.

Table 5.13   Examples of commonly used tests of hemostasis

Test	Assesses
Tourniquet test	Platelet function. Vascular stability of small vessels
Platelet count/platelet function test	Platelet number and function
Bleeding time	Platelet function and vascular stability of small vessels
Clotting time	Whole coagulation mechanism
Thrombin time	Conversion of fibrinogen to fibrin polymer
Prothrombin time	Adequacy of factors 2, 5, 7 and 10
Partial thromboplastin time	Adequacy of factors 8, 9, 11 and 12

Table 5.14   Hemostatic disorders

Condition	Abnormality
Hemophilia A	Factor 8 deficiency
Hemophilia B (Christmas disease)	Factor 9 deficiency
Other factor deficiences	Factors 11 and 12
Von Willebrand's disease	Factor 8 deficiency and reduced platelet adhesiveness
Parahemophilia (Owren's disease)	Factor 5 deficiency
Hemorrhagic disease of the newborn	Reduced activity of factors 2, 7, 9 and 10
Congenital afibrinogenemia	Absent fibrinogen
Idiopathic thrombocytopenic purpura	Reduced platelet number and function

Von Willebrand's disease is inherited in autosomal dominant mode. In this disorder, factor 8 deficiency is compounded by defects in platelet adhesiveness. Clinical presentation is usually with epistaxis, bleeding from the gums, prolonged oozing from cuts and increased bleeding after trauma or surgery. Management is similar to that of hemophilia.

Hemorrhagic disease of the newborn is now rare following the widespread use of the prophylactic vitamin K1 in neonates. Such treatment reduces the risk of depletion of factors 2, 7, 9 and 10 seen in a minority of newborn infants and potentially exacerbated by the absence of vitamin K from the breast milk. Prothrombin time is prolonged. Treatment involves the administration of parenteral vitamin K1 and support of the circulation with replacement transfusion when necessary.

Congenital afibrinogenemia is a rare, recessively inherited disorder associated with unexpectedly prolonged bleeding following trauma or surgery. Thrombin time is prolonged. Management is supportive and also involves the administration of replacement fibrinogen.

Thrombocytopenic purpura is characterized clinically by small hemorrhages into the superficial layers of the skin inducing purple discoloration. Tiny extravasations are designated petechiae and more extensive 'bruised' areas as ecchymoses. Bleeding may also occur into mucous membrane, brain or viscera. The commonest platelet disorder in childhood is *idiopathic thrombocytopenic purpura* (ITP) (Fig. 5.5), which is thought to be caused by sensitization owing to virus infection, following a latent period of 2 to 3 weeks. Antiplatelet antibodies can be demonstrated. Generalized ecchymoses and a petechial rash are typical with lesions, particularly prominent over the extremities. The tourniquet test is positive and the bleeding time is prolonged beyond 10 minutes.

Very occasionally, thrombocytopenia may be drug induced; *Wiskott–Aldrich syndrome* (eczema, thrombocytopenia and susceptibility to infection) is described in a previous section. Another rare association of thrombocytopenia is aplasia of the radii and thumbs which may be coupled with congenital cardiac and renal abnormalities.

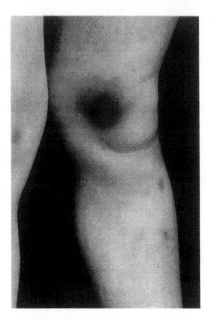

Figure 5.5 Typical ecchymoses in idiopathic thrombocytopenic purpura.

ITP should not be confused with *Henoch–Schönlein (anaphylactoid) purpura* (Fig. 5.6) which is a disorder in which vasculitic lesions affect small blood vessels, frequently following an upper respiratory infection. Boys are affected more than girls with peak incidence in the age range 3 to 5 years. Skin blood vessels are surrounded by cellular reaction of polymorphs and round cells and IgA deposits may also be seen. In distinction from ITP, skin lesions develop as small wheals or as red maculopapular lesions which occur in crops particularly over the pretibial areas, buttocks and extensor surfaces. Such lesions may develop petechial or purpuric qualities but frank ecchymoses are uncommon. Signs of multisystem involvement include abdominal pain, hematemesis, melena, hematuria, hemiplagia, seizures and arthritis. Renal involvement is potentially the most serious complication and may lead to chronic renal failure. Diagnosis of Henoch–Schönlein purpura is usually made on clinical grounds and treatment is supportive. Steroid therapy is reserved for the more serious complications or for cases of particularly severe skin involvement.

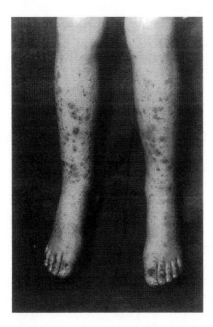

Figure 5.6 Typical rash of Henoch–Schönlein purpura.

Disorders of the lymphatic system

The mononuclear and phagocyte population of the spleen, liver and bone marrow acts as an immunological filter mechanism for the blood circulating through them. A large number of foreign antigens invade the body via the skin, respiratory and gastrointestinal tracts and then enter the lymphatic system rather than the blood. In this situation, the first line of cellular defense is represented in the lymph node system. Lymph nodes represent separate anatomical units distributed along lymphatic channels and are surrounded by a connective tissue capsule perforated at several points by feeding lymphatics which deliver antigens, lymphocytes and macrophages. Circulating lymph is actively 'filtered' within the node whose efferent vessel exits via the hilus containing sensitized B and T cells and antibody-secreting plasma cells (see above). The outer part of the node is designated the cortex and contains lymphoid follicles which are centers of B-cell activity. Antigenic stimulation causes primary follicles to become secondary follicles by enlarging to form pale staining germinal centers containing activated B cells, T cells, macrophages and reticulum cells. The paracortical areas between the primary and secondary follicles and the central medullary portion of the node are centers of T-cell activity. This structure provides a suitable system for delivering and exposing antigens to the immune system. Following such immunological stimulation, node size may increase tenfold within 1 week. After birth and following continuing exposure to environmental antigens, the mass of lymphoid tissue steadily increases during childhood to reach its peak in early puberty. Palpable lymph nodes are a common finding in children compared to adults, particularly in the cervical, inguinal and axillary regions. It is unusual to find parallel enlargement affecting the popliteal, mediastinal or supraclavicular regions in the absence of significant pathology.

Normal lymph node enlargement in childhood rarely exceeds 1 inch (2.5 cm) diameter in the neck, axilla or inguinal region although enlargement above 0.06–0.09 inches (2–3 mm) should be treated with suspicion when affecting other areas. Other causes for concern are when lymphadenopathy affects more than two regions or when nodes are associated with local heat (inflammation), pain, erythema, fluctuance, 'rubberiness' or a tendency to mat together or to become adherent to surrounding tissues. The causes of generalized and significant lymphadenopathy are summarized in Table 5.15.

Localized, isolated 'regional' lymphadenopathy is most often due to infection. Nodes in inguinal and iliac groups drain the lower extremities, perineum, genitalia, buttocks and lower abdominal wall. A small number of moderate-sized, discrete inguinal nodes are a common finding in children. Readily overlooked sources of infection producing such lymphadenopathy include insect bites, napkin dermatitis, injection site inflammation and low-grade infected eczema or seborrheic dermatitis. It is important to differentiate between enlarged lymph nodes and other inguinal swellings such as ectopic testes, hernias and lipomas.

Lymphatic vessels collect lymph from almost all tissues and organs except the central nervous system, muscle and non-vascular structures such

Table 5.15 Causes of generalized lymphadenopathy in childhood

Viral infections (Epstein–Barr, cytomegalovirus, HIV, rubella, varicella, measles, upper respiratory viruses)
Bacterial infection (tuberculosis, typhoid, staphylococcal or streptococcal bacteremia)
Protozoal infection (toxoplasmosis)
Fungal infection (coccidioidomycosis)
Immune mediated disorders (systemic lupus erythematosus, serum sickness, drug allergy, juvenile chronic arthritis)
Storage disorders (Gaucher's disease. Niemann–Pick disease)
Neoplasia (leukemia, lymphoma, Hodgkin's disease, neuroblastoma, histiocytosis X)

as cornea and cartilage. Essentially, lymph represents extracellular fluid loaded with lymphocytes and material of molecular size which is too large to cross capillary endothelium. This fluid is first delivered into lymph 'capillaries' and is then carried to regional lymph nodes via larger thin-walled transparent lymph vessels. Eventually, body lymph enters the thoracic duct and then the great veins via the right lymphatic duct.

When infection is not contained locally it may enter the lymphatic vessels as an *ascending lymphangitis* which is characterized by erythematous linear streaks along the course of a given group of lymphatics. This is usually followed by painful swelling of the appropriate regional nodes and may be followed by local edema where there is associated lymphatic obstruction. Bacteremia or septicemia may ensue unless infection is treated promptly.

Lymphedema refers to the diffuse pitting type of edema which results from obstruction of lymphatic flow. The most common site is in the lower extremities where it may be accompanied by firm thickening of skin and by susceptibility to cellular infection. The commonest causes of acquired lymphedema are post-inflammatory (lymphadenitis), surgical obliteration of nodes or lymph channels or post-therapeutic irradiation. Congenital pedal edema is a feature of Turner's syndrome (Bonnevie–Ullrich syndrome).

Congenital (early onset) lymphedema or *Milroy's disease* is an extremely rare, dominantly inherited disorder characterized by chronic pitting edema of the lower limbs. Variability of genetic expression ranges from minimal ankle swelling to greatly enlarged feet, legs and thighs. Overlying skin is attenuated but otherwise normal and there is usually slow asymptomatic progression of edema with time. Attempts to visualize lymphatics in involved areas have proved unsuccessful and the defect has therefore been thought to be due to an abnormality in lymphatic development rather than secondary to increased output of interstitial fluid. This defect is largely cosmetic with minor degrees of disability resulting in cases of gross lower limb edema. Resection of subcutaneous tissue and skin autographs have been performed with variable results and the use of diuretics and bed rest are only temporarily and partially effective.

Obvious care should always be taken to differentiate lymphedema from the commoner phenomenon of pitting edema caused by diseases such as hypoproteinemia, hepatic, renal and cardiac failure and venous obstruction.

DISORDERS OF THE ENDOCRINE SYSTEM (DIABETES MELLITUS)

Kathryn Noyes and Christopher Kelnar

The child with diabetes

Diabetes in children is a challenging condition, and is the commonest endocrine disorder of childhood. It is a permanent condition in which the body gradually ceases to produce the hormone insulin, which is normally secreted from beta cells of the islets of Langerhans in the pancreas. Despite considerable advances in management, childhood diabetes remains a disorder with significant long-term morbidity and reduced life expectancy and one which poses extreme stresses and strains on family life.

Insulin is a key anabolic hormone and is synthesized as a precursor molecule pro-insulin, which undergoes splitting to form insulin and the peptide, C peptide.

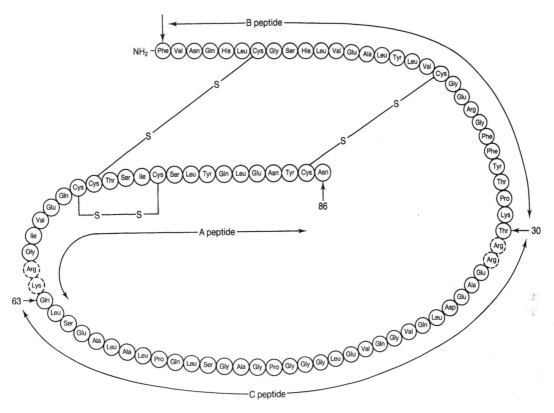

Figure 5.7 Schematic diagram of an insulin molecule.

Insulin has a direct effect to reduce blood glucose and it also inhibits release of stored glucose. This action is necessary to maintain glucose homeostasis. The symptoms and signs of childhood diabetes are the result of a lack of insulin.

In the healthy state, the carbohydrate content of ingested food is broken down into simple sugars and absorbed into the bloodstream from the intestinal tract. The glucose in the circulation then reaches the pancreatic beta cells and insulin is released.

Insulin allows entry of glucose into cells, particularly muscle and adipose tissue and it stimulates protein, glycogen and fat synthesis. Insulin decreases glucose output from the liver (which itself does not require insulin to allow glucose into its cells).

The lack of insulin in children with diabetes causes hyperglycemia. Muscle and adipose tissues are unable to utilize glucose, and glycogenesis and gluconeogenesis all contribute to the extracellular excess of glucose. Glucose is a powerful osmotic agent and the sustained elevation of blood glucose, as diabetes develops, leads to an osmotic diuresis. The subsequent marked polyuria leads to significant polydipsia, despite which dehydration soon becomes a major feature. The dehydration may be exacerbated by vomiting, itself often a result of gastric stasis owing to hyperglycemia and ketonemia (produced by increased fat breakdown as an alternative energy source).

Type I diabetes

Incidence

The incidence of type I diabetes (previously known as insulin-dependent diabetes mellitus or IDDM) is increasing rapidly in Europe, with the rate in many countries roughly doubling over the last 20 years.[8,9] The incidence in Finland at 42.9/1 000 000 per year is compared with one of the lowest type I diabetes incidence rates in China at 0.7/1 000 000 per year.[10] Whereas the incidence in some countries has reached a plateau, one Canadian study indicating that the annual incidence for all age groups between 0 and 14 years has been stable over the past decade,[11] there is a statistically significant increase of 2% a year in Scotland. The variation within a nation can also be striking and a higher incidence in urban over rural populations has been reported.[12]

The mean age of onset of childhood diabetes is 12 years with 25% presenting below the age of 5 years and 10% below the age of 2 years. The increased incidence during early puberty reflects hormonal changes that may exacerbate the islet cell damage.

Etiology

The development of diabetes in a child is multifactorial with both genetic and environmental factors playing a part. The wide geographical variations in incidence stress the importance of these environmental factors. Seasonal variation in the onset of type I diabetes has been observed worldwide, increasing commonly during the winter months. Overall, the risk of developing childhood diabetes is equal for both sexes, but interestingly there is a slight male excess in those countries with a high incidence and an excess of females in those countries with a low incidence.

Genetic associations with diabetes are well recognized. There is strong association between developing diabetes and histocompatability (HLA – human leukocyte antigen) markers and gene loci responsible for their synthesis on the short arm of chromosome 6 – loci DR3 and DR4 have particularly strong associations. 90–98% of all children with type I diabetes express DR3, DR4 antigens or both, but less than 1% of healthy subjects with such markers will ever develop diabetes.[13] This highlights the importance of the environmental trigger in the generally susceptible individual. Children with diabetes from

Table 5.16 Risks for childhood diabetes mellitus in Caucasians

Situation	Risk
General population	1 in 500
No family history but HLA DR3/DR3 or DR4/DR4	1 in 150
No family history but HLA DR3/DR4	1 in 40
Sibling with diabetes	1 in 16
Sibling with diabetes and	
–0 HLA haplotypes in common	1 in 100
–1 HLA haplotypes in common	1 in 20
–2 HLA haplotypes in common	1 in 8
Identical twin with diabetes	1 in 3
Offspring of affected mother	1 in 50
Offspring of affected father	1 in 20

families with a parent who has type I diabetes are significantly more likely to have an affected father than mother (Table 5.16).[14]

Cellular immunological mechanisms are also involved. Antibodies against islet cell cytoplasmic antigens (ICAs) and the enzyme glutamic acid decarboxylase (GAD) have been reported in type I diabetes.[16] However, it is unclear whether they play a direct role in the disease process or serve as a marker of tissue damage initiated by other etiological agents.[17]

Studies on identical twins have shown that the risk for the other twin to contract diabetes is in excess of 50%. The risk for diabetes in nonidentical twins was 11% in the same study.[18] If the etiology of type I diabetes was entirely due to genetic factors, the concordance rate in identical twins would be expected to be near 100%.

Environmental factors that trigger the disease process may start early in life, many years before the onset of diabetes.[19] Viruses, toxins, psychosocial factors and nutritional intake have all been implicated as potential environmental factors. Rubella, mumps, cytomegalovirus and Coxsackie B viruses have been implicated most often; 15–40% of cases of congenital rubella develop type I diabetes.

The risk of developing type I diabetes seems to be higher in babies of heavier birthweight in contrast to the common finding that non-insulin-dependent diabetes (type II) is associated with low birthweight. Some studies indicated an increased risk of acquiring diabetes if a child is not breast-fed at all or only for 3 months or less.[20]

The time that a child is first introduced to cow's milk seems to be of importance as it is the early introduction to cow's milk that increases the risk for diabetes.[20]

While the evidence still remains unclear as to the true cause of diabetes, it is important to explain to the parents of the newly diagnosed child with diabetes that it was not caused by something that the family could have avoided.

Clinical features

The clinical onset in most children is usually relatively acute although, in retrospect, parents may feel their newly diagnosed child with diabetes has 'not been right' for several months with poor appetite and malaise (Table 5.17).

A finding of glycosuria or hyperglycemia is a pediatric emergency and telephoned referral to a pediatrician on the day of diagnosis is mandatory. Any delay in referral may lead to the decompensated state of diabetic ketoacidosis (DKA), which is life-threatening. A child in DKA – i.e. 'diabetes out of control' – is dehydrated, hyperglycemic, ketonemic and acidotic (with a blood pH < 7.3 mmol/L and/or a serum bicarbonate < 10 mmol/L). This child may look less unwell than the biochemistry results soon reveal and the child is typically flushed (as a result of the ketonemia) and is bright eyed with deep sighing breathing – acidotic Kussmaul respiration.

Diagnosis

There is rarely any doubt about making a diagnosis of type I diabetes when the typical symptoms are found. The child with type I diabetes will have a raised venous plasma glucose

Table 5.17 Signs and symptoms of diabetes at the time of diagnosis

Polyuria and secondary polydipsia
Nocturnal enuresis (in previously trained child)
Weight loss – a feature of dehydration, loss of fat and muscle wasting
Lethargy
Behavioral changes – 2° to hyperglycemia
Infection, especially genital candidiasis

(random sample > 11.1 mmol/L or a fasting value of > 7.8 mmol/L – normal range 3.3–6.4 mmol/L), glycosuria, +/– ketonuria. This child will then require lifelong insulin therapy. Insulin is given by subcutaneous injection to a newly diagnosed child who is mildly symptomatic, i.e. not acidotic and not vomiting.

Unfortunately, DKA is still a common presentation of diabetes with one study showing 26% of new cases of pediatric diabetes presenting in DKA.[21] In this study, the incidence of severe DKA was significantly higher in children under 5 years of age. Cerebral edema is the unpredictable complication of DKA, with resulting significant morbidity and mortality.

Management of diabetic ketoacidosis

Priority is given to the resuscitation of the child. The further treatment aims are to replace the fluid losses, to correct the acidosis and to achieve normoglycemia.

Insulin

Subcutaneous insulin therapy

Insulin is inactivated in the gut by gastrointestinal enzymes, therefore insulin injections are given subcutaneously by means of a disposable syringe and needle, or via a pen device (Fig. 5.8).

It is important to use the correct injection technique as insulin injected intramuscularly is absorbed too quickly causing significant hypoglycemia.

Insulin can be extracted from animal sources (beef or pig) but it is usual to employ 'human' insulin in childhood diabetes. Most currently available human insulin is made biosynthetically by recombinant DNA technology using *Escherichia coli*. Physiologically, insulin is secreted into the portal circulation in monomeric form. Current commercial insulins exist in hexamer formation, which distorts in the presence of diminishing insulin concentration to dimeric and then monomeric insulin that circulates in the peripheral circulation and is bioactive. Therefore, there is a time delay after the insulin injection before the

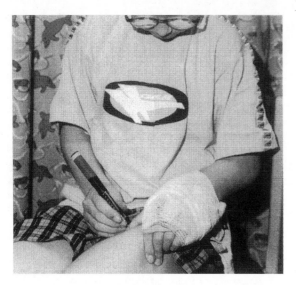

Figure 5.8   Child injecting insulin by means of pen device.

appearance of insulin activity because of this dissociation.[22] The aim of insulin therapy is to reproduce physiological insulin secretion but, as yet, all currently practicable regimens do so relatively poorly.

There is now a rapidly acting monomeric insulin analogue available. This is insulin lispro, which has superior pharmacokinetic properties for postprandial blood glucose control. It is injected immediately before the meal but enhances the risk for early postprandial hypoglycemia if the meal is delayed or if exercise is taken immediately afterwards. There is only limited data on the use of insulin lispro in the pediatric population.[23]

There are three main types of insulin which vary in the rapidity of their onset and in their duration of action.

1. The most rapid in onset is 'soluble' insulin, e.g. Actrapid, Humulin S, which takes effect after 30 to 60 minutes and has a peak action between 2 and 4 hours and a duration of up to 8 hours.
2. Intermediate-acting insulins. The commonest strategies to prolong insulin activity are to bind insulin to a simple peptide, protamine, to form the isophane insulins, e.g. Insulatard,

Humulin I, or to crystalize the insulin in the presence of zinc to form the lente insulins, e.g. Monotard. Their onset of action is 1 to 2 hours after injection, with a peak action between 4 and 12 hours and a duration of 16 to 35 hours.
3. Longer-acting insulins with slower onset, e.g. Ultratard.

Insulin is administered in units, abbreviated U (international units) and the most common insulin concentration is 100 units/mL.

Insulin regimens

Insulin injections must be given into sub-cutaneous tissue – not into the muscle below the dermis – to ensure that the insulin is reliably absorbed. Children are often thin, and their sub-cutaneous fat layer is also very thin. The upper outer area of the arms is the least preferred site for this reason and other more favored sites are anterior and lateral thighs, abdomen and buttocks. Insulin is most rapidly absorbed from abdominal injection sites and most slowly from the buttocks.

It is important to rotate the injections around the various sites to avoid the complication of lipohypertrophy or, more rarely, lipodystrophy. Repeated injections into the same site cause extra growth of fat and fibrous tissue. This unsightly lypohypertrophied 'lumpy' injection site then leads to variable glycemic control as a result of slower and more erratic absorption of insulin from it. However, children prefer injecting into these sites as it is less uncomfortable. Therefore, these children need frequent encouragement to move their injection sites.

Maintaining normoglycemia

In healthy children without diabetes, blood glucose levels dictate insulin output. In children with diabetes, normoglycemia (4–10 mmol/L in a child with diabetes) is maintained by balancing administered insulin, carbohydrate intake and exercise.

A balanced diet

Children with type I diabetes have the same basic nutritional requirements as other children and an adequate energy intake is needed to achieve and maintain normal growth. The diet should be reviewed regularly to meet the changing needs of growth and physical exercise without obesity. Regular distribution of meals and snacks throughout the day remains the most important way to avoid extremes of hyperglycemia and hypoglycemia.[24,25]

Diabetes UK, the former British Diabetic Association, recommends that small amounts of sucrose (simple sugar) can be taken as part of an overall healthy diet, particularly if taken as part of or after a meal. There is no evidence that sucrose is an etiological factor in the development of diabetes and studies have shown that eating small amounts of sucrose does not worsen glycemic control in individuals with well-controlled diabetes.[26] Reduction of fat intake, especially of saturated fats, is expected to reduce the risk of coronary heart disease and of stroke in later life. After 5 years of age, fat intake should be reduced to around 35–40% of total energy.

There is evidence that adolescents with type I diabetes have mildly disturbed cardiovascular risk profiles compared with non-diabetic siblings.[25] Reduction of fat intake in the schoolchild with diabetes should be a priority. Moderation in salt intake should be the aim for people with diabetes of all ages.

Exercise

In children with diabetes, the blood glucose response to physical exercise is variable. Hypoglycemia is the commonest unwanted reaction, and may occur during or shortly after a bout of exercise or importantly several hours later. It is not uncommon for the young person with diabetes to experience significant nocturnal hypoglycemia after a strenuous period of daytime activity. Hyperglycemia can also occur, especially if the blood glucose and total ketones are abnormally high at the start of exercise.[27]

Home blood glucose monitoring

Home blood glucose monitoring, using a finger-pricking device and a blood glucose meter, aids the process of maintaining good glycemic control. A finger prick blood test will reflect the immediate blood glucose reading. A blood glucose reading can change significantly within 15 to 30 minutes and isolated readings may therefore be of little benefit. However, blood glucose readings performed frequently and at different times provide useful information about glycemic control.

The aim is to keep most of the test results between 4 and 10 mmol/L and children are asked to check their blood glucose readings twice a day, at varying times pre-meals. The child and parents also need to know the indications and the process to check for urinary ketones. Ketostix – a reagent strip – dipped in the urine will detect a trace of urinary ketones up to large amounts of ketonuria. Ketonuria may be present during periods of relative insulin insufficiency and hyperglycemia (e.g. during a recurrent viral illness) or during prolonged hyperglycemia (e.g. vomiting) following the counter-regulatory glucagon hormone response. It is always important to check for ketones when the child with diabetes is unwell. It is not to be expected that a child with diabetes has more illness than a peer without diabetes but once unwell such a child can quickly decompensate metabolically and become seriously ill if the appropriate insulin therapy and intravenous fluids are not given.

Measurement of glycosylated hemoglobin

The measurement of glycosylated hemoglobin currently provides the best index of glycemic control. The reaction in which glucose binds to hemoglobin is non-enzymatic. The higher the blood glucose concentration and the longer the red blood cells are exposed to it, the higher the glycosylated hemoglobin. Of all the forms of glycosylated hemoglobin, it is HbA1c which best reflects glycemic control over the preceding 2 to 3 months. Although the HbA1c result is related to the lifespan of the erythrocyte (120 days), a large shift in blood glucose control is accompanied by a significant and rapid change in HbA1c, which may be observed within 2 weeks.[28]

The advantages of HbA1c as a test of diabetes control are that it is objective, independent of the patient's cooperation and independent of the time of the last meal. The major disadvantage is the lack of standardization in assay methodology between laboratories.[29]

It is normal for people with diabetes to have a slightly higher HbA1c result than in people without diabetes. However, the nearer the HbA1c result is to the normal value for people with diabetes, the lower the risk of developing the complications of diabetes.

It is equally important to avoid HbA1c results that are too low as this is likely to be the result of periods of significant hypoglycemia.

An elevated HbA1c result, particularly when the correct amount of insulin is prescribed, indicates a chronic problem with poor compliance of diabetes management.

Long-term goals

The Diabetes Control and Complications Trial (DCCT) has shown that improved glycemic control can positively affect the long-term risk of developing nephropathy, retinopathy and neuropathy. In the DCCT, over 1400 subjects with type I diabetes aged between 13 and 39 years were followed for up to 9 years.[30] There were two groups of patients; those receiving intensive insulin therapy and very regular telephone and clinic support and carrying out monthly HbA1c measurements achieved a steady mean HbA1c of 7%, the other group received conventional insulin therapy and 3-monthly clinic visits, and achieved a mean HbA1c of 9%. The intensive therapy group demonstrated the following outcomes:

- 62% reduction in the progression of retinopathy
- 27% reduction in the appearance of retinopathy in the cohort with no retinopathy at entry
- 56% reduction in the development of clinical albuminuria
- 61% reduction in clinically significant neuropathy.

It should be emphasized that the DCCT did not study children under the age of 13 years. The major adverse outcomes of the DCCT were a 300% rise in severe hypoglycemic episodes and a 10 lb (4.6 kg) weight gain.

Hypoglycemia

Hypoglycemia may be defined as a blood glucose level less than 4 mmol/L and is also known as a 'hypo'. It remains the most feared therapeutic complication of diabetes management by both children with diabetes and their families. Under normal circumstances, the brain relies exclusively on glucose for energy and is significantly compromised when the blood glucose level falls below 4 mmol/L. Different individuals experience different symptoms of hypoglycemia, yet the symptoms are usually the same from time to time for a given individual. It is important that the child and parents recognize the symptoms and act appropriately, as without treatment the child may become unconscious and convulse, and occasionally this may prove fatal. Fortunately, mortality is very low as the counter-regulatory response will generally revert blood glucose to normal.

Hypoglycemia may result from:

- not enough food, i.e. missed or delayed meal or snack
- extra exercise
- too much insulin.

Counter-regulatory hormones are released when the blood glucose level falls below 4 mmol/L. The resulting sympathetic stimulation leads to increased hepatic output of glucose, decreased peripheral uptake and increased cardiac output manifesting as tachycardia. These changes cause the mainly autonomic feelings of sweatiness and shakiness associated with a 'hypo'. When the glucose level falls further, then neuroglycopenia ensues leading to confusion, incoordination and odd behavior.

Mild and moderate hypoglycemia can usually be treated with oral quick-acting carbohydrate followed by starchy carbohydrate. Severe hypoglycemia often requires parenteral glucagon and intravenous glucose.

Blood glucose levels will rise within 10 minutes of giving glucagon[31] and once the child is conscious and able to drink, further carbohydrate should be given by mouth. However, a child may experience vomiting and headaches after hypoglycemia and parenteral glucagon may also cause vomiting. Intravenous dextrose may then be required to maintain normoglycemia. Unrecognized nocturnal hypoglycemia may also lead to the rebound hyperglycemia or Somogyi phenomenon. It is important to realize that despite a high-fasting blood glucose, a reduction in evening insulin dose is required.

The diabetes team

It is recommended that young people should be seen in a designated children's diabetes clinic. There should be an annual review clinic visit incorporating all aspects of diabetes control, management and education. Minimum routine follow-up should be every 4 months but more frequently following diagnosis. There should be an annual review appointment with a pre-arranged format. It is important for the child to see various team members including the podiatrist and not just the doctor at the clinic. Ideally, the team should have pre- and post-clinic meetings to discuss known or anticipated problems and possible interventions. Such an arrangement keeps all diabetes team members well informed and should ensure that the child with diabetes and the family are not given conflicting advice. Assessment of diabetes self-care issues is important and includes examination of injection sites and technique.

There is growing evidence that raised blood pressure has a role in diabetic renal disease[32] and it is good practice to make an annual record of blood pressure in all children attending the clinic. Optimizing diabetes control is known to decrease the incidence of diabetes complications and the devastating effects of some of these may be minimized when they are detected early, e.g. laser therapy for proliferative retinopathy. Therefore, annual screening should include examination of urine for microalbuminuria, plasma thyroid-stimulating hormone (TSH) measurement and examination of skin state and inspection of feet.

The child with diabetes requiring elective surgery

The aim is to manage the child with minimal disruption to the child's normal routine. Ideally, a child should be first on a morning theater list to avoid the need for intravenous glucose necessary during fasting. Owing to the lack of controlled trials, there is little evidence to support any particular method of management of children with diabetes in the peri-operative period.[33]

Complications of type I diabetes

The pathogenesis of complications is complex. We know from the DCCT results that glycemic control has a significant effect on the development of late complications but some patients with very poor control have no complications whereas others, who are apparently well, develop significant complications. Genetic susceptibility, gender differences and lifestyle factors all have an important role to play.

Specific complications

Vascular complications may involve large and/or small blood vessels. Diabetes is associated with a two- to threefold increased risk of coronary heart disease in men and a four- to fivefold risk in pre-menopausal women. Atheromatous changes in large blood vessels are widespread and are earlier in onset in people with diabetes. The increased risk for arteriosclerosis and cardiovascular diseases is thought to be caused by both high blood glucose levels and hyperinsulinism. Occlusion of large blood vessels with atheroma is common and may lead to ulceration and gangrene of the lower limb. The main factors responsible for foot problems in adults with diabetes are combinations of ischemia and neuropathy, with infection as both a provoking and complicating factor. Ulcers can develop as a result of mechanical trauma to the foot. This highlights the need in the pediatric diabetes clinic for the prevention of some future problems by good basic foot care and by full biomechanical assessment and subsequent management when appropriate.

Sustained periods of hyperglycemia lead to accumulation of glucose in the walls of the blood vessels causing thickening of the basement membrane of the capillaries together with proliferation of the capillary endothelium. This produces diabetic microangiopathy and affects mainly those cells which do not require insulin for glucose transport, i.e. the eyes, kidneys, nerves and blood vessels. Microangiopathy also affects skin circulation, especially the feet, and may lead to gangrene with wedge-shaped artifacts.

Smoking is an independent risk factor for nephropathy, neuropathy and retinopathy[34] and any child with diabetes should be actively discouraged from smoking. Nicotine will also cause an increased insulin resistance, i.e. a poorer blood glucose lowering effect of a given dose of insulin.[35]

Retinopathy

Retinopathy refers to damage to the retina, the light-sensitive part of the back of the eye that is responsible for transmitting visual images to the brain. Retinopathy is a condition that progresses slowly at first without causing any visual symptoms. The retina is affected by two main types of pathological changes – background retinopathy and proliferative retinopathy. There is a definite association between poor glycemic control and the onset/progression of retinopathy. The DCCT confirms that interventions that improve glycemic control delay the onset and slow the progression of this condition. The prevalence of retinopathy is highest in young-onset insulin-treated individuals, and steadily increases with duration of diabetes.

Background retinopathy is due to increased capillary permeability and is characterized by hemorrhages and microaneurysms (seen as bulges in the capillary wall), which leak plasma to produce hard exudates. Background retinopathy does not threaten vision and can remain stable/harmless indefinitely.

Proliferative retinopathy is due to capillary non-perfusion and growth of new blood vessels causing blindness through vitreous hemorrhage, fibrosis and renal detachment. Proliferative retinopathy is a post-pubertal event.

It is now possible to prevent much of the visual loss in diabetes by regular screening and treatment. Proliferative retinopathy can be treated using laser photocoagulation. When left untreated, proliferative retinopathy will progress to blindness within 5 years in 50% of such cases.

Background and preproliferative retinopathy have been found in children before puberty[36] and it is recommended that children are screened annually for diabetic retinopathy from the age of 10 years. The use of stereoscopic fundus photography has helped significantly in retinal examination, and is a useful adjunct to ophthalmoscopy.

Nephropathy

Microalbuminuria is an early predictor of overt nephropathy in diabetes. A maximum of 40% of the population with diabetes develop this complication even in those with poor glycemic control. The incidence of nephropathy appears to increase up to 15 years from diagnosis of diabetes and then declines. The influence of hereditary factors on the development of nephropathy is strong.

Screening for microalbuminuria should only be undertaken after the onset of puberty, since microalbuminuria is rare beforehand and its predictive significance in children has not been established. The pathogenesis is multifactorial and associated factors are; type I diabetes for longer than 5 years, elevated blood pressure, poor glycemic control and lipid abnormalities. There is now clear evidence that treatment of hypertension can slow the progression of early nephropathy to end-stage renal failure. Controversy persists about the value of lipid-lowering therapy, especially in young patients.

Care is required when interpreting the clinical relevance of microalbuminuria in children with an intercurrent urinary tract infection, immediately post-exercise or during menstruation. In those children with significant and persistent microalbuminuria, all attempts at improving glycemic control should be tried.

Neuropathy

This term refers to damage to the nerves and develops in approximately 30% of all adults with diabetes. The most common test to detect subclinical neuropathy in children with type I diabetes is motor nerve conduction velocity. Using this technique, abnormalities have been detected early after the onset of diabetes, suggesting a functional metabolic abnormality.[37] The pathogenesis is unclear but it is thought to involve microvascular changes involving the endoneuronal capillaries and metabolic changes as a result of hyperglycemia.

Peripheral sensory neuropathy is the commonest form and presents as numbness, paresthesia and loss of pain sensation. Peripheral sensory neuropathy itself is not a feature of pediatric diabetes.

The autonomic nervous system may become affected and may lead to male impotence, nocturnal diarrhea and postural hypotension. Patients with autonomic neuropathy are also at risk of unexpected hypoglycemic episodes as the autonomic nervous system is responsible for producing many of the warning signs of hypoglycemia (pallor, sweating and tachycardia). Again, the DCCT shows evidence of benefit in the intensive treatment group, where clinical neuropathy was reduced.

Thyroid autoimmunity

Autoimmune thyroid disease is the most common form of autoimmune disease occurring in families with type I diabetes. 5% of children and young adults with diabetes develop hypothyroidism.[38] Its onset is insidious and is easily missed before poor growth, deteriorating school performance, lack of energy and excess weight gain become apparent. Hypothyroidism is easily screened for with a measurement of plasma TSH on a fingerprick sample, and the test should be part of the annual clinic review. Hypothyroidism is treated with a once-daily dose of oral thyroxine.

It is known that there are many autoimmune associations with type I diabetes. Addison's disease is rare in the general population (1:50 000) but is five times more common in those with type I diabetes in adult life.

Celiac disease

Children with diabetes have a prevalence of 3–5% of celiac disease identified on antibody screening and confirmed on jejunal biopsy.[39] These patients were largely symptom-free, compared with the classical mode of presentation with marked gastrointestinal disturbance, and therefore diagnosis may be difficult. However, it is known that there are a number of complications of untreated celiac disease, e.g. growth retardation, late menarche, male and female infertility, disturbances of bone and calcium metabolism[40] and implications for the future development of small bowel lymphoma and gastrointestinal carcinoma.

Diabetes management – the future

The delivery of insulin more physiologically is an important goal but a satisfactory clinical and commercial development is not likely in the foreseeable future. However, insulin analogues with extended action are being developed.

Cure by transplantation is the hope of many children with diabetes and of their families. However, studies in adults with diabetes undergoing this procedure show disappointing and potentially hazardous results. Transplantation or implantation of pancreatic islet cells directly into the hepatic system would be extremely advantageous and may prove of value in the future.

The child with diabetes as an individual

It is too easy to forget the physiological burden of diabetes in childhood. Children must have their diabetes therapy tailored to their individual needs taking into account knowledge of their domestic situation and their psychological and physiological health.

REFERENCES

1. Nelson K, Holmes L. Malformations due to presumed spontaneous mutations in newborn infants. N Engl J Med 1989;320:19.
2. Graham JM. Smith's recognizable patterns of human deformation. 2nd ed. Philadelphia: WB Saunders;1988.
3. Jones KL. Recognizable patterns of human malformation: genetic, embriologic and clinical aspects. 5th ed. Philadelphia: WB Saunders;1996.
4. London Dysmorphology Database. Oxford: Oxford University Press. http://www.oup.co.uk/omd
5. Uddhav K, Detan S. Advances in the human genome project. A review. Mol Biol Rep 1998;1:27–43.
6. Online Mendelian Inheritance in Man (OMIM). Catalog of human genes and genetic disorders, authored and edited by McKusik VA et al, based at Johns Hopkins University and elsewhere. http://ww.ncbi.nlm.nih.gov/Omim/
7. Miller D, Weber J, Green J. The management of AIDS patients. Basingstoke: Macmillan;1986.
8. Green A, Gale EAM, Patterson CC. Incidence of childhood onset insulin dependent diabetes mellitus: the EURODIAB ACE study. Lancet 1992;339:905–909.
9. Bingley PJ, Gale EAM. Rising incidence of IDDM in Europe. Diabetes Care 1989;12:289–295.
10. Bao MZ, Wang JX, Dorman JS, et al. HLA-DQ beta non-Asp-57 allele and incidence of diabetes in China and the USA. Lancet 1989;ii:497–498.
11. Blanchard JF, Dean H, Anderson K, et al. Incidence and prevalence of diabetes in children aged 0–14 years in Manitoba, Canada, 1985–1993. Diabetes Care 1997;20(4):512–515.
12. Lamb WH. Aetiology, epidemiology, immunology: environmental factors, genetics and prevention. In: Court S, Lamb W, eds. Childhood and adolescent diabetes. Chichester: Wiley;1997:1–15.
13. Kelnar CJ. Endocrine gland disorders and disorders of growth and puberty. In: Campbell AGM, McIntosh N, eds. Forfar and Arneil's textbook of paediatrics. 5th ed. Edinburgh: Churchill Livingstone; 1992; 996–1098.
14. Wagener DK, Sacks JM, La Porte RE, et al. The Pittsburgh study of insulin dependent diabetes mellitus: risk for diabetes among relatives of IDDM. Diabetes 1982;31:136–144.
15. Connor JM. Inheritance/genetics of childhood diabetes. In: Kelnar CJH, ed. Childhood and adolescent diabetes. London: Chapman and Hall;1995:161–167.
16. Baekkeshov S, Aanstoot HK, Christgau S, et al. Identification of the 64K autoantigen in insulin dependent diabetes as the GABA-synthesising enzyme glutamic acid decarboxylase. Nature 1990;347:151–156.
17. Dorman JS, O'Leary LA, Koehler AN. Epidemiology of childhood diabetes. In: Kelnar CJH, ed. Childhood and adolescent diabetes. London: Chapman and Hall;1995:161–167.
18. Kyrik KO, Gren A, Beck–Nilsen H. Concordance rates of insulin dependent diabetes mellitus: a population based study of young Danish twins. BMJ 1995;311:913–917.
19. Leslie RD, Elliot RB. Early environmental events as a cause of IDDM. Diabetes 1994;43;843–850.
20. Verge CF, Simpson JM, Howard NJ, et al. Environmental factors in IDDM. Diabetes Care 1994;17;1381–1389.
21. Pinkney JH, Bingley PJ, Sawtell PA, et al. Presentation and progress of childhood diabetes mellitus: a prospective population-based study. Diabetologia 1994;37:70–74.
22. Wales J. Insulin strategies. In: Court S, Lamb W, eds. Childhood and adolescent diabetes. Chichester: Wiley;1997:166–185.
23. Mohn A, Dunger DB. Insulin therapy in children and adolescents with type 1 diabetes. Curr Paediatr 1999;9(3):158–163.
24. Magrath G, Hartland BV and the Nutrition sub-committee of the British Diabetic Association's Professional Advisory Committee, London, UK. Dietary recommendations for children and adolescents with diabetes: an implementation paper. Diabet Med 1993;10:874–885.
25. Brenchley S, Govindji A. Dietary management of children with diabetes. In: Kelnar CJH, ed. Childhood and adolescent diabetes. London: Chapman and Hall;1995;271–281.
26. Bantle JP, Laine DC, Thompson C. Metabolic effects of dietary fructose and sucrose in types I + II diabetic subjects. JAMA 1986;25:3241–3246.
27. Greene SA, Thompson C. Exercise. In: Kelnar CJH, ed. Childhood and adolescent diabetes. London: Chapman and Hall;1995:283–293.
28. Goldstein DE, Malone JL, et al. Tests of glycaemia in diabetes. Diabetes Care 1995;18:896–909.
29. Matthews D. The concept of control. In: Court S, Lamb W, eds. childhood and adolescent diabetes. Chichester: Wiley; 1997:125–136.
30. DCCT Research Group. The effect of intensive treatment of diabetes on the development and progression of long term complications in insulin dependent diabetes mellitus. N Eng J Med 1993;329:977–986.
31. Aman J, Wranne L. Hypoglycaemia in childhood diabetes. Effect of subcutaneous or intramuscular injection of different doses of glucagon. Acta Paediatr Scand 1988;77:548–553.
32. Robertson K, Lamb B. The point and purpose of the clinic – personnel and practical aspects. In: Court S, Lamb W, eds. Childhood and adolescent diabetes. Chichester: Wiley;1997.
33. Milaszkiewicz RM, Hall GM. Peri-operative management of the diabetic child. In: Kelnar CJH, ed. Childhood and adolescent diabetes. London: Chapman and Hall;1995:345–350.

34. Mühlhauser I. Cigarette smoking and diabetes: an update. Diabetes 1994;11:336–343.
35. Attvall S, Fowelin J, Lager L, et al. Smoking induces insulin resistance – a potential link with the insulin resistance syndrome. J Intern Med 1993;233:327–332.
36. Kernell A, Dedorsson I, Johansson B, et al. Prevalence of diabetic retinopathy in children and adolescents with IDDM. A population based multicentre study. Diabetologia 1997;40:307–310.
37. Becker DJ, Orchard TJ et al. Control and outcome: clinical and epidemiologic aspects. In: Kelnar CJH, ed. Childhood and adolescent diabetes. London: Chapman and Hall;1995:519–538.
38. Court S, Parkin JM. Hypothyroidism and growth failure in diabetes mellitus. Arch Dis Child 1982;57:622–624.
39. Sigurs N, Johansson C, Elfstrand PO, et al. Prevalence of coeliac disease in diabetic children and adolescents in Sweden. Acta Paediatr 1993;82(9):748–751.
40. Holmes GKT. Non malignant complications of coeliac disease. Acta Paediatr Suppl 1996;412:68–75.

FURTHER READING

Asherson GL, Webster ADB. Diagnosis and treatment of immuno-deficiency diseases. Oxford: Blackwell; 1980.

Brook CGD, ed. Clinical paediatric endocrinology. Oxford: Blackwell 1995. Growth disorders. Clinics in Endocrinology and Metabolism 1986;15(3):411–713.

Esterly JR. Congenital hereditary lymphoedema. J Med Genet 1965;2:93.

Hanas R. Insulin-dependent diabetes in children, adolescents and adults. Uddevalla: Piara HB;1998.

Horowitz SD, Hong R. The pathogenesis and treatment of immunodeficiency. Basel: Karger;1977.

Hosking CS, Roberton DM. The diagnostic approach to recurrent infections in childhood. Clin Immunol Allergy 1981;1:631–639.

Kelnar CJH, ed. Childhood and adolescent diabetes. London: Chapman and Hall;1995.

Kelnar CJH, Savage MO, Stirling HF, Saenger P, eds. Growth disorders – pathophysiology and treatment. London: Chapman and Hall;1998.

McKusick V. Mendelian inheritance in man; Catalogs of autosomal dominant, autosomal recessive and X-linked phenotypes. 5th ed. Baltimore: Johns Hopkins University Press;1978.

Marshall WA. Human growth and its disorders. London: Academic Press;1977.

Miller DR. Blood diseases in infancy and childhood. Oxford: Blackwell Scientific;1994.

Nathan DG. Hematology of infancy and childhood. 5th ed. Philadelphia: WB Saunders;1997.

Schroeder E, Helweg-Carson HF. Congenital hereditary lymphoedema (None–Milroys–Meiges disease). Acta Med Scand 1950;137:198.

Shannon KM, Ammann AJ. Acquired immune deficiency syndrome in childhood. J Paediatr 1985;106:332.

Tanner JM. Foetus into man. Physical growth from conception to maturity. London: Open Books;1990.

Warkany J. Congenital malformations. Chicago: Year Book Medical Publishers;1971.

Willoughby MLN. Paediatric haematology. Edinburgh: Churchill Livingstone;1977.

World Health Organization. Acquired immunodeficiency syndrome. WHO/CDC. Case definition for AIDS. Wkly Epidemiol Rec 1986;61:69–73.

6

Rheumatic diseases of childhood and adolescence

Kevin Murray and Jill Ferrari

Chronic inflammatory conditions that affect connective tissue may have profound effects when they occur in childhood. This group of conditions includes juvenile idiopathic arthritis (JIA), dermatomyositis, systemic lupus erythematosus and linear scleroderma. Pediatric rheumatologists who care for such patients also care for children with other musculoskeletal disorders including joint hypermobility and reflex sympathetic dystrophy. This chapter will describe the basic clinical features of these different conditions and will focus upon the implications for lower limb involvement and function. In particular, the effects upon the ankle and foot apparatus will be highlighted as will the role of the podiatrist in the treatment of such problems.

JUVENILE IDIOPATHIC ARTHRITIS

Previously termed juvenile chronic arthritis (in Europe) or juvenile rheumatoid arthritis (in North America), this group of disorders has been renamed and classified in order to reflect a unity of description and better understanding of the multiple and unique chronic arthropathies that may start in childhood.[1] Although originally thought of as one disease, in the last several decades it has been clear that many distinct forms of chronic arthritis occur in childhood with unique clinical features, predisposing genetic factors and most likely underlying pathogenesis. The current classification of these arthropathies is as follows:

1. oligoarticular JIA
2. extended oligoarticular JIA

3. polyarticular JIA – rheumatoid factor negative
4. polyarticular JIA – rheumatoid factor positive
5. systemic JIA
6. enthesitis-related arthritis (juvenile-onset spondyloarthropathy)
7. psoriatic arthritis
8. unclassified – having features of more than one of the above categories.

Oligoarticular JIA

Oligoarticular JIA is the commonest type of arthritis to affect children, and occurs in 60–70% of all JIA patients. It predominantly affects children under the age of 8 years, and is much more common in females. By definition, this form of arthritis involves four or fewer joints in the first 6 months of the disease and it is this period of time that defines which type of arthritis a child has. Commonly, oligoarticular JIA affects the lower limbs with the knee joint being the most frequently affected, followed by the ankle and subtalar joint. Occasionally, a small joint of the hand or foot, or the elbow is involved.

Children often present with a swollen joint, stiffness and some pain. They may also present with a deformity of the joint with the other symptoms having gone unnoticed, particularly in early childhood. A flexion deformity of the knee is one of the common modes of presentation. Although oligoarticular JIA is perhaps the mildest type of arthritis in terms of severity, it may have profound effects on individual joints. Since this form of arthritis occurs in young children, it has significant effects upon modeling and upon the growth of young joints. Peculiar to childhood, the phenomenon of overgrowth of joints is seen particularly in oligoarticular JIA. Most commonly, this occurs at the knee where enlargement of the ends of the long bones (comprising the tibial and femoral epiphysis) may be observed. Overgrowth is usually asymmetric and is more commonly found on the medial side, which leads to a significant valgus deformity. In addition, there is often overall lengthening of the limb leading to a leg-length discrepancy. Such a discrepancy clearly has significant effects upon ambulation in terms of gait pattern and cadence.

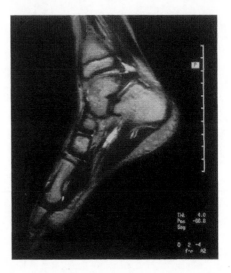

Figure 6.1 A magnetic resonance imaging study of the foot/ankle in a patient with oligoarticular JIA. In this T_2-weighted image, areas of synovial fluid accumulation are seen in the posterior tibiocalcaneal joint region and below the subtalar joint (© Institute of Child Health and The Hospitals for Sick Children).

Consequently, the change in forces through the knee has effects upon the more distal joints. These effects may vary depending on whether the ankle and/or the foot are involved.

The ankle is the second most commonly involved joint in this form of arthritis and overgrowth may also be seen here. The overgrowth may lead to alterations such as lengthening of the distal fibula epiphysis and/or the tibial epiphysis, together with abnormal modeling and shaping of the talus. These changes lead to marked limitation and function of the ankle joint. Once again, the overgrowth and remodeling may be asymmetric leading to abnormalities such as a varus or valgus hindfoot.

A recent study using magnetic resonance imaging (MRI) revealed that the subtalar joint is frequently involved on those occasions when the ankle joint has clinically documented inflammation.[2] Although the inflamed subtalar joint is often limited in motion, this is rarely appreciated by many clinicians. MRI may accurately identify areas of joint involvement and of fluid accumulation (Fig. 6.1).

Involvement of the subtalar joint may also lead to significant abnormalities in growth and in par-

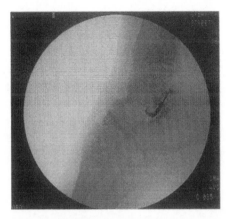

Figure 6.2 Radioopaque dye injected into the subtalar joint under image intensification in a child with oligoarticular JIA of the ankle and foot.

ticular in the incongruity of joint surfaces and in marked limitation of motion. Such loss of motion at the subtalar joint is more commonly seen than limitation of the ankle joint in childhood arthritis.

Tarsal involvement is less common in this form of arthritis. However, it is frequent in other forms of disease including polyarticular JIA and juvenile spondylarthropathy as described below. Similar changes upon growth and modeling as previously described are seen in the tarsus with loss of mobility, function and integrity of the joints.

Persistent chronic arthritis in the ankle or foot joints will eventually result in damage to cartilage and loss of joint space. Such damage occurs significantly later in the oligoarticular form of the disease compared with other diseases such as polyarticular and systemic JIA. It is clear that early intervention with anti-inflammatory or disease-modifying drugs can alter the course of such joint disease.[3] However, it is the institution of long-acting intra-articular steroid treatment in the last few decades that has had the most profound effect in this form of arthritis. The injection of intra-articular medication such as triamcynolone, hexacetonide or acetonide has been shown to significantly reduce the incidence of overgrowth and deformity in JIA.[4] Repeated injections into either the ankle, subtalar or midfoot joint may be required over several years

and provide a good alternative to the necessity for regular administration of non-steroid anti-inflammatory drugs (NSAIDs) and even disease-modifying anti-rheumatic drugs (DMARDs) (Fig. 6.2).

Physical therapy and occupational therapy remain an integral part of managing children with chronic joint disease and include not only stretching and strengthening regimens but also splinting techniques including the use of knee splints and ankle/foot splints which are worn in bed at night or during ambulation in some cases. Wrist and hand splints are also worn at night for rest and in order to maintain a functional position. It is likely that splints contribute to the prevention of significant deformities such as fixed flexion of the knee and to loss of dorsal flexion at the ankle. The use of in-shoe devices, such as custom-made insoles and ankle/foot orthotics, has a significant role and will be discussed below. Footwear modifications, e.g. shoe raises and 'rockers', are also important treatment considerations.

Extended oligoarticular JIA

Approximately 30% of patients who start with oligoarticular onset (" 4 joints) JIA will develop more extensive disease after the first 6 months. This is not predictable in the onset phase, although some genetic risk factors have been described.[5] Children in whom this occurs follow a course very similar to that of rheumatoid factor negative polyarticular JIA (see below). The disease may be rapidly progressive in some patients and just as destructive as the more polyarticular forms of disease. The specific interventions are as those described for the other forms of arthritis.

Polyarticular JIA – rheumatoid factor negative

This is the commonest form of polyarticular disease to affect children. As rheumatoid factor is not detected, it is termed seronegative. This disease is completely distinct from the other polyarticular arthritis affecting children in which rheumatoid factor is found (see below). This disease is also more common in young girls although it occurs throughout childhood and may even extend well into adult years (as seronegative rheumatoid arthritis).

By definition, the disease starts with more than four joints involved in the first 6 months of the disease. In practice, many more joints become progressively involved over time unless disease-modifying treatment is introduced early. There is a particular predilection for lower limb involvement just as in oligoarticular-onset JIA. Similarly, joint involvement tends to be asymmetric (unlike rheumatoid factor positive polyarticular JIA). Ankle, hind and midfoot involvement is relatively common, second only to knee involvement in frequency.[6] The hip joint may be involved and occurrence of disease in this location may produce early overgrowth and deformity, including shortening of the femoral neck and persistent anteversion with predictable effects upon posturing of the lower limb and on gait (Fig. 6.3).

Characteristic involvement of small joints occurs, particularly the metatarsophalangeal (MTP) and proximal interphalangeal (PIP) joints

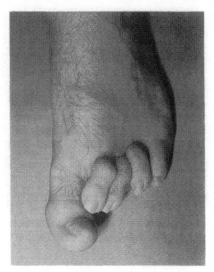

Figure 6.4 Growth abnormalities of the toes in an adolescent with JIA from early childhood.

and may lead to either over- or undergrowth of the toe with occasionally spectacular deformities in the foot. Hallux valgus or varus may also be seen owing to either overgrowth or destructive disease. Similar effects may be seen in the other toes on occasion (Fig. 6.4).

In the upper limbs and axial skeleton, involvement of the elbows and wrists is not uncommon and involvement of the cervical spine early in the disease with a tendency to fusion is characteristic. Temperomandibular involvement with subsequent micrognathia leads to a characteristic facial appearance in many patients. Many of the potential deformities and joint damage may be prevented or delayed by the early introduction of disease-modifying drugs such as methotrexate and sulfasalazine together with the aggressive and early use of intra-articular steroids. Corticosteroids also have a role in controlling the inflammatory joint disease but with a risk of overall growth suppression and vascular necrosis later.

Involvement of the foot and ankle joints in this form of JIA is similar to that described in oligoarticular JIA, but it may progress much more rapidly. Once more, the subtalar joint and midfoot joint involvement is commonly seen when ankle involvement has occurred early in the disease.[2]

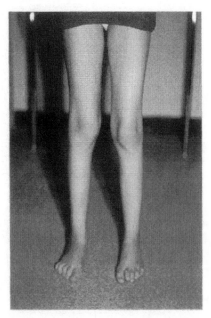

Figure 6.3 Anteversion of the right hip leading to foot pronation.

It is important to note that traditional radiological studies (plain X-rays) underestimate the extent of disease involvement. Early changes in cartilage status and underlying bony changes together with synovial hypertrophy and invasion may be documented early in the disease on MRI studies of joints, particularly with the co-administration of gadolinium (see Fig. 6.1). These studies suggest that clinical examination often underestimates either the degree or the extent of joint involvement in a number of patients. Studies in adults with rheumatoid arthritis where biopsies were performed in the apparently uninvolved other knee, in addition to the active knee, indicate that synovitis is often present at a level where involvement was not clinically obvious.[7]

It is clear that from a very early stage the involvement of physical therapists, occupational therapists and podiatrists is mandatory in the optimal care of such patients. The prevention of deformity may be enhanced by early use of orthoses. The use of such devices is widely believed to have a significant role to play in terms of pain relief in childhood forms of chronic arthritis. The maintenance of mobility is essential in order to prevent the occurrence of deformities, which are so commonly seen when these children do not mobilize.

Polyarticular JIA – rheumatoid factor positive

This seropositive disease essentially represents the childhood onset of 'classic' rheumatoid arthritis. Fortunately, this is one of the less frequent types of disease seen in childhood, accounting for approximately 5–10% of cases. However, along with systemic onset arthritis, seropositive polyarticular JIA accounts for a large proportion of those patients with high levels of functional disability in later life.[3] It has previously been termed juvenile-onset rheumatoid arthritis. The disease manifests uniquely in childhood since it occurs in the growing child and has many different potential effects on the joints. Just as in the adult form of the disease, it starts as a symmetrical inflammatory polyarthropathy

(>4 joints but usually many more). It is typical to see involvement of the small joints of the hands and feet early in the disease. The involvement of wrists, knees and ankles also occurs early. Involvement of all the foot joints is common in the disease though it may manifest somewhat later clinically than in other forms of JIA.

By definition, children with this form of disease have detectable rheumatoid factor in their blood. This antibody is classically described as an anti-immunoglobulin IgG antibody (of the IgM subtype). Although the specific role of this antibody is uncertain, generally it is seen as a marker for more severe disease, with a greater likelihood of joint destruction, particularly when treated late or untreated. The involvement of the ankle and foot in this condition is similar to that described above but it is usually symmetrical. Early intervention with disease-modifying drugs and intra-articular steroids is mandatory, along with physical therapy and podiatry.

Systemic JIA

This form of JIA, as originally described by George Frederick Still in 1896, is characterized by the occurrence of high fevers, a macular evanescent erythematous rash and a tendency to cause inflammation of the serosal surfaces (pericarditis, pleuritis and peritonitis). It is this form of the disease that is associated with the marked elevation of inflammatory markers such as erythrocyte sedimentation rate and C-reactive protein, together with severe anemia in many patients. Although 50% of these patients will have a disease remission after a number of years, the other 50% will tend towards a progressive and often very destructive symmetrical polyarticular arthropathy requiring treatment with corticosteroids, DMARDs and NSAIDs. Early treatment of patients with physical therapy, occupational therapy and podiatry is required.

The arthritis tends to be a symmetrical disease with a striking proliferation of bulky and deforming synovium. These patients have characteristically marked swelling of the tenosynovium of both hands and feet. Children who develop the progressive arthropathy in systemic

JIA demonstrate early evidence of joint damage such as joint space narrowing and erosions. Although they may develop localized overgrowth, rarely is there significant overgrowth in length. More frequently, there may be found an overall loss of growth owing to the profound effects of this disease and specifically on linear growth because of the use of corticosteroids.

Enthesitis-related arthritis (juvenile-onset spondyloarthropathy)

This condition occurs predominantly in boys over the age of 8 years and is related to the 'adult form' of ankylosing spondylitis. The arthropathy characteristically involves the large joints of the lower limb in an asymmetric fashion. The knee and ankle joints are commonly involved but it is the involvement of the tarsal region and on occasion the first MTP joint that most characterizes this form of arthritis in childhood. Early involvement of the hip is not uncommon and may be destructive.

One characteristic feature of this particular arthritis is the occurrence of enthesitis. Inflammation of the enthesis (ligaments and tendons as they insert into joints or joint regions) is frequently underestimated in such patients. Typical areas to be involved include the insertions of the Achilles tendon into the posterior calcaneus, the proximal and distal plantar fascia and the insertion of the patella tendon into the tibial tubercle. However, multiple other sites may be documented in patients including the anterior iliac crest, the peripatella regions of the quadriceps muscle insertions, and the peroneal muscle insertion into the fifth metatarsal (Figs 6.5, 6.6, 6.7). It has been argued that the synovitis in the joints is in fact secondary to the adjacent enthesitis and periarticular inflammation.

In a number of patients, the degree of synovitis may be limited with enthesitis being the predominant symptom. In many cases, this is exquisitely painful leading to great difficulties with weightbearing, particularly when it occurs in the plantar fascia or Achilles tendon insertion. A number of children have been labeled as being malingerers or having school refusal as the subtle

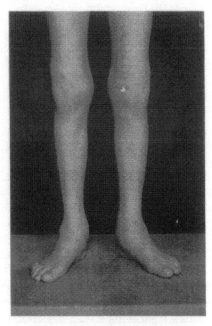

Figure 6.5 Severe bilateral involvement of both ankles and feet (in addition to knees) in a child with JIA. Synovial swelling in addition to bony overgrowth of the ankles is seen.

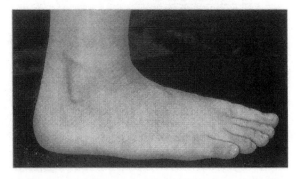

Figure 6.6 Inflammation of an enthesis at the base of the right fifth metatarsophalangeal joint in enthesitis-related arthritis in a 10-year-old girl (© Institute of Child Health and The Hospitals for Sick Children).

swelling and exquisite tenderness are often not obvious and missed by clinicians. Where there is enthesitis of the proximal plantar fascia, the patient will have great difficulty weightbearing on the hind foot and will develop a toe-walking pattern. Frequently, plain radiographs are normal although bone scans may on occasion show significant inflammation in the location of the

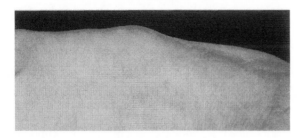

Figure 6.7 Close-up of the lesion in Figure 6.6 (© Institute of Child Health and The Hospitals for Sick Children).

enthesis. MRI studies and ultrasound can show the inclination of the involved enthesis in exquisite detail. The occurrence of such enthesitis has profound implications for ankle and foot function.

This disease is managed in a similar fashion to JIA. The medication sulfasalazine would appear to have an important role, but the potent disease-modifying drug, methotrexate, is also commonly used. Cortiocosteroid joint injections are also frequently employed in this form of the disease. Occasionally, entheses may be injected, particularly the proximal plantar fascia insertion with significant benefits.

The synovitis in this form of arthritis may also lead to local overgrowth in the tarsal region of the foot and occasionally to general overgrowth of the ankle joint.

Psoriatic arthritis

Much like adults, children may also develop arthritis in association with psoriasis. The arthritis that occurs in this situation has some unique features. Psoriatic arthritis has a predilection for the involvement of the whole of the fingers or toes rather than inflammation of the discrete joints such as the interphalangeal or metacarpal phalangeal (MCP) or MTP joints. Often the inflammation may cause dactylitis which comprises contiguous inflammation of tenosynovium (usually of the flexor tendons) together with arthritis in MTP (MCP), PIP and characteristically distal interphalangeal joints. Involvement of the distal interphalangeal joints of the hands and feet is thought to be characteristic of

psoriatic arthritis, although it may occur in other forms of juvenile arthritis. The basis for inflammation of the joints in this disease has also recently been postulated as being due to an initial underlying enthesitis, similar to that of enthesitis-related arthritis described above.

The typical psoriatic skin rash (erythematous and scaly) is particularly seen over the extensor surfaces of the knees, elbows and MCP joints. However, it may occasionally be seen behind the ears and in the scalp and on the soles of the feet. The rash may occur at the same time as arthritis but more commonly occurs much later in children.

The pattern of arthritis overall may be very similar to oligoarticular JIA or to rheumatoid factor negative polyarticular JIA. Occasionally, it is a symmetrical polyarthritis. The treatment is similar to that of other forms of JIA but deformities of the toes in particular may be more profound and may require more specific intervention from the podiatrist.

OTHER RHEUMATIC DISORDERS OCCURRING IN CHILDHOOD

Inflammation of the joints may occur in many other connective tissue diseases and, in particular, dermatomyositis, systemic lupus erythematosus, localized and generalized scleroderma and, rarely, sarcoidosis. An acute inflammatory arthritis may also occur as part of a viral infection such as rubella, enteroviral infection (such as Coxsackie) or parvovirus B19. In most of these cases, the arthritis is transitory, resolving without sequelae. However, in certain patients, the arthritis may become chronic. Specific infections such as Lyme disease may also progress to a chronic arthritis, especially in untreated patients.

Systemic lupus erythematosus

This multisystem disease occurs in children as well as in adults. Its manifestations are not unique to childhood, although the effects upon a growing child may be different and more profound than that seen in adults. The disease is characterized by a systemic inflammation with involvement of multiple organs. This includes the occurrence of skin rash, mucosal ulceration, myositis, arthritis, nephritis and central nervous system inflammation. Other characteristic features include fatigue, weight loss and general debility. The arthritis itself is rarely deforming in the early stages. Treatment usually involves corticosteroids and hydroxychloroquine and occasionally methotrexate. Serious organ involvement may indicate the use of immunosuppressant drugs such as cyclophosphamide and azathioprine. The joint involvement in certain cases may be persistent and painful and require similar interventions for the chronic joint diseases as described above.

Dermatomyositis

Juvenile-onset dermatomyositis is a rare disease of childhood but an important cause of significant long-term disability. It is characterized by chronic inflammation in the skin and muscle. An inflammatory arthropathy may occur in as many as 50% of cases, and in 10–20% of these this may become chronic and potentially destructive. However, the primary abnormality is now thought to be endothelial inflammation or damage allowing the ingress of inflammatory cells. Involvement of the gastrointestinal tract and other organs may be seen in certain patients.

Although the disease may follow a monophasic course over a number of years and go into remission in one-third of patients, in another third it follows a chronic relapsing course with the development of significant disability. In a further third, it is potentially a severe disease with a tendency to cutaneous ulceration and, on occasion, gastrointestinal ulceration with a high risk of calcinosis in the muscles and skin later in the course of the disease. In the last group, there is still a significant mortality associated with the disease.

The condition is treated similarly in children and adults with high-dose steroids and immunosuppressive drugs. In the acute phase, significant weakness, particularly of the proximal muscles, is noted. On occasion, this proximal muscle weakness may be severe enough to result in respiratory failure. In the acute phase of the disease, splinting of particular joints such as the knees, ankles and wrists may be required in order to prevent the rapid development of contractures. Similar contractures may also occur in these joints in the chronic phase owing to shortening of muscle fibers or the replacement of muscle tissue with scar tissue, or because of chronic arthritis within the nearby joints. The role of the physical therapist and podiatrist is clearly important in both early and later phases of this disease in order to help prevent deformity. In certain patients, a polyarthritis may also develop which adds to the risk for significant joint impairment. Involvement of the physical therapist early in the disease is usually limited to gentle passive stretching. More aggressive physical therapy during acute inflammation is felt to be associated with aggravation of the underlying condition although this is unproven. Protection of joints and soft tissues in the early phase is thought to be important as trauma may predispose to development of subsequent calcification.

Hypermobility syndromes

While it is clear that the range of motion of the joints of children is significantly greater than that of adults (Fig. 6.8), some children are considered to have what is termed as 'hypermobility'. The arbitrarily defined Beighton criteria[8] describe a scoring system designed to document generalized

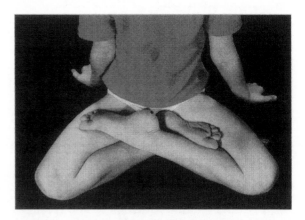

Figure 6.8 An 8-year-old girl complained of pain in her knees and ankle demonstrating generalized joint hypermobility (© Institute of Child Health and The Hospitals for Sick Children).

hypermobility. The following joints are scored thus:

a. the ability to hyperextend the MCP joints to 90° or beyond (1 point for each side)
b. hyperextension of the elbows beyond 10° (1 point each side)
c. hyperextension of the knees beyond 10° (1 point each side)
d. the ability to appose the thumb to the forearm on flexion of the hand and wrist (1 point each side)
e. the ability to place the hands on the floor with forward bending, with knees straight (1 point).

Patients are considered to have generalized hypermobility if they have a score of ≥ 4 out of 9. In practice, many patients have a score of between 7 and 9. It is clear that many people have more localized forms of hypermobility which may be restricted, for example, to the hands and feet or to the lower limbs in general.

Patients are termed as having benign joint hypermobility syndrome if they have a symptom complex involving arthralgia, occasional joint effusions and musculoskeletal dysfunction which is related to the joint hypermobility (such as subluxation or dislocation episodes). It has been estimated that up to 10% of children may have 'hypermobility' of their joints as so defined, but far fewer of these have the benign joint hypermobility syndrome. Possible clinical manifestations in childhood include arthralgias of the knees, ankles and feet. A number of these patients have been diagnosed as having 'growing pains' in childhood. In early infancy, a number of these patients may have a history of 'clicky hips' or occasionally of congenital dislocation of the hips. Throughout their childhood, these patients have a tendency to suffer sprains or strains of their joints and, in the adolescent years, back pain appears to be a common phenomenon.

With regard to the feet and ankles, the majority of these children have a significant pes planus related to their hypermobility (Fig. 6.9) with an associated valgus deformity of the hindfoot on standing. It is the altered transmission of weight-bearing forces that is thought to produce

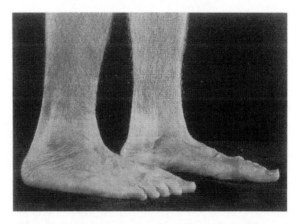

Figure 6.9   Marked pes planus and skin abnormalities seen in a 14-year-old girl with Ehlers–Danlos syndrome who has severe joint hypermobility (© Photography, Illustration and Audiovisual Centre, UCL, London).

symptoms in the lower limb and, in particular, anterior knee pain in certain patients. Empirically, it has been shown that many patients will benefit from orthotic interventions such as the provision of custom-made insoles or from specific footwear. The majority of patients, however, benefit greatly from specific exercise programs. Usually coordinated by a physical therapist, such programs focus on maintaining the range of joint motion, while specifically strengthening the muscles which cross joints (see Ch. 13).

The etiology of this condition is not completely understood. It has been argued that such patients represent one end of the 'spectrum' of joint mobility but family studies seem to suggest that there is an inherited pre-disposition similar but less severe than the related genetic conditions, Ehlers–Danlos syndrome and Marfan syndrome. These syndromes can present in childhood with the severe effects of joint hypermobility. It has been postulated that the benign joint hypermobility syndrome may represent a mild genetic variant of Ehlers–Danlos syndrome although without the risk for significant internal organ involvement from connective tissue derangement.

Reflex sympathetic dystrophy

This syndrome, also known as algodystrophy or complex regional pain syndrome type II, occurs in both children and adults. It predominantly affects the extremities with lower limb involvement being more common than upper limb. Reflex sympathetic dystrophy has been reported in other body areas including the neck and trunk. The classic history is of a limb that suffers a minor trauma or other incident. Subsequent to this, intense pain is experienced and the patient finds great difficulty in moving the limb. There is associated difficulty with either weightbearing or upper limb use over days to weeks. Edema of the soft tissues may be noted with associated development of allodynia and hyperesthesia. Subsequently, alterations in vasomotor tone occur and the limb may appear dusky or pale at various times. Increase in sweating is noticed in some patients. The latter phenomenon has led to the use of the word 'sympathetic' in the name of the condition. Research has yet to prove that there is any defined abnormality of the sympathetic nervous system.

Patients with this syndrome are often markedly disabled and distressed. Psychological issues are felt to be important either in the causation or manifest subsequently and require specific treatment in the overall management of this condition.

Involvement of the lower limb is commonly from the mid lower leg downwards and it affects the whole of the ankle and the foot. Commonly, symptoms pre-date the diagnosis by weeks or months. A diagnosis is usually made when the signs become more evident. Radiological investigations may reveal some osteoporosis, thought to be secondary to immobility and disuse. Bone scans may show either reduced or increased uptake. Patients frequently require admission, analgesia and intervention with intensive desensitization and remobilization (usually performed by a physical therapist or podiatrist). Hands-on physical therapy and hydrotherapy are felt to be of great benefit, particularly in children.[9] Patients may require splinting in order to encourage the foot and ankle into a more functional or anatomical position, particularly at rest or during the night. Alterations to footwear may be required.

In general, the outcome in both children and adolescents is reasonably good with resolution in many cases. In adults, the outcome is less certain. It appears that the longer the delay to diagnosis, the lesser the chance of an optimal outcome. Although it appears there are no definite underlying etiological factors, conditions which predispose to this syndrome may include hypermobility of the joints, previous trauma to the limb and psychosocial factors.

ROLE OF THE PODIATRIST IN PEDIATRIC RHEUMATOLOGY

The treatment of JIA

Since there are a number of different forms of this disease affecting many or just a few joints, the child with JIA may present to the podiatrist with a diversity of problems. However, the deformity seen at any affected joint is usually predictable, regardless of disease subgroups. The function of the lower limb will be affected when there is involvement of any lower limb joint and although some variation in individual gaits may be expected, the children frequently present with very typical features. It is the role of the podiatrist to work with the pediatric rheumatology team, particularly the physical therapist, to correct or maintain joint positions in order to maximize function and reduce pain.

Changes to gait and joint position

There is very little documented evidence on the altered gait patterns seen in JIA. Those studies undertaken have been confused by the use of unsuitable control groups. However, some of the information provided in the studies does reflect clinical observation, i.e. a shortened single stance phase, increased heel contact time and reduced toe-off.[10,11] These three changes occur as a consequence of joint stiffness or deformity and as the result of the effort to minimize pain.

The hips, when affected, frequently move into a position of flexion and internal rotation. If the child has been immobile, for example, spending too much time in a chair during the active phase of the disease, marked fixed flexion deformities may be seen (typically up to 50°). When mobility

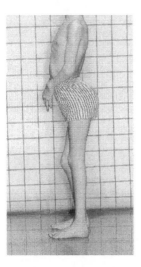

Figure 6.10   Fixed flexion at the hip joint resulting in increased anterior pelvic tilt and lumbar lordosis.

has been maintained, flexion deformities of 5–10° are more common. A flexed hip position will nearly always lead to knee-flexion during stance and gait. The knees can only remain straight if a severe lumbar lordosis occurs (Fig. 6.10). The lack of extension reduces the child's ability to make a normal stride thus shortening step length and reducing cadence. After an improvement in joint range of motion, the step length may be slow to improve with habit preventing a rapid change in gait. The internal hip rotation impacts on function throughout the limb, influencing both knee and foot position. With hip disease, the surrounding musculature weakens. Loss of power in gluteus maximus prevents active hip-extension; weakness in the abductors results in a Trendelenburg gait. Again, this lateral sway quickly becomes habitual, and is seen long after muscle strength returns.

When the knees are involved in the disease process, flexion and valgus deformities are seen. Such deformities become fixed if daily muscle building and stretches are not undertaken, or if correct resting positions are not maintained. The child may be in severe pain when the joints are inflamed, but it is essential that, unlike in the treatment of an adult, the joints are not rested. Although perhaps initially distressing for both

the parents and the child, the joints must be both strengthened and stretched when inflamed. This is best performed in the morning after a hot bath, when the joints are at their stiffest. Stretching at this stage will allow an improved range of motion and thus better function throughout the day. Although the podiatrist may not be directly involved with these exercises, the podiatrist should reinforce the need for this regimen to the patient and add in specific foot mobilizations where required.

With knee-flexion deformities, secondary hip-flexion may occur as previously mentioned and, in order to maintain an upright posture, the child may develop a lumbar lordosis. With either hip or knee involvement, an immediate change in gait may be seen. When standing with the hips and knees in flexion, the child tries to maintain a plantargrade foot position. Since the anterior aspect of the tibia is tilted forwards as a result of the knee flexion, the ankles are placed in a relatively dorsiflexed position. As range of movement is lost, absence of further dorsiflexion prevents heel contact at the start of the stance phase and whole foot contact occurs instead.[12] Plantarflexion at the ankle is lost with the decrease in hip- or knee flexion and extension. In order to make up for the loss of ankle joint movement, a plantarflexion deformity at the forefoot has been noted with an excessively dorsiflexed ankle joint. The resultant high-arched foot position has been termed a 'heelfoot' or pseudo-cavus.[12] Alternatively, excessive foot pronation occurs in order to compensate for the lack of dorsiflexion.

A valgus knee deformity would be expected to have the predictable effect of causing foot pronation, however, occasionally this is not the case and a marked inverted foot position is seen as the child compensates for the valgus leg by developing a varus heel.

In oligoarthritis and extended oligoarticular disease, the asymmetrical knee involvement leads to a leg-length discrepancy. One study has found that all children included had a leg-length discrepancy at some point during their illness.[13] Although discrepancies are no doubt common in the healthy population, they do not seem to have

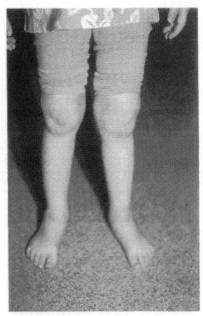

Figure 6.11 Genu valgum with synovitis leading to increased foot pronation.

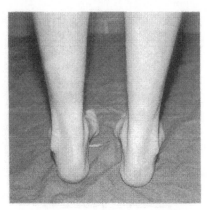

Figure 6.12 Pes cavus with increased external tibial torsion and forefoot adduction.

such a marked influence on the lower limb function, even when the discrepancy is small. In the early stages of the disease, the affected limb is always longer. To prevent pelvic tilt and functional scoliosis, the knee flexes and may move into a valgus position and the foot pronates (Fig. 6.11). Without treatment, these positions become fixed. During gait, the upper body compensates with an increase in lateral sway.

The foot and ankle position during stance is influenced by joint changes in the hip and knee as well as by local joint disease. With hip flexion, the femur moves into an internally rotated position. Secondary compensation within the tibia may be seen by an increase in external tibial torsion. This compensation has been noted in healthy children in the absence of joint disease, but its development in JIA is often rapid. In a healthy child, an increased tibial torsion would be associated with an out-toed gait and foot pronation. In JIA, the opposite position frequently evolves. The increased malleolar position takes the ankle joint mortise into an externally facing position (Fig. 6.12). The talus is therefore held in abduction, which causes the heel to invert under-

neath and the forefoot to adduct relative to the talus. A cavoid foot position develops (see Fig. 6.11) but with a greater degree of forefoot adduction than seen in the healthy child.[12] The reason that this compensation is seen only in JIA is not clear. However, it may be related initially to subtalar joint stiffness and reduced eversion since the foot is frequently rigid and resistant to correction.

Clinically, it is quite difficult to identify subtalar joint disease. However, it should be remembered that the ankle and subtalar joint share many ligaments. Therefore, active disease in the ankle will impact upon subtalar joint function. It is rare to find a normal subtalar joint range of motion when the ankle is involved.

A pronated foot position is seen more commonly in JIA.[14] The reason for this remains unclear but slowing of the normal developmental changes is a possibility since both general and local growth may be altered in JIA. Because of the need to compensate for a rearfoot and forefoot varus in the early years, most young children function around a pronated foot position. This will be true in JIA. However, the presence of synovitis within the ankle and subtalar joint complex will stretch supporting ligaments and allow the pronated foot position to worsen rather than improve with age, particularly if muscle power is reduced.

The disturbance of growth plays a role in the development of other deformities. The overall linear growth of the child may be reduced at

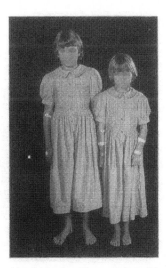

Figure 6.13 Identical twin girls – one has JIA, which has resulted in a slowing of overall growth (© Institute of Child Health and The Hospitals for Sick Children).

times of prolonged active disease (Fig. 6.13). In addition, growth at individual epiphyses may also be disrupted. Conversely, active local disease may increase growth and at the knee joint this may result in a genu valgum deformity. Disruption of the epiphysis of the ankle may lead to a varus or valgus tilt of the talus thus influencing the position of foot (Fig. 6.14).

Not all of the subgroups of JIA involve active synovitis. Children with spondyloarthropathies may present with features seen in adult disease such as enthesiopathies affecting the Achilles tendon and the insertion of the plantar fascia. Gross foot deformities are less common in such children. However, treatment is often a challenge since the entheses may be extremely painful and reducing the stress through the insertions can be difficult. In addition, the feet may be very stiff and function may be poor because of the stiffness and pain.

The podiatric treatment of JIA involves maintaining the foot in a good functional position, encouraging correct posture and gait with full muscle strength. A comprehensive lower limb and gait assessment of the child needs to be undertaken so that the podiatrist can record accurately joint ranges of motion, muscle strength and those joints with active disease. Tenosynovitis is often missed when the feet are generally swollen. As a result of limited joint movement, tenosynovitis or bursitis, children with JIA develop poor gait patterns in an effort to reduce stress on painful joints. Frequently habitual gaits are seen when joints are no longer swollen or painful and a normal range of motion is present. Walking is a learned process and it is not uncommon for the child to regress during active disease. Whenever it is planned to change the patient's foot or gait position, the effect on other lower limb joints should be borne in mind.

While using plaster serial casts to correct abnormal foot positions has been reported successful,[15] the muscle wasting that occurs with such techniques must be considered. Foot orthoses, full-length shoe raises, rocker sole adaptations and gait re-education are the mainstays of treatment. The type of material used in the manufacture of the orthoses will vary depending upon the disease pattern presenting. A more rigid material may be desired if the aim is to control or change the foot position. These are generally well tolerated by children provided they fit well and are accommodated by the shoe. The child with a spondyloarthropathy may benefit from a more shock-absorbing device. Where ankle or foot disease is present, orthoses should generally be prescribed in order to control abnormal foot positions. Even when the foot position is good, regular reviews should still be

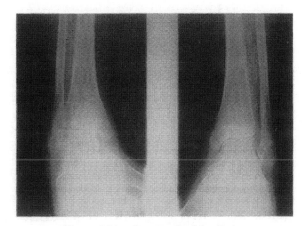

Figure 6.14 Overgrowth of the fibula.

undertaken since deformity may occur rapidly in these children. The decision to treat a child who has an abnormal foot position, but no ankle or foot disease is more difficult. The podiatrist needs to decide whether or not the position is sufficiently poor that pathological changes are likely in later life; whether or not the foot position is contributing to deformity in other joints that have active synovitis; or whether or not the foot functions well and only requires more frequent reviews. It should be borne in mind that small joint disease within the foot is quite difficult to identify clinically. Low-grade synovitis and grumbling disease may slowly erode the joint and although there is no evidence to show that orthoses prevent foot deformity, maintaining a good position and function is unlikely to be detrimental.

At all times, the child and the parents should be educated with regard to the condition being treated and the aims of the treatment should be explained. Compliance with orthotic management will be poor unless their use in preventing future deformity is stressed. Most children with JIA will be regularly following a muscle strengthening and stretching program. Specific foot exercises may be added to these programs. However, it must be remembered that it will be necessary for the child and the parents to commit large amounts of their time to such therapy and therefore unrealistic exercise programs should be avoided.

The subject of footwear should be addressed with advice given on the correct type, regardless of the need for orthoses. Footwear adaptations may be used in order to aid gait. Rocker soles are particularly useful for re-training gait

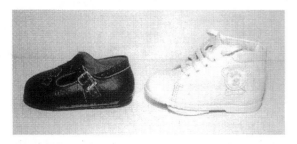

Figure 6.15 Addition of a rocker sole to a toddler's shoe.

when the heel–toe action has been lost (Fig. 6.15). Full-length shoe raises are invaluable in correcting deformities related to the leg-length discrepancies.

Other rheumatic conditions

The podiatrist is less frequently involved in the treatment of other juvenile rheumatic conditions such as dermatomyositis and systemic lupus erythematosus. This is because such diseases are less likely to affect the feet in the same way as JIA does. When involving an arthropathy, the joint positions that are observed are similar to those of JIA and therefore foot position and function will need to be addressed. Leg-length discrepancies are less common, but equinus deformities are seen in dermatomyositis as the proximal muscle weakness is frequently accompanied by contracture of the calf muscles. Heel raises and night splints may be required until muscle balance has been regained. In dermatomyositis, rest is indicated during active disease; exercise at this stage may increase the breakdown of muscle. Orthoses may be indicated as they improve lower limb mechanics sufficiently in order to aid recovery of the muscles. In systemic lupus erythematosus, joint deformity is less common but vasculitis affecting the digits may put the patient at risk of breakdowns. Attention to footwear is important in the prevention of pressure areas.

Certain children (and adults) possess a greater range of motion than would be expected in the normal population and they may be termed 'hypermobile'. This hypermobility may be part of a more generalized condition or it may affect only peripheral joints. Although the term benign joint hypermobility syndrome is relatively new, it may be applied to any patient who has chronic musculoskeletal symptoms related to hypermobile joints (see above). The arch of the foot is maintained on standing by the bony architecture and by the ligaments. Very little support is given to this arch by the muscles until the foot functions. It is therefore not surprising that foot deformity is seen in patients who exhibit increased stretch within their ligaments even in the absence of obvious biomechanical malalignment. Foot pronation is most frequently seen and this has a 'knock-on' effect on lower limb function. Muscle fatigue is common when the joints are not well supported by the ligaments. Treatment involves attention to posture and foot position. The child should be encouraged to adopt a good upper body posture, utilize the gluteal muscles to control the position of the femur and thus control pronation by core stability and limitation of internal leg rotation. Crouched gaits should be corrected with specific quadriceps exercises and foot orthoses should be used to correct the foot position. Since hypermobility may last throughout their lifetime, these children should concentrate on re-training their gait in order to control foot position through muscle strength rather than relying on a lifetime of orthoses.

Team approach to treatment

The treatment of children with rheumatic conditions can be extremely rewarding. A sound knowledge of biomechanics is required as well as a knowledge of the developing foot, upper body posture and muscle testing. The rheumatology team quickly embraces the specialist information that a podiatrist can bring and the podiatrist benefits from the exchange of knowledge from the other medical and paramedical specialists within the team.

REFERENCES

1. Petty RE, Southwood TR, Baum J, et al. Revision of the proposed classification criteria for juvenile idiopathic arthritis: Durban, 1997. Br J Rheumatol 1998;25(10): 1991–1994.
2. Remedios D, Martin K, Kaplan G, et al. Juvenile chronic arthritis: diagnosis and management of tibio-talar and sub-talar disease. Br J Rheumatol 1997;36(11):1214–1217.
3. Levinson JE, Wallace CA. Dismantling the pyramid. J Rheumatol Suppl 1992;33:6–10.
4. Sherry DD, Stein LD, Reed AM, et al. Prevention of leg length discrepancy in young children with pauciarticular juvenile rheumatoid arthritis by treating with intraarticular steroids. Arthritis Rheum 1999;42(11): 2330–2334.
5. Van Kerckhove C, Luyrink L, Taylor J, et al. HLA-DQA1*0101 haplotypes and disease outcome in early onset pauciarticular juvenile rheumatoid arthritis. J Rheumatol 1991;18(6):874–879.
6. Cassidy J, Petty R, eds. Textbook of pediatric rheumatology. 2nd ed. Philadelphia: WB Saunders; 1995.
7. FitzGerald O, Soden M, Yanni G, et al. Morphometric analysis of blood vessels in synovial membranes obtained from clinically affected and unaffected knee joints of patients with rheumatoid arthritis. Ann Rheum Dis 1991;50(11):792–796.
8. Beighton P. 1999 Hypermobility scoring. Clin J Path 1999;15(3):218–223.
9. Murray CS, Cohen A, Perkins T, et al. Morbidity in reflex sympathetic dystrophy. Arch Dis Child 2000;82:231–233.
10. Lechner DE, McCarthy CF, Holden MK. Gait deviations in patients with juvenile chronic arthritis. J Am Physical Therapy Assoc 1987;67:1335–1341.
11. Dhanendran M, Hutton WC, Klenerman L, et al. Foot function in juvenile chronic arthritis. Rheum Rehab 1980;19:20–24.
12. Truckenbrodt H, Hafner C, Von Altenbockum C. Functional joint analysis of the foot in juvenile chronic arthritis. Clin Exp Rheumatol 1994;12 (suppl.10):S91–S96.
13. Simon S, Whiffen J, Shapiro F. Leg-length discrepancies in monoarticular and pauciarticular juvenile rheumatoid arthritis. J Bone Joint Surg Am 1981;63(2):209–215.
14. Spraul G, Koenning G. A descriptive study of foot problems in children with juvenile rheumatoid arthritis. Arthritis Care Res 1994;7(3):144–150.
15. Mavidrou A, Klenerman L, Swann M, et al. Conservative management of the hindfoot in juvenile chronic arthritis. The Foot 1991;1:139–143.

7

Pediatric neurology*

Edwin J. Harris

INTRODUCTION TO THE NERVOUS SYSTEM

Neurons and neuroglia (nerve supporting cells) are all produced from embryonic neuroectoderm, which has become specialized on the dorsal surface of the embryo during the third week of gestation (Fig. 7.1). The lateral margins of this neural plate invaginate and close dorsally to form the central nervous system (CNS). At the same time neural crest cells proliferate and migrate through the mesoderm and later differentiate into the dorsal roots, sensory and motor nerves, autonomic ganglia and Schwann cells which make up the peripheral nervous system (PNS). The first point of fusion of the neural tube is in the medulla and fusion progresses rostrally and caudally until week 7. Differentiation at the rostral and caudal ends of the developing nervous system then commences. Disturbances around this time produce such problems as anencephaly and myelomeningocele.

Between weeks 8 and 16 neural proliferation occurs. Chromosomal abnormalities, teratogens (irradiation, toxins, e.g. alcohol) or infections may prevent proliferation. Migration of cells to specific sites producing nerve tracts and nuclei occurs mainly between weeks 12 and 22. Incomplete migration of cells results in such clinically recognizable entities as agenesis of the corpus callosum and severe abnormalities such as schizencephaly. Organization of neurons occurs from week 20

* The editors and Edwin J Harris wish to acknowledge the contribution made by Dr Robin Grant as the co-author of the chapter in the first edition upon which this revision is based.

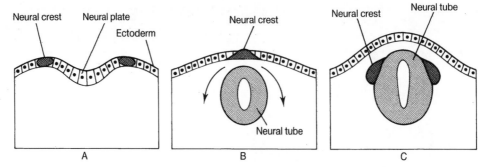

Figure 7.1 Transverse section through the dorsal structures of the embryo at 3 weeks (A) to 7 weeks (C) gestation demonstrating development of the neural tube and neural crest.

onwards and continues for several years after birth. The major changes that occur are alignment and orientation of cortical neurons, sprouting of dendrites and axons, and development of synapses. Failure of complete organization is usually the result of perinatal insults but also occurs in Down syndrome and primary mental retardation. Myelination of axons starts around the second trimester, occurring first in the PNS, in motor then sensory roots, and next in the CNS in the major sensory and then motor tracts. Myelination in the cerebral and cerebellar hemispheres starts well after delivery, continues over the first two decades and is necessary for the development of fine motor and sensory control, refinement of balance and coordination, and for development of reasoning and intelligence. The gray matter contains nerve cell bodies and the white matter contains myelinated axons. The neurons are supported by glial tissue (astrocytes and oligodendrocytes). Afferent (sensory) neurons transmit action potentials from peripheral receptors (e.g. in the skin) to central neurons (e.g. in the sensory cortex). Efferent neurons send axons from central cell bodies (e.g. in the motor cortex) to peripheral effector organs (e.g. in muscle).

CONTROL OF POSTURE AND MOVEMENT

Voluntary movement is initiated from the cerebral cortex, although there is some evidence that deeper structures such as the thalamus, cerebellum and basal ganglia aid in initiation of movement by their actions on the motor cortex.

Descending tracts

Corticospinal tracts

The upper motor neurons (UMNs) descend via the posterior limb of the internal capsule in the corticospinal tracts and corticobulbar tracts. At the level of the medulla most of the corticospinal fibers cross the midline and descend as the lateral corticospinal tracts. A smaller percentage of these fibers do not decussate and they descend as the anterior corticospinal tracts and only cross at their segmental levels. Most corticospinal fibers end on interneurons in lamina VII of the spinal cord. These pathways are concerned with fine movements.

Reticulospinal and vestibulospinal tracts

The reticulospinal tracts start in the pons and medulla and partially decussate and synapse with interneurons in lamina VII. Reticulospinal tracts control movements that do not need conscious attention. Vestibulospinal tracts from the vestibular nuclei in the medulla descend uncrossed and end on interneurons in the spinal cord. These neurons mediate extensor tone and allow us to maintain an upright posture.

Basal ganglia and cerebellum

The basal ganglia and cerebellum do not have descending tracts, but they do modify movement and possibly store learned patterns of behavior. The basal ganglia (caudate nucleus, putamen and globus pallidus) are concerned with posture, truncal movements and gross limb movements. The role of the cerebellum is to smooth and to coordinate movement. The cerebellum has extensive afferent input from the motor cortex (via the pontocerebellar tracts), spinal afferent systems (spinocerebellar), and vestibular (vestibulocerebellar) receptors. The efferents from the cerebellum relay to the thalamus (and brain-stem nuclei) which in turn influence the motor cortex (thalamofrontal projections). These supraspinal projections ultimately affect the rate and pattern of discharge from the lower motor neurons (LMN) in the brain stem (cranial motor nuclei) and spinal cord (anterior horn cells).

Peripheral nervous system

Axons from the anterior horn cells exit the spinal cord via the anterior (motor) nerve roots and then join with the sensory nerves to form a mixed nerve (Fig. 7.2). Mixed nerves contain large and small diameter fibers. The somatic motor nerves and sensory nerves subserving joint vibration

and position sense are well myelinated and conduct action potentials quickly, while the smaller fibers subserving pain and temperature or to muscle spindles are poorly myelinated and have slower conduction velocities. At the distal end of the mixed peripheral nerve, motor and sensory elements once more part company, the former to muscle and the latter to specialized sensory nerve endings. The LMN terminates at the neuromuscular junction by forming the presynaptic terminal that lies over a specialized motor end plate. Motor control is finely controlled by a feedback loop in the PNS via gamma efferent neurons to muscle spindles and via Ia afferent fibers from muscle spindles that provide information about small changes in muscle stretch.

Neurotransmitters

Neurotransmitters are chemicals released at synaptic junctions and are present in the CNS and the PNS. These chemicals are different from hormones in that they produce their effect locally (i.e. at a synapse) rather than at a distant site. There are many different types of neurotransmitters and many subsets of each type. The neurotransmitters that have most effect on movement and posture are acetylcholine (Ach), dopamine (DA) and gamma-aminobutyric acid (GABA). Acetylcholine acts through two types of receptors: nicotinic and muscarinic. Cholinergic neurotransmission in the cortex and subcortical areas is mediated through both types of receptor whereas in the spinal cord and at the neuromuscular junction neurotransmission is through nicotinic receptors. In the CNS its action is still ill defined but it may be important in memory. Stimulation of the LMN causes release of Ach from presynaptic vesicles and this binds to postsynaptic nicotinic receptors, which results in the release of calcium from muscle sarcoplasmic reticulum, which in turn causes muscle contraction. Ach is also the neurotransmitter present in all preganglionic neurons, parasympathetic postganglionic neurons and sympathetic postganglionic neurons. Stimulation of these causes bradycardia, bronchoconstriction, small pupils, vasodilation and sweating.

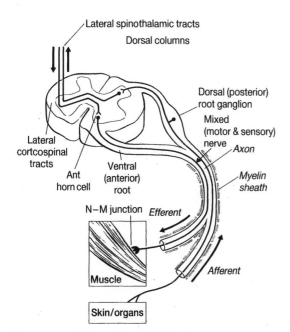

Figure 7.2 Afferent pathways from sensory end organs in the periphery to the spinal cord and efferent (motor) pathways from spinal cord to the neuromuscular junction.

Dopaminergic neurons in the basal ganglia are necessary to enable proper control of posture, tone and speed of movement. There is a relative balance of action of DA and Ach in basal ganglia and when there is a net reduction of DA, a Parkinsonian state is produced with flexed posture, increased tone (rigidity), slowed movement (hypokinesia) and tremor. When there is relative excess of DA, movement disorders such as dyskinesia may predominate.

GABA is an inhibitory transmitter within the brain, spinal cord and cerebellum. Activation of the GABAa receptor produces a postsynaptic inhibitory action potential. The GABAb receptor is inhibitory to norepinephrine, glutamate, DA and serotonin. Following any damage to the UMNs in the brain or spinal cord, excitatory influences predominate. Benzodiazepines and valproate facilitate GABA binding and thus produce an anticonvulsant action. Baclofen is a GABAb agonist and therefore acts as a muscle relaxant.

HISTORY AND PHYSICAL EXAMINATION

Neurological evaluation starts with a history of the presenting complaint, past medical history, maternal obstetric history, birth history, developmental history, family history, drug and social history and a review of systems. Most neurological diagnoses can be made from history alone and examination and investigations only confirm what is usually apparent.

Careful documentation of the presenting complaint is critical to the understanding of the problem. Many diagnostic errors occur because of misunderstanding the complaint. Terminology can be a major problem. Since the child is rarely the historian, a third party expresses the chief complaint. Although it is often parents, it may also be appointed caregivers lacking critical details. Their interpretation of events is colored by their own experiences, conception of the problem, fears of the diagnosis and information given to them by friends, relatives and other healthcare personnel. The historian may use ter-minology that has specific medical meaning. The historian's understanding of these terms may radically differ from that of the clinician.

The past medical history may contain information needed for the diagnosis. Parents and other custodians do not always appreciate the relevance of some of this information and may even conceal information from the physician. Medication history must be probed for prescription, non-prescription and alternative medications.

Developmental history may contain items of importance. History of the pregnancy may contain clues suggesting fetal distress. Cesarean section can never be accepted without explanation because elective cesarean sections are infrequently performed. The history of acquisition of the developmental landmarks outlines the child's neurological progression and maturity. Sequential acquisition of landmarks is necessary since they build on each other.

Development of head control starts with the ability to raise the head from the bed, first in the prone and then in the supine position. This is followed by rolling over, first from the prone position and then from the supine position. Sitting balance is a marker for trunk stability. Crawling marks the development of reciprocal limb control. Standing upright is a marker of ability to balance the center of gravity over a small surface area. Independent walking integrates all of the skills into patterns of purposeful locomotion. Bowel and bladder control mark more advanced neurological maturity, although there are social factors involved in acquisition of these two landmarks. Cerebral dominance in the form of hand preference acquired very early is an indication of cerebral dysfunction on the opposite side.

Neonatal examination

The most important aspect of the neonatal neurological examination is observation. Level of alertness, ability to suck and to swallow, morphological features such as weight and length, head shape and circumference, symmetry and position of all limbs and digits and normal spinal and facial features should all be recorded. Level of alertness varies with time of feed and examination is best performed prior to a feed when the baby is active and unlikely to vomit. When the baby is held upright, the hips are usually flexed and the head hangs limply forward. When the baby is supported under the abdomen, it may momentarily lift the head up, and when laid supine the head will turn to one side. The hands are usually fisted at rest but during feeding the arms may partially extend and the baby will try to grasp the breast. Eye contact with the mother during breast-feeding occurs early. A healthy baby will startle at a loud noise and will have an active cry when hungry. Muscle tone may be slightly increased and various primitive reflexes such as the grasp, Moro, sucking, rooting and tonic neck reflex are present. The plantar reflexes are extensor.

By 3 months, the baby produces vigorous movements at rest with the hands open or loosely fisted. When the baby is held upright, its head will bob. When prone, the baby's head will be held up for a few seconds. When the baby is supine, the head is in the midline. The baby will be able to hold a toy for a short time. The Moro, tonic neck reflex and grasp reflex may now be suppressed. The baby will smile, vocalize and follow an interesting object. At 6 months, the baby, when supine, can lift the head up, roll from supine to prone and can maintain the head and chest up in this position. The baby can support its weight when in the standing position, transfer a toy from hand to hand with a rather coarse grasp and recognize familiar faces and voices. At 9–10 months, infants can pull themselves into an upright posture and, by 12 months, can usually stand for a moment unassisted and walk when led. By 15 months, the infant can walk with a broad-based gait and by 18 months can manage a rather stiff run with only occasional falls. At 2 years, the child can run without falling and can usually walk up and down stairs without help. It is also valuable to observe simple motor tasks, e.g. rising from a squatted position, walking on the heels to test the ankle dorsiflexors and on the toes to test gastrocnemius. Balance may be assessed by asking the child to stand with feet together with eyes open, in order to test cerebellar function, and then with eyes closed, to test joint position (Romberg's test). By 3 years, the child can balance momentarily on one foot; at 4 years, the child can run and jump; and by age 5, the child can skip and balance on one foot for a short time with the eyes closed. Testing tandem gait will often identify subtle cerebellar signs. Hopping is a good, quick, non-discriminative test, which if accomplished, usually means that the lower limb motor, sensory and cerebellar functions are normal.

The upper limbs can be quickly screened by means of five observations:

1. The child is asked to hold both hands out with the palms upward. Proximal weakness is likely to be present if the arms cannot be raised or if they drift downwards.
2. The child is asked to touch the nose with the eyes open. Failure to do so may indicate cerebellar dysfunction.
3. The child is asked to touch the nose with the eyes closed. When the maneuver can be performed with the eyes open but not closed, there is usually a sensory issue.
4. The upper extremity is evaluated for tone and range of motion. Palmarization of the thumb and fingers, decreased pronation and supination as well as elbow flexion contractures are the more common abnormal observations. Size and proportion of muscle masses can be easily observed.
5. A valuable reproducible test of dexterity or for clumsiness is the timed nine-hole peg test (timed at putting nine pegs in nine holes, using one hand at a time).

These simple, quick, screening tests usually identify children who require a more detailed neurological examination.

Formal neurological examination

Limb symmetry, muscle bulk, tone, strength and reflexes should be compared on each side, both proximally and distally. Both upper extremities and lowers should be tested. Muscle strength can be tested in groups. Interpretation is based on knowledge of muscle innervation. In the lower limbs, L1, 2, 3 supply the hip flexors (iliopsoas); L4, 5, S1 innervate the hip extensors (glutei); L2, 3, 4 supply the knee extensors (quadriceps); L5, S1, 2 innervate the knee flexors (hamstrings); L4, 5 supply ankle dorsiflexion (tibialis anterior) and S1, 2 plantar flexion (gastrocnemius). Subtalar inversion is mediated by L4 nerve root and eversion by L5, S1.

The reflex levels may be remembered by: ankle jerk S1, 2; knee jerk L3, 4; supinator jerk C6; triceps jerk C7.

The plantar response should be tested last by drawing an object from behind the lateral malleolus along the lateral border of the foot and then across the metatarsal heads (Chaddock's test). This is as effective as Babinski's method and is less likely to produce a withdrawal response.[1] The physiological response is downgoing movement of the toes. Extension of the toes may be physiological extensor withdrawal or a frankly positive Babinski's sign. This distinction is important. Extensor withdrawal is normal up to age 2, but Babinski's sign is pathological at any age. The cremasteric reflex in males and the abdominal skin reflexes in both sexes round out the most commonly performed superficial reflexes.

Testing sensation requires patient cooperation. If there are no sensory complaints, a brief screening examination should suffice. When there are complaints of numbness or tingling, the patient should be asked to map it out and the distribution should be confirmed and localized (i.e. nerve root, single nerve or glove and stocking). In order to prevent transmission of disease, pain sensation should be tested using a safety pin that is then disposed of after the test. Testing vibratory sense evaluates for peripheral neuropathy and posterior column involvement.

The dermatomes can be quickly tested.[2] In the lower limbs, anterior thigh is supplied by L1, 2, 3, the lower leg by L4 anteromedially, L5 anterolaterally, S1 the outer border of the foot and sole, S2 up the back of the leg and S3, 4, 5 over the buttock.

Joint position sense is tested by moving the toes while the eyes are closed and asking the patient to identify the direction of movement. Vibration sense is tested by placing a vibrating tuning fork over a bony prominence and asking if the patient feels vibration and testing for extinction by asking when the child no longer feels the vibratory sensation. Examiners can use themselves as the control. Cerebellar function should be tested last because the presence of motor or sensory problems makes it is difficult to comment on coordination. Slurred speech (dysarthria), jerky eye movements (nystagmus), finger–nose–finger test, smoothly running the heel up and down the shin (heel–shin test), rapid alternating movements and tandem gait are tests for cerebellar function.

ABNORMAL NEUROLOGICAL PATTERNS AND PHYSIOLOGICAL ABERRATIONS

Some clumsiness during walking is considered normal. As many as 10% of children may be clumsy to a degree. Abnormal clumsiness with delay in reaching the appropriate motor milestones merits full neurological examination.

Certain movement disturbances correlate with specific anatomical neurological lesions: UMN damage produces weakness of extensor muscle groups in the upper limb and of flexor groups in the lower limb associated with spasticity, hyperreflexia and extensor plantar response. When spasticity is unilateral, the arm is held flexed and the leg extended. The hips circumduct and the toes and outer aspect of shoes are often scuffed. When there is bilateral UMN damage, the gait is scissored and abductor tone results in the knees rubbing when walking coupled with plantarflexion and inversion of the feet. There may also be lordosis and a rather festinant, precarious gait as is seen in cerebral palsy (CP).

Damage to the basal ganglia produces tremor, increased tone (rigidity), slowed movement (hypokinesia) and flexed posture.

Cerebellar damage results in slurred speech, nystagmus, and incoordination in the upper and lower limbs and a wide-based, ataxic gait.

Muscle disorders (e.g. polymyositis or Duchenne muscular dystrophy) produce weakness and wasting proximally in the lower and upper limbs. Reflexes are normal, and there are no sensory abnormalities. The gait is characteristically swaggering, with rolling at the hips (Trendelenburg gait) because of the lower girdle weakness. Some dystrophies (e.g. myotonic dystrophy) result in distal weakness and wasting, producing a gait similar to that of peripheral neuropathy but without sensory signs.

Loss of cerebral control modulating inhibition of the simple reflex arcs results in hypertonicity and hyperreflexia. Purposeful movement is affected, acquisition of motor landmarks is delayed and abnormal posturing leads to contractures.

LMN disorders produce wasting, fasciculations (spontaneous contraction of motor units), hypotonia, weakness, areflexia and flexor plantar responses without sensory changes. Loss of anterior horn cells results in denervation of muscle. Severity of weakness reflects the degree of denervation, and eventually atrophy of muscle with flaccid paralysis develops. Weakness interferes with balance of the center of gravity and maintenance of articular stability. Walking is abnormal and contractures frequently occur.

Fatigable muscle weakness, worsening with activity, may reflect failure of neurotransmission at the neuromuscular junction, resulting in the finding of myasthenia. There are no fasciculations, reflex changes or sensory loss. Myotonia is the inability to relax muscle after a sustained contraction and it produces problems ranging from minor annoyance to significant loss of function. Motor and sensory dysfunction may occur as the result of degenerative peripheral and CNS pathology. Neuropathies produce sensory and motor signs. Loss of vibration distally in the lower limbs with reduced ankle jerks is often an early sign of a peripheral neuropathy and precedes numbness and weakness. Peripheral neuropathies produce weakness of ankle dorsiflexion that results in foot drop and a high steppage gait. Many of these syndromes are hereditary. Sensory involvement is frequently minimal and since it does not produce marked impairment, patients are frequently unaware of sensory change. The motor component dominates with muscle weakness and imbalance resulting in severe interference with locomotion.

PATTERNED RESPONSES

There are a number of patterned activities that indicate maturation of the CNS. These produce movement that is counterproductive to trunk and extremity function and interfere with appropriate postures that are needed for the activities of daily living.[3,4]

Some patterns are cord mediated. They are present at birth, but involute rapidly with maturation by about 2 months of age. Flexor withdrawal occurs when the sole of the foot of a fully extended limb is stimulated. Flexion of the hip and knee on the stimulated side is considered to be an abnormal response, but is physiological up to about 2 months of age.

Extensor thrust is tested by stimulating the sole of the foot while the hip and knee are flexed. Extension of the stimulated limb is considered abnormal after 2 months.

Crossed extension is tested by flexing the limb to be tested first. The opposite limb is then flexed. Spontaneous extension of the originally flexed limb is considered pathological after 2 months of age. Similarly, with both legs in extension, tapping the medial side of one limb may produce abduction, internal rotation and foot plantarflexion on the opposite side.

Certain other patterns are mediated at the brain-stem level. Such patterns are considered static postural reflexes. They change tone throughout the body, and are elicited by position of the head and neck. They usually involute by 6 months of age.

The asymmetrical tonic neck reflex is elicited by placing the infant supine with the head in midline and the extremities extended. The head is turned to one side. The test is positive if there is extension of the arm and leg on the side of the body that the face is turned and flexion of the arm and leg on the occiput side.

The symmetrical tonic neck reflex is tested with the child prone on the examiner's lap. The head and neck are flexed ventrally. If the reflex is present, there is increased flexor tone in the upper extremities and extensor tone in the lower extremities. Reversing the maneuver by dorsiflexing the head will produce upper extremity extensor tone and lower extremity flexor tone if the reflex is positive.

Midbrain-level-mediated reflexes also occur. Rotating the head passively tests the neck-righting reflex. A positive reaction results when the body rotates as a unit in the same direction as the head. This phenomenon should disappear by 6 months.

Other reflex patterns are automatic-move-ment-patterned reactions to stimuli. The best known of these is the Moro reflex. The child is placed supine. The stimulus can be a loud noise, a blow to the sides of the examining table or allowing the head to drop an inch or two (2.5 or 5 cm) to the examining table. When positive, abduction with extension of the arms and legs is followed by movement of the extremities to midline. Its presence is abnormal after 6 months of age.

The Landau reflex is elicited by suspending the child prone by holding at the thorax. In the abnormal response, dorsiflexion of the head and neck produces extension movement in all four extremities. This is physiological from 6 months to about 30 months.

Holding the child prone at the pelvis and allowing the body to drop toward the ground tests the parachute reflex. When positive, the arms extend to protect the face. This reflex becomes positive at about 6 months and persists throughout life.

Some of these (such as the parachute reflex and the righting reflex) are beneficial when they persist. Others (such as the Moro, symmetrical and asymmetrical reflexes) produce destructive movement patterns that interfere with normal activities. These destructive patterns are likely to be found in quadriplegic (total body) CP.

ORTHOPEDIC TREATMENT ISSUES

Within the scope of this text, it is not possible to discuss therapy for all of the individual diseases.

Fortunately, a number of therapeutic issues are shared by many different conditions. Although accurate diagnosis is necessary to predict prognosis, it is possible to approach the subject from the standpoint of clinical symptom management. In order to illustrate the management of these therapeutic problems, four models will be specifically highlighted: CP, muscular dystrophy, the hereditary sensorimotor neuropathies and myelomeningocele. Therapy for the others will be discussed in less detail in separate sections.

SPECIFIC CLINICAL PROBLEMS

Neuromuscular diseases have their greatest impact on motor skills and ambulation. Problems with maintaining head control, trunk stability, effective sitting postures and mobility make it impossible for children to realize their intellectual potential and to lead a socially useful life. In keeping with the goal-oriented approach to therapy, a number of clinical problems are common to the various neuromuscular diseases and form the basis for clinical therapy.

Contracture

Permanent shortening of muscle is a common complication of many neuromuscular diseases. Muscle grows in length by adding sarcomeres to the myotendinous junction stimulated by repetitive stretching of the muscle to its maximal length. In the early stages of contracture development, it is possible to regain some length by careful stretching of the muscle through physiotherapy. Once a contracture develops, no amount of stretching can recapture the lost length (myostatic contracture). Attempts to stretch in the presence of a contracture will result in muscle or tendon injury.

Shortening of a muscle results in limited range of joint motion. Eventually the capsule and peripheral soft tissue structures also become contracted resulting in decreased range of motion for two reasons:

1. decreased range of motion produced by the short muscle

2. decreased range of motion produced by soft tissue contractures.

Prevention is the most important therapeutic goal in the management of contractures. Physiotherapy can do much to prevent the development of these deforming and disabling changes (see Ch. 13). Once these changes occur, the only successful management is surgical lengthening of the contracted soft tissues. Lengthening of the tendon increases the range of joint motion, but at the expense of weakening the muscle. It does not increase the length of the muscle.

Imbalance

Purposeful coordinated movement and quality activity require balanced joints. This allows smooth, efficient movement and prevents the development of joint and muscle contractures. Balance may be upset in two ways. First, balance is affected by unequal strength in the agonists and antagonists. Second, balanced activity may be disturbed when selective muscles fire out of phase.

Imbalance results in joint subluxations and dislocations. Digital deformities serve as good examples of this process. Hammertoes are most likely to develop when the long toe flexors attempt to overcome weakened ankle plantar flexors. This may be complicated by spasticity or weakness of the intrinsic muscles that should normally stabilize the proximal phalanges of the lesser toes.

Calcaneus deformity

Calcaneus deformity occurs when the heel is on the ground and the toes are not (Fig. 7.3) This is rarely seen naturally in CP, but it may occur as an iatrogenic complication in association with crouch gait following overlengthening of the Achilles tendon.[5] The ankle remains in calcaneus but the forefoot and midfoot plantarflex in global fashion so that the metatarsal heads reach the ground. The calcaneus change at the ankle causes limitation of ankle dorsiflexion. The posterior

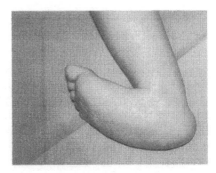

Figure 7.3 Calcaneus deformity. This deformity is rarely seen as a primary deformity in CP. However it may occur as an iatrogenic complication following overlengthening of the tendo Achilles.

and lateral compartments assume some of the load through flexor augmentation (flexor substitution), and the hindfoot–midfoot complex takes on a cavoid configuration (Fig. 7.4). Careful preoperative evaluation and attention to preoperative muscle strength assessment best prevent this problem. Joint contractures can be prevented by well though-out bracing plans or by appropriate muscle transfer designed to support and to strengthen the activity of the weakened muscle.

Managing imbalance caused by out-of-phase muscle activity is an entirely different problem. Surgical transfer of a strong muscle to support out-of-phase activity usually fails even in the

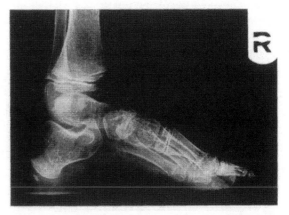

Figure 7.4 Cavus deformity resulting from overlengthening of the Achilles tendon. The ankle is maximally dorsiflexed in the ankle mortise and the forefoot is plantarflexed through the midtarsal joints.

neurologically intact individual. These transferred muscles ultimately function as tenodeses.

Volitional control

Some central nervous diseases cause total or incomplete loss of voluntary control over muscle activity. The child lacks the ability to perform purposeful, coordinated movements and may have difficulty in locating body parts in space. Destructive movement patterns may take place. Physiotherapy may help the child to suppress these patterns and may also assist the child to recruit new neuronal pathways in order to develop some purposeful activity.[6,7] When this does not occur, bracing is needed to overcome the loss of purposeful activity.

Persisting primitive reflexes

Primitive reflexes that persist into childhood may produce movement pattern activities that are triggered by an appropriate stimulus. In certain cases, mass activity is evoked by body part position, e.g. the symmetrical and asymmetrical tonic neck reflexes. These reflex activities are counter-productive to smooth efficient locomotion.

Seven of these reflexes are significant because they may be used to predict walking ability. Bleck[8] has designed a grading system that uses seven of these primitive reflexes as predictors of independent ambulation (Table 7.1).

Table 7.1 Predicting walking potential according to Bleck

Detrimental reflexes (score 1 point if present)	Favorable reflexes (score 1 point if absent)
Asymmetrical tonic neck reflex	Foot placement reaction
Neck righting reflex	Parachute reflex
Symmetrical tonic neck reflex	
Moro reflex	
Extensor thrust	

Prognosis
0 points = good prognosis
1 point = guarded prognosis
2 or more points = poor prognosis

SPECIFIC FOOT AND ANKLE PROBLEMS

Equinus

Ankle equinus is the most common problem shared by CP, Duchenne muscular dystrophy and a number of other neuromuscular conditions. Equinus deformity exists when there is insufficient dorsiflexion of the ankle to allow toe clearance during swing phase of the gait cycle and for heel contact at the initiation of stance phase (Fig. 7.5). Equinus may produce excessive knee and hip flexion as compensatory mechanisms to allow the toes to clear the ground during the swing phase (Fig. 7.6A–D). More commonly, equinus deformity of the ankle produces major gait alterations during stance phase. There are three patterns that are frequently seen. The first pattern is one in which the beginning of stance phase is initiated by toe contact. This is then followed by a modified full flat pattern which operates through the remaining one-half of stance phase (toe–heel gait). A second gait pattern in stance phase is limited to toe contact with the heel never coming to the ground (toe–toe pattern). The third pattern, premature heel-off, may be the only finding in mild equinus.

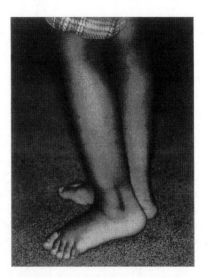

Figure 7.5 Equinus deformity due to insufficient dorsiflexion of the ankle during swing phase and for heel contact at the initiation of stance phase.

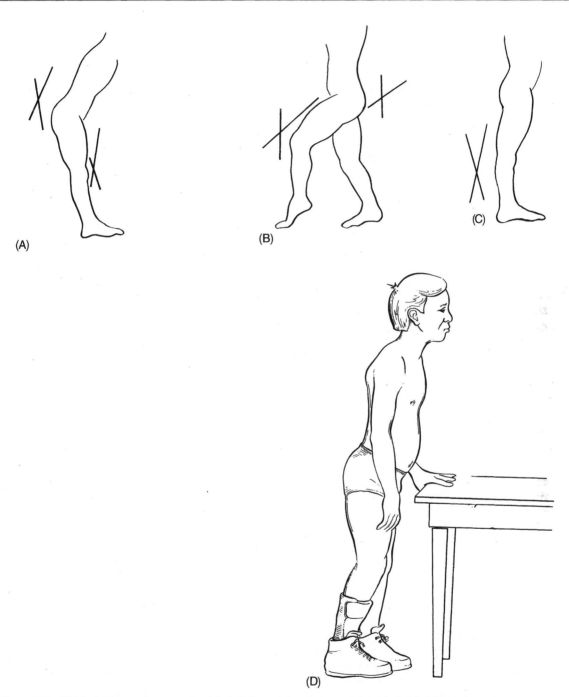

Figure 7.6   (A) Unyielding equinus may result in inability to bring the center of gravity behind the hip joints. This makes it impossible for the child to stand or walk without crutches. (B) Excessive knee and hip flexion may be necessary to allow toe clearance during swing. (C) Genu recurvatum may result when equinus is unyielding and uncompensated. (D) In the presence of knee or hip flexion contracture, the child may 'stand or walk on the toes' – even in ankle–foot orthotics.

There are two potential mechanisms for dorsiflexing the foot above neutral. The major excursion of motion (and most physiological) is at the level of the ankle. However, subtalar and midtarsal joint pronation can allow just enough dorsiflexion of the distal and lateral portions of the foot to clear the ground. When there is high gastrocsoleus tone and low body weight, the toe-to-toe pattern predominates. When increased body mass becomes great enough to overcome the hypertonicity and the stretch reflex, an equinovalgus deformity is produced.

Long-standing equinus results in myostatic contracture of the triceps mechanism. The altered gait pattern becomes fixed and permanent. Flattening of the talar dome develops as the result of body weight transmitted to it through the tibia, the action of the triceps tendon posterior to it and ground reactive force operating distal to it.

With the addition of tibialis posterior spasticity, a pattern of equinovarus results. There may be some associated adduction of the forefoot and midfoot, and the whole picture may be complicated additionally by a forefoot varus deformity when tibialis anterior is also involved.

The treatment of equinus should begin before the child starts walking and before the deformity becomes fixed by contracture. Early physiotherapy maintains range of motion and prevents the development of contracture. This should be started at time of diagnosis without delay in order to prevent fixation of the deformity. For as long as an appropriate range of motion can be achieved, the mainstay of therapy is bracing. Subtalar control can be achieved by designing an ankle–foot orthosis (AFO) with the heel bisection in the same plane as the long axis of the tibia. The ankle is maintained at sagittal plane neutral. This is possible as long as there are no hip- and knee-flexion contractures. Failure to take hip- and knee-flexion contractures into account will result in a persisting toe-walking gait when the child wears the AFO (Fig. 7.6D). Knee-flexion may also be managed by adding a ground reaction plate to the proximal portion of the AFO as long as knee extension is complete. Bracing the ankle in slight plantarflexion or dorsiflexion respectively may control knee-flexion or hyperextension in gait.

Equinovalgus patterns may be managed in much the same way as simple equinus. An AFO incorporating a well-molded heel seat and a well-contoured medial longitudinal arch will control this deformity as long as there is range of motion of the ankle to allow enough dorsiflexion above neutral that the patient is not required to pronate the subtalar and midtarsal joint.

Equinovarus patterns are almost impossible to brace. The equinus component is fairly straightforward but attempting to use orthotics to pronate the subtalar and midtarsal joints in the presence of spasticity almost always fails. Fractional lengthening of tibialis posterior (with lengthening of the Achilles tendon when a fixed contracture coexists) works well.[9–15] This is followed by an AFO to maintain the correction.

When equinus becomes fixed by myostatic contracture, physical therapy and bracing will not help. At this point, surgery is indicated to bring the patient to a state in which the patient can then be braced.

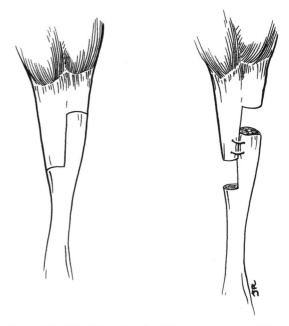

Figure 7.7 The Z-plasty of the Achilles tendon. The slide is constructed by creating a longitudinal splint in the tendon along its long axis. Peripheral cuts are then made as indicated. The separated segments of the tendon are allowed to slide. Integrity is maintained by suture of the arms of the cut tendon.

Surgical success requires selection of the proper procedure. Although there are a number of procedures described, all may be classified into two categories. The first includes all that are designed to lengthen the Achilles tendon. This may be accomplished by sectioning the tendon longitudinally and then by making proximal and lateral cuts in different directions so that when the tendon is subjected to stretch, the ends separate and slide along each other. The Z-plasty is the best example of this procedure (Fig. 7.7). Multiple hemisections of the tendon may also be made according to the technique of Hoke. When the tendon is then subjected to longitudinal stretch, these hemisections separate, and the tendon will separate longitudinally. The sliding component of the repair allows the tendon to remain in continuity (Fig. 7.8). This latter procedure may be performed percutaneously. In many cases of children with CP, the Hoke-type procedure has been found to be more satisfactory than the Z-plasty technique because such children have less postoperative muscle spasm. The disadvantage of the

Hoke-type procedure is that only a comparatively small lengthening can be achieved by this technique. When the surgeon underestimates the amount of lengthening required, tendon continuity may be lost and this will result in excessive scarring in the tendo-Achilles and also convalescence will be delayed significantly.

Overlengthening produces a calcaneocavus deformity. Attempts to shorten an overlengthened tendo-Achilles rarely succeed. Radical plantar release and transfer of functioning tendons to the posterior calcaneus may be of some benefit but the advantages and disadvantages must be weighed carefully in individual cases. It must be remembered that muscles that are to be transferred are actually out-of-phase in function.[16–18] Calcaneocavus deformity is best managed by preventing its occurrence in the first place. Careful preoperative assessment and strict adherence to technique are therefore mandatory for all cases in which tendo-Achilles lengthening is contemplated.

When tibialis anterior is involved, it occasionally becomes necessary to balance its effect on the forefoot. This may be accomplished in one of two ways: (i) the tendon can be moved laterally. It is important to move the tendon only as far in a lateral direction that it no longer inverts (supinates) the forefoot. When it is moved too far laterally a deformity in the opposite direction will result. (ii) Tibialis anterior may be split, with the lateral half being transferred to the area of the cuboid.[19] When performed properly, this procedure will balance the forefoot satisfactorily (Fig. 7.9A, B).

Hallux varus

Adduction deformity of the hallux may occur with neuromuscular disease. It is caused by contracture of the abductor hallucis. Non-operative therapies (such as physiotherapy, straight and outflare last shoes) fail. Treatment becomes surgical. Thomson described a procedure in which he excised the entire abductor hallucis.[20] This procedure may result in injury to the plantar neurovascular bundles, iatrogenic hallux valgus and a cosmetically unacceptable appearance.

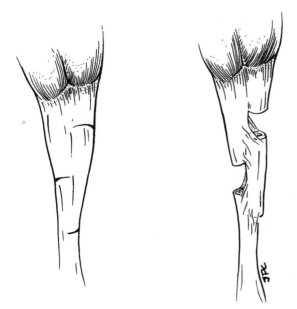

Figure 7.8 Tendon lengthening by the technique of Hoke. The transverse incisions are made in the tendon from the periphery to midline as indicated. The tendon is stressed longitudinally and the cut ends are allowed to slide. No sutures are used and the procedure can be performed through percutaneous stab incisions.

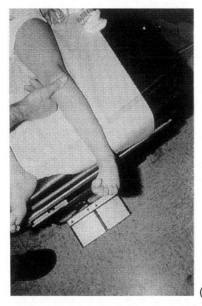
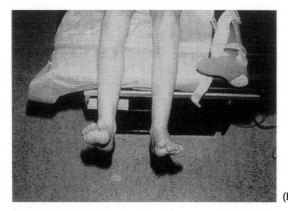

(A)

(B)

Figure 7.9 (A) The left equinus with hindfoot and forefoot varus deformity in a child with spastic diplegia. (B) Following Achilles tendon lengthening, fractional lengthening of tibialis posterior at the myotendinous junction and split tibialis anterior transfer.

Tenotomy at the level of the first metatarsal base has also been described,[21,22] although the possibility of contracture through the cut section of the muscle must be taken into consideration. Either lengthening or transfer of the distal abductor tendon with release of the muscle from the plantomedial skin and the medial first metatarsal has been very successful.

Hallux abductovalgus

Hallux abductovalgus is common in patients with neuromuscular disease. It begins in the pre-teen years and progresses rapidly. There are no successful non-operative treatments. Since the condition is caused by muscle imbalance, soft tissue procedures (which are usually successful in the neurologically normal population) almost always fail. Adaptive changes in the first metatarsophalangeal joint also occur early in the disease. Surgery for this deformity must be extremely aggressive. In order to prevent progression or recurrence, it is frequently necessary to perform an arthrodesis of the first metatarsophalangeal joint.

TREATMENT
Bracing in neuromuscular disease

There are a number of issues common to many of the neuromuscular diseases. These include muscle weakness and inability to control and coordinate muscle activity. Such problems cause difficulties with gross and fine motor skills, joint instability and balance issues. All of these are detrimental to walking.

Not all problems are responsive to bracing. In order for bracing to succeed, a problem amenable to bracing is identified and a solution is planned.

Lower extremity orthoses are named according to the joints covered. Foot orthoses are frequently called in-shoe orthotics. The University of California Biomechanics Laboratory (UCBL)-type orthotic is the most efficient non-pronating orthotic. It exerts its effect on the midtarsal and subtalar joints. It has no effect on ankle motion. The main indication for the use of UCBL orthotics is to control subtalar joint pronation (Fig. 7.10).

On those occasions when the subtalar joint needs controlling, frontal plane problems may

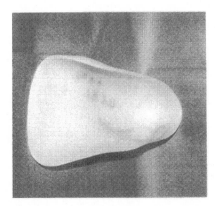

Figure 7.10 University of California Biomechanics Laboratory (UCBL) orthotic.

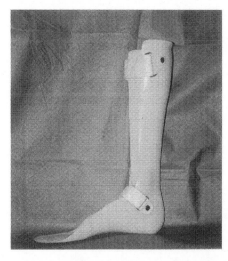

Figure 7.12 An Ankle–Foot orthotic (AFO) is used when control of the subtalar and midtarsal joint as well as control of the ankle joint in the sagittal plane is required.

also need to be addressed. This situation requires trim lines on the orthotic that come above the malleoli but do not restrict sagittal plane motion. Such an orthotic is called a supramalleolar orthotic (SMO) (Fig. 7.11). Its use is limited, but in those children who have hypotonia, ligamentous laxity or paralysis with resulting instability in the frontal plane, an SMO does have the advantage of controlling both the joints of the foot as well as the frontal plane. Control should be restricted to the fewest number of motion segments necessary.[23] Treatment failure may occur when the clinician mistakes primary ankle valgus or tibia valga for frontal instability.

AFOs control the subtalar and midtarsal joints as well as the ankle in the sagittal plane (Fig. 7.12). The ankle motion may be rigidly locked at neutral, or the position of the ankle can be varied by adding ankle joint articulations to allow varying amounts of ankle joint motion (Fig. 7.13). Stops and locks may be added as the circumstances dictate. Both solid ankle and articulated AFOs assist in toe clearance in swing.[24]

Ground reaction orthotics (GROs) combine the features of an AFO in order to allow control of the knee in the sagittal plane. An anterior component in front of the tibial tubercle extends up above the patella (Fig. 7.14). By carefully adjusting the amount of plantarflexion at the ankle, the modified AFO will force the knee into full extension – even in the presence of a grossly weakened quadriceps.

Knee–ankle–foot orthotics (KAFO) are used when both the ankle and the knee need control in the sagittal plane. These devices have a number of features that may be added as needed. Uprights may be single or double. The knees can be fitted with a number of locking mechanisms.

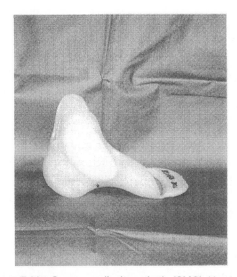

Figure 7.11 Supra – malleolar orthotic (SMO). Use is limited but it will control both the joints of the foot and motion in the frontal plane.

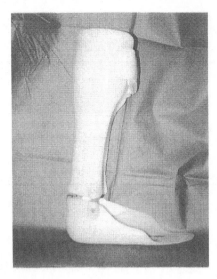

Figure 7.13 The addition of articulations to an AFO will allow control of ankle joint motion.

A simple drop lock allows the child to lift the locking mechanism in order to allow full knee-flexion as needed. If manual dexterity is an issue, the locking mechanism can be fitted with a large ring and spring mechanism. Other knee mechanisms allow a specified range of unrestricted motion. Ratchet mechanisms are also available. These devices allow virtually unlimited knee activity.

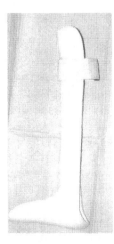

Figure 7.14 By extending the anterior component of the AFO to above the patella and by carefully adjusting the amount of plantar flexion at the ankle, the AFO will now force the knee into full extension.

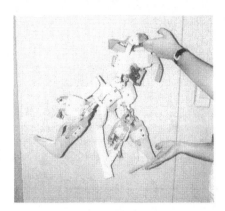

Figure 7.15 Reciprocal gait orthoses (RGO)

Reciprocal gait orthoses (RGOs) are a special form of hip–knee–ankle–foot orthoses (HKAFOs) (Fig. 7.15). They are designed to produce an opposite flexion or extension hip movement on one side when activity in the opposite direction occurs on the other side of the orthotic. This is accomplished through a series of cables or levers that work the hip joints of the orthotic. In order for the device to be useful, the child must have strong hip flexors that are under voluntary control. These are most commonly used by children who have upper or middle lumbar level myelomeningocele. Katz et al report a study of RGOs compared to HKAFOs, and noted that many patients favored RGOs.[25]

ADDITIONAL COMPLICATIONS IN NEUROLOGICAL DISEASE

There are a number of orthopaedic problems that are common to many of the neuromuscular diseases. These include (a) osteopenia, (b) fractures, (c) antetorsion and (d) internal and external tibial torsion.

Osteopenia

Disuse produces osteopenia in both the appendicular and axial skeletons. The problem is partially managed by producing stress loading of the extremities. When functional ambulation is not anticipated, placing the child in the upright position is critical in developing strong bone in the extremities and spine. Considerable effort is made both by physical therapy and orthotic management to ensure that the child will spend some time in the upright position.

Fracture

Fractures occur very frequently in children with neuromuscular disease. These may occur during therapy, or may occur from otherwise insignificant trauma.

Complete, incomplete and fatigue fracture patterns are all encountered. Sudden onset of pain without associated trauma or pain following what should have been insignificant trauma usually means fracture. Occasionally the fracture patterns are occult. Such fractures resemble stress fractures in other areas of the body and they may not show positive X-ray changes for 5 to 15 days following the actual insult. Occasionally the fracture pattern may be purely cancellous. The cortex is not involved and the true nature of the problem becomes evident only when cancellous bone condenses in the repair process. Although the possibility of trauma is well known, the diagnosis is frequently missed.

Equinus deformity is frequently associated with calcaneal fractures in children with neuromuscular disease. This may occur at any time but it often follows periods of immobilization for medical or surgical procedures. Body weight directed from above through the tibia into the talus is countered by ground reactive force against the forefoot as well as the upward vector produced by activity of the Achilles tendon. When the ankle will not allow sufficient dorsiflexion for neutral position to be reached, fracture of the posterior body of the calcaneus may result. This may happen spontaneously or it may follow minimal trauma. The physical examination shows edema in the retrotibial triangle behind the ankle. There is moderate to severe pain when the medial and lateral sides of the posterior calcaneus are compressed. X-ray changes may not be evident for 2 weeks. Such injuries are best treated by immobilization for as short a time as possible to allow both for relief

of pain as well as for consolidation of the fracture. Prolonged immobilization worsens osteoporosis and predisposes the patient to additional fracture.[26]

Children with myelomeningocele have a high fracture rate. However, their problem is compounded as they lack sensation in most of or the entire limb. Fractures usually follow immobilization for medical and surgical procedures.[27–29] Short orthoses pose a particular risk (e.g. an AFO may become so small that the proximal portion of the orthosis is located midcalf). This produces significant stress at that point and fracture of the tibia can result.

Salter–Harris type I fractures occur frequently in children with myelomeningocele[29] and such fractures may or may not displace. These fractures heal but they do so with very exuberant callus formation. The periosteum may be stripped for some distance away from the cortex and extensive subperiosteal hemorrhage results. Since the patient cannot feel pain, it is the physical findings that draw attention to the injury. The child may develop local swelling, increase in temperature and may become irritable. Hyperpyrexia frequently occurs and the child may develop a leukocytosis. These findings complicate the picture and make it difficult to distinguish early infection from fracture.[30] The risk of osteomyelitis and septic joints is already high in these patients.

Antetorsion

Antetorsion occurs frequently in children with neuromuscular disease. Incidence is especially high in CP. It is beyond the scope of this chapter to discuss antetorsion in great detail except to say that angles above the upper norm for the age produce intoeing. Coxa valga is frequently associated with antetorsion. Coxa valga does not influence the position of the limb in the sagittal or transverse plane but does influence the amount of femoral head coverage by the acetabulum. Excessive coxa valga is a risk factor for subluxation and dislocation of the hip.

Intoeing produced by femoral antetorsion cannot be managed by physiotherapy, exercise or bracing. Unlike the normal child, antetorsion occurring in neuromuscular disease does not reduce with age. It may interfere enough with ambulation that a proximal femoral derotational osteotomy may be needed.

Internal and external tibial torsion

Internal and external tibial torsion are frequently seen in patients with neuromuscular disease.[31] These problems do not regularly occur with muscular dystrophy, but are frequently associated with CP, myelomeningocele and other paralytic conditions. The most likely explanations for both internal and external tibial torsion are hamstring imbalance and abnormal propulsion. Internal or external tibial torsion adversely modifies toe-off. As a consequence of this abnormal gait pattern, the problem tends to worsen. Unlike the normal child, spontaneous correction of tibial torsion is unlikely to occur. Derotational osteotomy of the tibia will usually provide sufficient correction to justify its performance.

SPECIFIC NEUROLOGICAL AND MUSCULAR DISEASES

Friedreich's ataxia

The most common hereditary ataxia is Friedreich's ataxia.[32] This is an autosomal recessive condition with a high spontaneous mutation rate. Degenerative changes occur in the cerebellum, posterior columns and lateral corticospinal tracts.

The classical presentation is with a clumsy ataxic gait in a child slow to achieve motor milestones. In the space of a few years, the ataxia is more obvious and clumsiness in the upper limbs becomes apparent. The ataxia is initially due to a mixture of cerebellar and dorsal column damage but later it is also complicated by UMN involvement. Tendon reflexes in the lower limbs are nearly always absent owing to peripheral sensory involvement, but the plantar responses are extensor. Vibration sense is lost early in the lower limbs and joint position sense becomes impaired later in the disease. Truncal instability may occur late in the disease. This will likely require spinal support. Skeletal abnormalities, such as pes cavus and talipes equinovarus, are seen in 75% of sufferers and kyphoscoliosis will develop in nearly all cases. Cardiac murmurs and hypertrophic cardiomyopathy are common.[33]

While classical Friedreich's ataxia is clinically easy to diagnose, there are many atypical cases where separation from other forms of hereditary ataxia such as Roussy–Levy syndrome (wasting in lower limbs and no cerebellar signs), hereditary cerebellar ataxia (no skeletal or spinal cord signs), or olivopontocerebellar ataxia (later onset, no spinal cord signs) may be difficult. Magnetic resonance imaging (MRI) may demonstrate atrophy of the cerebellum and spinal cord. Nerve conduction studies (NCS) reveal severely slowed or absent sensory conduction with normal motor conduction velocities. Cerebrospinal fluid (CSF) shows mild elevation of protein and the electrocardiograph (ECG) and echocardiography are frequently abnormal. There is usually a steady decline in function with death in 10 to 20 years. However, some patients with an autosomal dominant form have been reported to live a normal lifespan. Cardiac abnormalities along with diabetes mellitus, kyphoscoliosis and recurrent chest infections significantly contribute to morbidity and mortality.

Friedreich's ataxia may also be mistaken for Charcot–Marie–Tooth syndrome in the early stages. Differential diagnosis is based on the absence of ataxia and upgoing plantar responses in patients with Charcot–Marie–Tooth syndrome. In addition, most patients with Charcot–Marie–Tooth syndrome do not show profound loss of vibratory sense.

Guillain–Barré syndrome

Guillain–Barré syndrome is an acute postinfectious demyelinating motor neuropathy that predominantly involves the anterior spinal roots. The segmental demyelination is probably due to a cell-mediated immune response against PNS myelin but when severe it can result in some irreparable axonal damage as well. Approximately 50% of patients describe a preceding upper respiratory tract infection or diarrheal illness that has occurred 1 to 3 weeks before the onset of the weakness. Back pain is often an early symptom and although there may be sensory symptoms, motor weakness predominates. Reflexes are lost early in the course of the disease. Commonly the initial onset of weakness occurs distally and ascends. However, often the weakness is generalized and progresses over the next 3 to 4 weeks. Guillain–Barré syndrome becomes life-threatening when the respiratory or bulbar muscles are involved or when there are autonomic disturbances producing swings in blood pressure and tachycardia. The inflammation of the motor roots results in a marked increase in CSF protein with little or no elevation in CSF white cells. NCS may be normal initially as most of the demyelination occurs proximally in the nerve roots rather than distally in the nerve. Virological tests sometimes demonstrate elevations in titers of Epstein–Barr virus or cytomegalovirus.

Recovery of strength in this condition takes place over some months as remyelination occurs slowly. There is a 10% mortality rate in even the best series. Treatment is supportive with ventilation when required, control of autonomic disturbances and physiotherapy. In severe cases, plasmapheresis reduces the amount of time spent in an intensive treatment unit on a ventilator and improves the grade of weakness sooner than in those who do not require plasmapheresis.

Some very mild cases may be encountered at the community level. It may be very difficult to prove these mild cases, and diagnosis is based on the clinical history and the ascending pattern of weakness. Such cases are not life-threatening, and these children may present with lower extremity disturbances. Dropfoot is the most common presenting symptom. The child may be presented for evaluation because of the development of a slapping gait owing to loss of anterior compartment deceleration. Complete recovery can be anticipated, and the dropfoot is managed with an appropriate AFO until recovery is complete. Unless contracture has already developed, a solid ankle variant of the AFO is appropriate because it will permit ambulation. Involvement of the patient in a physiotherapy program is essential to prevent the development of equinus ankle contracture.

Myasthenia gravis

Myasthenia gravis (MG) is a relapsing and remitting autoimmune disease where acetylcholine receptor autoantibodies (AchR ab) are directed against the patient's own postsynaptic AchRs at the neuromuscular junction. There are also abnormalities in the thymus gland, most commonly hyperplasia but occasionally neoplasia (thymoma). Myasthenia gravis may be divided into neonatal (NMG), congenital (CMG), juvenile (JMG) and adult (AMG) forms.

NMG appears transiently in 10–20% of infants born to myasthenic mothers and is probably due to placental transfer of AchR ab from the mother. These babies present within 48 hours of birth, with a poor cry and a poor ability to suck as a result of fatigable bulbar weakness. Less commonly there is generalized weakness or respiratory failure. The condition may last several weeks and the spontaneous improvement is paralleled by a steady reduction in neonatal AchR antibody titers. CMG is rare and never life-threatening. It is usually present at birth but is so mild it may go unnoticed until adulthood. There is a high familial incidence, but mothers do not have AchR antibodies.

JMG is similar to the adult form and usually presents at about 8 years of age. It affects females three to four times as often as males and generally affects the cranial nerves first, with ptosis, diplopia or facial weakness.

Diagnosis is based on the symptoms of fatigable muscle weakness, the demonstration of AchR antibodies in the serum, electromyographic evidence of a decremental response in amplitude of action potentials to repetitive muscle stimulation and a response to edrophonium chloride, a short-acting anticholinesterase which prevents the destruction of Ach by cholinesterase at the neuromuscular junction.

In life-threatening situations where there is respiratory or bulbar involvement, removal of circulating AchR ab by plasmapheresis can produce a short-lived improvement in muscle strength.

Longer-acting anticholinesterases and steroids that suppress the autoimmune response occurring at the neuromuscular junction are the mainstay of treatment and may lead to long-term remission. Removal of the thymus may also produce improvement or even long-term remission.

Cerebral palsy

CP is defined as abnormal control of movement or posture of a patient beginning early in life as a result of a CNS lesion, damage or dysfunction and not the result of a recognized progressive or degenerative disease.[34] The lesion causing CP does not progress, but the clinical findings are likely to change with time.[35]

CP can be classified by movement disorder into spastic, ataxic and dyskinetic forms, and the spastic form may be subclassified into quadriplegia, diplegia and hemiplegia.[36]

Although regarded as a movement disorder resulting in orthopedic implications, CP is a global CNS problem. Cognitive dysfunction, expressive and receptive speech issues, pervasive developmental disorder, attention deficit and seizures frequently are issues that complicate the child's rehabilitative effort.

Expansion of the definition of CP has broadened the list of causes. Etiologies now include genetic abnormalities, infections, toxins, prematurity, trauma, CNS malformations and metabolic abnormalities affecting the immature CNS. The insult may occur from the beginning of the prenatal period to age 2 years. Common causes in years past are now uncommon. For instance, massive hemolysis resulting from Rh incompatibility is rarely seen.

The diagnosis of CP is usually made during the first 2 years of life. A common cause is intraventricular hemorrhage (IVH) in preterm infants in association with respiratory distress syndrome and cardiovascular difficulties, which alter cerebral blood flow. Hypotension causes periventricular leukomalacia.[37] Hypertension causes may be neurologically silent in up to 78% of these cases.[38] IVH occurs in 40% of infants weighing less than 3 lb 5 oz (1500 g) and in 40% of infants less than 35 weeks gestation.[38] One-third develop severe handicaps.

IVH can be identified by ultrasound scanning through the anterior fontanel. MRI of the brain also identifies hemorrhage, but the procedure requires anesthesia of the infant in order to give diagnostic imaging. MRI and computed tomography (CT) will also identify structural lesions within the CNS.

About 75% of cases of CP have predominantly spastic forms. Diplegia (40%) is slightly more common than quadriplegia (35%) or hemiplegia (25%). Ataxic and dyskinetic syndromes occur in about 18% and 7% respectively.[39] Patients may suffer from mental retardation (53%), epilepsy (50%), sensory deficits (hearing or visual), and emotional problems.

Patterns of movement disorders in cerebral palsy

The pattern of the motion disorder is named after the number and location of the limbs involved in the process. The limb involvement is dependent on the site and extent of the neuroanatomical insult.

Monoplegia. This is the simplest pattern with involvement of only a single upper or lower limb. Monoplegia rarely occurs in CP. The anatomical lesion must be very discrete and highly localized to produce such a focal neurological defect. Perinatal insults produce more global neurological lesions. Vascular malformations, stroke and tumor are more likely to exhibit monoplegic patterns.

Hemiplegia. Both limbs on one side of the body are involved in this pattern. The lower extremities are more severely affected. The involved extremities are located on the side opposite the CNS lesion (Fig. 7.16). Early development of cerebral dominance suggests hemiplegia because this motor skill is usually not acquired until at least age 18 months. Earlier development of hand preference suggests dysfunction on the opposite side. This is especially true when the left is the preferential side because only about 15% of the population are left-handed. Equinovarus is the most common lower extremity deformity.[40] Flexion

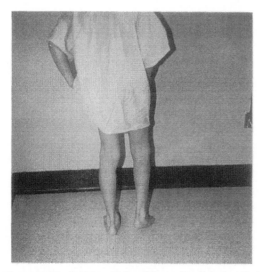

Figure 7.16   Patient with hemiplegia. Hemiplegia affects both limbs on one side of the body.

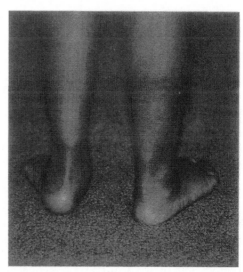

Figure 7.17   The most common foot and ankle deformity in diplegia is bilateral equinovalgus.

deformities of the hip and knee are commonly associated. These contractures must be recognized before the equinus deformity is treated.

Diplegia. All four extremities are involved in this pattern. The lower extremities are heavily involved. The upper extremities are very mildly affected. The severity is evenly balanced between the two sides. The most common foot and ankle deformity in diplegia is bilateral equinovalgus[40] (Fig. 7.17). The term double hemiplegia has fallen into disuse because of the similarity to diplegia. There is some limited usefulness in this term because some children have a pattern of diplegia with one side that has a different pattern or is more involved than the other side.

Quadriplegia. Total body CP may be a better term than quadriplegia. There are two reasons that make this change useful. First, the axial skeleton is also involved in this pattern. Second, primitive tonic reflexes remain long after they should have involuted. These reflexes are very destructive because they produce stereotyped movements and postures in response to body part position and often based on head and neck position. Some of these reflexes are the Moro, Landau, symmetrical and asymmetrical tonic reflex. The useful primitive patterned reflexes may be

absent. These include the righting reflex, the stepping reflex and the parachute reflex. Therapy for this particular form of CP is very disappointing. The movement patterns make sitting, walking and other simple tasks of daily living extremely difficult. Extensive braces do not help and they inhibit normal muscle function.[41]

Bobath developed a neurodevelopmental (NDT) treatment program which attempts to inhibit abnormal infantile reflexes and to facilitate more normal movement patterns.[42] This is popular in many rehabilitation centers but well-designed trials demonstrating objective benefit over other methods are still lacking. Bobath's program may stimulate the child and improve social integration into the family and for future life, although it may not significantly reduce the number of operations that the child will require. Physiotherapy, such as positioning of the patient to avoid contractures, and lightweight night splints may be useful to keep ankles in a neutral position but these are often ineffective or uncomfortable.

Surgical intervention for muscle contractures should be approached cautiously in patients with athetosis, dyskinesia or chorea, because there is often a tendency for overcorrecting – especially in the dyskinetic patient. Surgery to improve ambulation should be delayed until after the gait has matured (age 6 to 10 years) and the patient should be mobilized early with minimal casting. 68% of severely or profoundly retarded children survive for more than 5 years.

Treatment of equinus, equinovarus and equinovalgus in cerebral palsy

The initial treatment for these CP-associated deformities is prevention. Physical therapy should be started as soon as the diagnosis is made. The therapist will perform a detailed initial assessment for future reference as treatment progresses. Formal therapy sessions help achieve and maintain range of motion. This carries over in home programs supervised by the physiotherapist (see Ch. 13).

The basics of non-operative intervention for equinus and its variants are stretching and bracing. Bracing improves gait, decreases tone, stretches spastic muscles to allow growth,[43] improves standing and provides a broader base of support.[44] Bracing has both preventive and maintenance roles in the management of equinus. Once achieved, bracing will help maintain range of motion. Bracing is not a substitute for physiotherapy and will not create range of motion when it does not exist. Bracing above the ankle also provides sagittal plane stability. As the infant achieves trunk balance, ankle instability makes standing difficult. Stability of the ankle in both the coronal and sagittal planes facilitates standing.

In order to be effective, bracing must be used at all times during which limb positioning would favor equinus position. The child must use the orthoses during waking hours as well as during sleep.

AFOs may be articulated or of the solid ankle variety. Articulated AFOs allow unrestricted ankle dorsiflexion while controlling plantarflexion to a desirable position. They have some disadvantages. The addition of hinges makes them very bulky and makes shoe fitting difficult. When spasticity is present, forced dorsiflexion in an articulated AFO may elicit a plantarflexing deep tendon reflex.[45] This may make it difficult for the child to wear the device and may cause therapeutic failure owing to non-compliance. Carmick reported that gait was more efficient with articulated AFOs.[46] Radtka et al studied the effects of dynamic ankle–foot orthoses (DAFOs) and articulated and solid AFOs, and found that patients and parents preferred DAFOs.[47]

Certain forms of equinus are dynamic, in other words the plantarflexion of the ankle is due to increased tone and not due to contracture. Articulated braces may cause a 'crouch position' composed of stance in ankle dorsiflexion, knee-flexion and hip-flexion. The triad of hip and knee contractures associated with ankle equinus is a major problem in children with all forms of CP.

If hip and knee contractures are present when the ankle can be brought to neutral position, the child may walk in equinus in the AFOs with the knees and hips in flexion even though the brace controls the ankle at sagittal neutral.[46]

Tonal inhibition casting has been used on and off for several decades. The principle of tonal inhibition is that tone in the trunk and lower extremities can be reduced when the ankle is held at sagittal neutral with the calcaneus vertical and the toes hyperextended. Padding is placed on either side of the Achilles tendon. These are very difficult to apply. Any imperfection in technique leads to extensor thrust. Pain necessitates immediate removal of the casts. Although there is some subjective improvement in tone in the short term, there is no evidence that there is lasting carry-over after casting stops.[48]

Serial casting is used to help achieve a useful range of ankle motion if there is contracture. Like tonal inhibition casting, these casts are difficult to apply. When using stretching casts for equinus deformity, the position of the subtalar joint must be controlled so that pronation is not introduced into the final position. Casts remain on for periods of 1 to 2 weeks depending on the age of the child. If improvement occurs, it is rapid over 2 to 3 weeks. Additional range is not as rapidly achieved. The initial benefit may actually be produced by weakening the muscles by immobilization. It is unlikely that a myostatic (permanently shortened) contracture can be stretched by any means. Appropriate bracing is necessary following successful stretching casts.[40]

Recently, botulinum A toxin has been used in the management of dynamic contracture. It prevents release of Ach at the myoneural junction.[5] This weakens the muscle, decreases spasticity[35] and reduces tone.[49] Cosgrove et al note that botulinum A decreases tone and increases the ability to stretch muscle. This may encourage longitudinal growth to prevent contracture.[50] Flett et al concluded that botulinum A injections were of similar efficacy to serial casting in improving dynamic calf tightness.[5]

Unresponsive or recurring equinus is a surgical issue. When possible, surgery for equinus should be delayed until age 6 years to lessen the likelihood of recurrence.[49] Surgery for equinus alone should not be performed in the presence of hip and knee contracture. If these are present, the child should have surgery at all three levels in the same operative sitting to reduce the number of surgeries required.[51,52]

Treatment – equinovalgus

Treatment of equinovalgus parallels the treatment of equinus alone. There are two unique problems with this deformity. First, the heel is in valgus, and this position is made worse by body weight loaded through the limb. This produces a cantilevered deformity below the level of the subtalar joint. The short mechanical lever arm of the calcaneus makes brace control of the subtalar joint very inefficient. Second, some degree of forefoot varus often develops. This is difficult to control in an AFO. A calcaneal osteotomy may be necessary to reposition the heel.

Treatment – equinovarus

It is almost impossible to brace equinovarus. The problem is the varus deformity at the subtalar joint. Orthotics may be used in the short term to prevent additional deformity while the child is being readied for surgery. Tibialis posterior is dysfunctional and must be addressed.[40] Con-

trolled lengthening of the Achilles tendon and fractional lengthening of tibialis posterior above the medial malleolus are successful in managing the combined deformity. It may be necessary to modify the insertion of tibialis anterior. The entire tendon can be transferred, or the tendon can be split and the lateral limb transferred. Residual heel varus can be treated by calcaneal osteotomy.

Hereditary motor and sensory neuropathies (HMSN)

In 1968, Dyck and Lambert classified the combined sensory and motor neuropathies with heritable characteristics. Although several different authors have revised this classification, it is still very useful today.[53,54]

These diseases are characterized pathophysiologically by degenerative changes in the peripheral nerves which result from loss of myelin and also from fragmentation of the axons. These entities represent a spectrum of degenerating conditions induced and modified by inherited chromosomal abnormalities resulting in change in the peripheral and central nervous systems.[55,56] The classification of these varying syndromes is outlined in Table 7.2.

The most familiar and best studied of the hereditary motor and sensory neuropathies is Charcot–Marie–Tooth syndrome. Affected patients may either fully express this disease or present with formes frustes with varying degrees of neurological expression. Certain patients have early and severe disabling symptoms, while others run a much more benign course. The term Charcot–Marie–Tooth syndrome is used to

Table 7.2 The hereditary motor–sensory neuropathies (HMSN types)

HMSN type I	Hypertrophic neuropathy (peroneal muscle atrophy)
HMSN type II	Neuronal type of peroneal muscle atrophy
HMSN type III	Hypertrophic neuropathy of infancy (Dejerine–Sottas)
HMSN type IV	Hypertrophic neuropathy with excess phytanic acid (Refsum's disease)
HMSN type V	Peripheral neuropathy with spastic paraplegia

Table 7.3 Genetics of HMSN I and II

Disease	Mode of inheritance	Gene location
HMSN IA	Autosomal dominant	17p11.2
HMSN IB	Autosomal dominant	1q21–23
HMSN IC	Autosomal dominant	?
HMSN X-linked	X-linked recessive	Xq13
HMSN II	Autosomal dominant	1p35–36

describe Dyck and Lambert types I and II forms. The clinical progression, severity of symptoms and the age of onset help to separate these two. Types I and II may also be separated clinically on the basis of electrodiagnostic studies and by DNA analysis.

HMSN I and II (Charcot–Marie–Tooth syndrome)

Type I Charcot–Marie–Tooth syndrome (HMSN I) is a demyelinating neuropathy characterized by decreased nerve conduction velocities resulting from loss of myelin resulting in loss of saltatory conduction. Type I presents in the teens or 20s with slowly progressive pes cavus, gait changes, cramping and foot drop owing to wasting of the peronei. The peripheral nerves may be palpably enlarged. Sensory disturbances are not a prominent feature of the syndrome. In type I (HMSN I), nerve conduction velocities are less than 15 m/s (normal 50–60 m/s), CSF protein is elevated and sural nerve biopsy demonstrates segmental demyelination and remyelination. Genetic information is outlined in Table 7.3.

In type 2 (HMSN II) nerve conduction velocities are slowed to about 65% of normal velocity. CSF is normal and biopsy reveals axonal regeneration. In type 2, the onset of muscle weakness is not until adult life and nerves are not palpable. Pes cavus, hammertoes and ankle instability are common presentations and they may occur before the development of weakness. Hyporeflexia and a glove and stocking distribution of impaired sensation accompany distal weakness and wasting in the lower limbs. Progression is very slow in both these types of HMSNs and effective splinting may prolong ambulation for many years.[57] Surgical management for type II

differs from type I. In general, long-term results of posterior tibial tendon transfer as part of a staged procedure have been considered poor.[58] This consensus of poor result is probably due to the fact that tibialis posterior fails to remain active after a number of years. If the goal is to remove the deforming force of tibialis posterior in an attempt to prevent additional deformity, this procedure is highly successful.

HMSN II phenotype has three subdivisions. Types IIA and IIB begin during the second decade of life as distal weakness in the legs. It can be variable from side to side. Upper biceps and triceps as well as patellar deep tendon reflexes may be present, but the Achilles tendon reflexes are almost always absent. There is mild distal sensory loss. Type IIC has respiratory muscular and vocal cord paralysis.

Foot deformities in Charcot–Marie–Tooth syndrome (HMSN I & II)

The feet are almost always affected first. Both pes planus (Fig. 7.18) and pes cavus (Fig. 7.19A, B) have been reported as early foot findings.[59] This may be explained by varying patterns of calf muscle atrophy over time.[60] Clumsy gait or other walking abnormalities may be the initial complaints. Instability in walking is the common

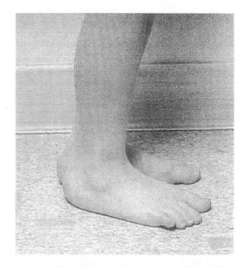

Figure 7.18 Pes planus deformity in a patient with Charcot–Marie–Tooth syndrome.

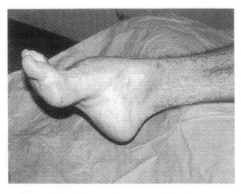

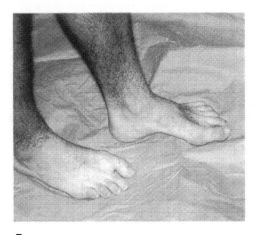

Figure 7.19 A & B   Pes cavus deformity may also be seen with Charcot–Marie–Tooth syndrome.

There are two patterns of cavovarus. In the first pattern, subtalar joint pronation becomes limited and a hindfoot varus deformity results. In the second variation, pronation of the subtalar joint is preserved but the forefoot develops a rigid forefoot valgus. In both cases, the subtalar joint abnormally supinates. The distinction between the two is important because the therapeutic approach to each is different. The Coleman Block Test helps to distinguish the two types (Fig. 7.20A, B).

The intrinsic muscles of the feet are involved early and the loss of stability normally provided by these muscles results in flexion deformity of the digits. Since flexor substitution is an important compensation for muscle weakness, early hammer and mallet toe deformities result.

Gait disturbances

Gait disturbances are difficult to manage and there are two components that need to be addressed: (i) mediolateral instability is a major problem. Such patients feel unstable, frequently develop supinatory ankle injuries, and wear shoes badly. (ii) In more advanced cases, anterior compartment weakness results in foot drop with

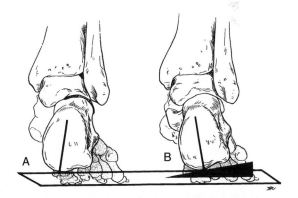

Figure 7.20   The Coleman Block Test is designed to separate fixed rearfoot varus deformity from the flexible type. (A) In stance, the heel is in varus. (B) A wedge or block is placed under the lateral heel and lateral forefoot.
If the hindfoot varus is flexible (sufficient range of motion of the subtalar joint complex), the heel will move into valgus when the foot is placed on the wedge as shown. If there is no subtalar range of motion, the heel will stay locked in varus.

factor in most disturbances and involves the invertor–evertor muscle pairs. Occasionally, there may be calf hypertrophy.[61] Although uncommon, equinus may be a presenting gait disturbance.

Cavus deformity

With progression, hindfoot varus becomes a major clinical finding. Since the anterolateral compartment muscles of the leg are affected early, the peroneals and tibialis anterior show early weakness but tibialis posterior is fairly well preserved. This muscle then becomes the deforming force that produces varus deformity. With further progression, cavoadductovarus pattern presents.

difficulty clearing the floor during swing phase. Posterior contractures result in fixed ankle equinus.

AFOs provide both frontal and sagittal stability for the foot and ankle. Although it is possible to articulate the ankle to allow some dorsiflexion, most patients initially do better with the ankle fixed at or near neutral in the sagittal plane. In milder cases, Schaffer plates are used to provide some symptomatic relief for pain and fatigue which occurs in the plantar musculature. Eventually, the cavus deformity becomes so advanced that surgical intervention is necessary.

There are two approaches in surgery for cavus foot caused by HMSNs. In early childhood, the goal is to slow down or stop the progression of the deformity even at the expense of incomplete reduction. Tibialis posterior remains strong during the course of Charcot–Marie–Tooth syndrome and becomes the principal deforming force. Transfer of tibialis posterior through the interosseous membrane into the dorsolateral aspect of the foot in the area of the third cuneiform is a logical approach to the problem.[62,63] Release of the contracted plantar fascia is also beneficial.

Dorsiflexion of the forefoot may be aided by transferring the digital extensors into the metatarsals using the techniques of Hibbs[64] and Jones.[65]

Adolescents require osteotomy of the midfoot. The Cole procedure[66] resects a wedge of bone from the lesser tarsus and when combined with a plantar release, the cavus component will effectively be reduced. This procedure excessively shortens the foot and may complicate an already small size. The Japas procedure,[67] when combined with a plantar release, reduces cavus architecture without producing additional shortening of the foot.

Digital deformities cause discomfort. The proximal and distal interphalangeal articulations become contracted early in the course of the disease and interfere with shoe fitting. These are managed by either resection arthroplasty or interphalangeal fusion.

HMSN III (Dejerine–Sottas disease)

HMSN III (Dejerine–Sottas disease) is also a demyelinating neuropathy characterized by cyclical demyelinization and repair. It is inherited as an autosomal recessive trait.[37,68] Motor milestone delay and hypotonia occur before 1 year of age. Weakness begins in the distal parts of the limbs and then extends proximally. In such cases, there is an associated loss of sensation and proprioceptive sense with resulting ataxia with an accompanying loss of deep tendon reflexes. Motor conduction velocity is delayed. Some children develop equinovarus deformity.

HMSN IV (Refsum's disease)

HMSN IV (Refsum's disease) is a metabolic hypertrophic neuropathy associated with abnormal amounts of phytanic acid.[37,68] It is a metabolic neuropathy. It is very rare and has few orthopedic issues.

Peripheral neuropathy with spastic paraplegia

This uncommon problem is characterized by lower extremity weakness with crouch gait leading to hip- and knee-flexion contractures and dorsiflexed feet associated with increased tone, hyperreflexia and clonus with an upgoing plantar reflex.[68]

Spina bifida

Spina bifida is defined as varying degrees of failure to close the neural tube and posterior vertebral elements. This ranges in severity from asymptomatic spina bifida occulta (affecting 5–10% of the population) to myelomeningocele (the spinal cord and roots lie in a cystic defect protruding through the skin) associated with hydrocephalus, Chiari 2 malformation, scoliosis and foot deformities. Myelomeningocele occurs in the lower spine (80%) or cervical area (20%). The incidence of myelomeningocele varies from

1 in 3000 in Japan to greater than 1 in 300 in parts of Wales. Antenatal diagnosis of severe dysraphic states is possible, either by elevated maternal serum alpha-fetoprotein levels or by ultrasound screening in the first trimester. When left unrepaired, infants with myelomeningocele will most probably die quickly from meningitis and other recurrent infections. Prompt closure of the spinal defect results in a very high survival rate. However, 33% of survivors are totally dependent and only 20% are independent. Of course, these data are strongly influenced by the level of function.

Myelomeningocele is obvious at birth. Spina bifida occulta may or may not be associated with cutaneous abnormalities such as lumbosacral dimple, sinus or hair tuft. These may point to an underlying dysraphic state such as diastematomyelia, lipoma or dermoid cyst.

There are two forms of spina bifida occulta. One type has failure of the posterior elements and associated cutaneous midline findings with or without neurological defects. The other is a finding on X-ray usually identified incidentally during imaging studies for problems unrelated to symptoms of neural tube defect. Bony element fusion failure with midline dimple, hair patch, hemangioma or soft tissue mass is indicative of dysraphism and these children need MRI of the cord to identify neurosurgical pathology. Children with fusion defect alone and no neurological symptoms are unlikely to have cord pathology and need no work-up.

Children with myelomeningocele have flaccid paraparesis or paraplegia with loss of sensation and bladder atonicity, leading to frequent infections and renal damage. Detailed neurological assessment is extremely important when considering management.[69]

Determination of functional neurological level is very difficult in neonates and very young infants. Flailing movements generated from the hips may give the illusion of purposeful distal movements, but their true origin soon becomes apparent. Unfortunately, the parents interpret these movements as evidence that the original bleak functional prognosis was incorrect. Func-

Table 7.4 Medical Research Council Muscle Testing Scale

Grade	Response
0	No movement
1	Flicker of activity
2	Movement with gravity neutralized
3	Movement against gravity
4	Almost full strength
5	Full strength

tion is often asymmetrical with very little correlation between motor and sensory levels. Motor level is determined by the innervation level that will produce a grade three movement pattern (movement against gravity) according to the Medical Research Council's grading system (Table 7.4).

Children with very low lumbar and sacral functional levels usually are community ambulators but are not guaranteed a good long-term prognosis for continued walking. Functional levels may actually deteriorate.[70,71] Most frequently, this is caused by tethering of the spinal cord producing symptoms with growth. Traction and resulting ischemia cause loss of neurological function in a child who is already severely compromised. Surgical release of the tether may prevent future neurological deterioration, but recovery of lost function is not expected. Hydromyelia, syringomyelia, progressing hydrocephalus and shunt failure may also cause deteriorating peripheral control, loss of trunk stability and milestone regression.

Obesity impacts negatively on continued walking. Muscle strength is already affected and the child usually does not exercise enough to keep weight under control. Independent ambulation requires high-energy expenditure, and requires an investment in patient time and effort. Teens entering high school often discover that speed in moving from classroom to classroom becomes a greater priority than walking with assistive devices at a slow speed. As a result many teenagers make the decision to stop community ambulation. Eventually, this decision carries over to household ambulation.

Patient management requires a multidisciplinary approach[72] involving pediatric, neurology, orthopedics, urology, rehabilitation and podiatric services.[73] The aims are to develop independence, promote ambulation where possible and prevent respiratory and urinary tract infections, pressure sores and flexion contractures.

Functional levels may be asymmetric comparing one side to the other. Segments of the cord below the level of the defect may remain intact. The simple reflex arcs at the cord level may remain intact but are unmodulated by higher areas of the CNS. This results in uncontrolled spontaneous activity which makes functional level determination more difficult for the inexperienced, raises false hope among the family and results in imbalance of muscle with deformity.

Rehabilitation and treatment

Rehabilitation begins when the spine lesion is closed. Since most patients with myelomeningocele have caudal lesions, much of the rehabilitation is directed towards the spine, hips, knees and feet. Lower levels have better prognosis for function and independent ambulation. In order to fully appreciate the complexities of these problems, it is important to review the relationship of muscle activities in the lower extremities and the functional neurological levels.[74] The level of function is the key to the understanding of deformity.[75] It must be remembered that there is some disagreement about the relationship between levels and function. Although innervation of an individual muscle may come from several levels, there is a threshold needed for useful function. This threshold is usually more caudal than the level required to produce deformity.

Patterns of muscle activity – dependence on functional level

The iliopsoas muscle is the major hip flexor deriving its innervation from L1, 2, 3. Some significant function of the iliopsoas is present when the child has functional activity down to the level of L1.

The quadriceps and the adductors may be considered together since they derive their innervations from L2, 3, 4. Although the quadriceps is considered to be an L4 muscle from the standpoint of deep tendon reflexes, considerable quadriceps function is present when L3 is intact.

Tibialis anterior derives its innervation from L4, 5. When L4 is intact, tibialis anterior is capable of producing major foot deformity since the remaining anterior compartment muscles are not functioning.

Extensor hallucis longus, extensor digitorum longus and brevis, gluteus medius and the medial hamstrings all derive their major innervation from L5.

Tibialis posterior and flexor digitorum longus derive their major innervations from L5 and S1. Flexor hallucis longus completes the posterior compartment and derives its innervation from L5, S1, 2.

Peroneus longus and brevis, gastrocnemius, soleus, gluteus maximus and the lateral hamstrings are all considered to be fundamentally S1 muscles.

The foot intrinsics are S2, 3, 4 muscles. An added advantage of function at this level is the acquisition of urinary bladder and anal sphincter control.

With this information, it is possible to consider the functional level as a predictor of both useful activity as well as static deformity when muscles remain unbalanced. It is important to remember that both motor deficits and sensory loss occur together. The patient has not only paralysis but also loss of protective sensation for the skin and joints. Additionally, vasomotor stability below the functioning level is frequently involved.

When L1 is the lowest functional level, there is usually no controlled activity at the hip, knee and ankle. There may be some flexion deformity at the hip owing to some activity at the iliopsoas, but the knees and ankles are flail. When L2 is the lowest functioning level, there is volitional flexion and adduction activity at the hips and also there is some partial extension of the knees. The ankles are flail. Since iliopsoas and the adductors are unopposed, there will be flexion and adduction deformity at the hip level. There is usually no deformity at the knee and the foot is usually flail. When L3 is the lowest functioning level, there is active hip flexion and adduction as well as extension activity of the knee. There is no ankle activity. Flexion, adduction and external rotation deformity at the hip are observed. The knee is fixed in extension and the ankle is flail. When L4 is the lowest functioning level, the child has active flexion and adduction at the hip. The knees will extend and the foot will dorsiflex and invert. The hip is fixed in flexion, adduction and lateral rotation and the potential for dislocation of the hips is high. The knees show extension deformity and the feet have dorsiflexion and inversion deformity. When L5 is the lowest functioning level, the hips have active flexion, adduction and abduction. The knees show active extension as well as partial flexion produced by activity of the medial hamstrings. The feet dorsiflex and invert. The hips show flexion deformity but they are balanced in the frontal plane. The knees are partially balanced by active extension from the quadriceps along with some flexion from the medial hamstrings. The feet show calcaneus deformity since the entire anterior compartment is now functional. The posterior compartment is still paralyzed. On occasion, the feet will show severe pronation deformity because of partially innervated but unopposed peroneals.

When S1 is the lowest functioning level, the hips have full activity. The hips are almost completely balanced by the addition of most of the gluteal maximus. The knees are fully balanced because of the addition of the lateral hamstrings. The feet show full dorsiflexion, inversion and eversion but there is only partial plantar flexion. The hips and knees are both balanced without resulting deformity. The incidence of toe deformities, calcaneovalgus and vertical talus is common at this level. When S2 is the lowest functioning level, the hips, knees and feet are almost totally functional except for some of the foot intrinsic muscles. The hips, knees and ankles are balanced. The absence of certain of the intrinsic foot muscles results in late onset cavovarus and flexion deformities of the toes.

Interventions

The therapeutic intervention for myelomeningocele may be divided into four periods: the immediate postnatal period; the period between birth and the onset of ambulation; the period of functional walking; and the decreasing ambulation period of late adolescence and adulthood.

The neonate. Before closure of the defect it may be difficult to assess the true functional level. Some additional loss may occur during operative closure. The effects of hydrocephalus add to the difficulty of determining functional level. Attention should be directed toward evaluating deformities of the extremities produced by muscle imbalance, spasticity and in utero molding. Much of the early care is provided by the neurosurgeon.[76]

Just prior to the beginning of ambulation. Equinovarus, equinus, calcaneus, calcaneovalgus, hallux valgus, digital deformities and metatarsus adductus should be identified and treated promptly so that they do not interfere with shoe fitting and ambulation. Even if it is determined that the child will never have any useful walking potential, plantigrade feet are necessary in order to allow shoe fitting for inclement weather as well as stable platforms for allowing the child to become upright in a standing frame.[77,78] Acceptable foot shape is also necessary to prevent the development of pressure lesions of the skin. Early management of foot and ankle deformities is complicated by the fact that the infant's medical condition may make it difficult to manage these problems effectively. For a period of time following closure, the infant must remain prone. It is impractical to have both feet unavailable for intravenous access and heel sticks for hematological testing. During this period, therapy is largely confined to manipulation. Once the infant is stable, plaster of Paris splinting may be applied as indicated.

Ambulatory considerations. Presuming the functional levels are appropriate, it will be some time before any independent ambulation is possible. During this period, continued splinting and physical therapy are used. Bracing provides stabilization, prevents contracture, allows the child to become upright, assists in acquiring motor milestones and prevents crouch.[77] Since sensation is impaired, meticulous care of the skin is necessary to prevent breakdown. Splints and orthotics must fit well and be adjusted for growth.

When the child can maintain hip and knee extension, some independent ambulation is expected. Even when the child cannot manage hip and knee extension alone, appropriate orthotics may perform this movement for the child. Orthotic management and physical therapy will allow children to maximize their potential for independent ambulation (Fig. 7.21A, B)

For those patients who have higher functional levels, the physiological burden of ambulation becomes so great that they choose wheelchair transportation for its ease and speed. Even these children need periodic upright posturing in order to develop some bone mass. Osteopenia of disuse is a major problem for these patients and fractures become a part of life.

Treatment for the feet. Foot problems are the most common orthopedic issues in spina bifida and are secondary to muscle imbalance. They include equinus and equinovarus deformity, vertical talus, ankle and subtalar valgus, and pes cavus.[77]

Specific treatment for the feet and ankles depends on the level of function. Muscles derive innervation over several levels but best function demands complete or almost complete innervation of the muscle in order to provide useful strength. Incompletely innervated muscles lack sufficient strength and their antagonists will produce deformity.

Certain fixed joint postures contraindicate independent walking. Ambulation requires hip and knee extension either from balanced musculature or from bracing. Flexion contractures of the hip and knee make walking impossible.

Children who have function at S2 and below have no major orthopedic problems. The child has protective sensation for the entire foot. Instability of the toes may result from incomplete innervation of the intrinsic muscles. Claw toes may develop later in childhood.

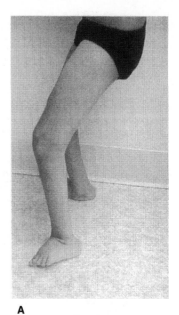

A

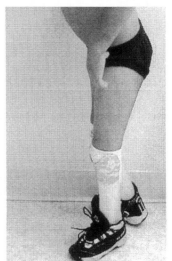

B

Figure 7.21 A & B Even in severe deformity orthotic management may substantially maximise the child's potential for independent ambulation.

Children who function at S1 usually have balanced knees and hips. The extrinsic muscles of the feet have sufficient strength to produce a normal heel-to-toe gait. There may be some weakness of the gastrocsoleus complex and cavus deformity may appear later in childhood. Flexion deformity of the toes is produced when the long toe flexors augment a weakened gastrocsoleus group. There is no specific bracing for this possible complication and significant cavus deformity ultimately becomes a surgical problem.

Pes planus is common in the gray area between functioning L5 and S1 levels. This is usually a significant deformity. The majority of these patients do well when UCBL-type orthoses are prescribed provided that the peroneals are not too strong. These devices maintain the heel vertical and prevent the secondary development of an independent forefoot varus.

When the lowest functioning level is L5, the anterior compartment muscles are generally intact and calcaneus deformity results. Crouch pattern with the hips and the knees flexed results. Calcaneus deformity is very difficult to brace but an AFO with an anterior clamshell will maintain the foot at right angles.[79] The posterior component of such an orthosis then serves to keep the knee extended.

However, it may occasionally be necessary to add a ground reaction component to the anterior of the AFO. In selected cases, transfers from very strong anterior compartment muscles to the tendo-Achilles will balance the ankle to near neutral.[80] Such procedures make it easier to functionally brace these children. At L5, the feet are partially insensate and special attention must be paid toward good brace fitting as well as periodic inspection in order to prevent the development of trophic ulcers. In spite of such problems, many of these children achieve a high degree of independent ambulation throughout adolescence.

Patients whose lowest functioning level is L4 have problems with frontal plane as well as sagittal plane balance. Tibialis anterior function results in a varus position of the forefoot. Frequently, there is also a calcaneus component and together the combination of forefoot varus and calcaneus deformity is extremely difficult to brace. A further complication is the fact that much of the foot is insensate. AFOs with carefully designed anterior clamshell components will help to prevent secondary deformity as well as allowing the child a degree of upright posture.

Regression. Factors such as hydrocephaly, syringomyelia and progressing tether of the cord result in loss of functional level over time.[81] In addition, extrinsic factors such as obesity and the need for mobility in the presence of weakness results in a conscious decision of the patient to cease walking.

Duchenne and Becker muscular dystrophies

Duchenne muscular dystrophy is the most common and severe of the progressive dystrophies. It is an X-linked recessive dystrophy caused by a mutation at position 21 on the short arm of the X chromosome resulting in a defective gene product (dystrophin).[82] It almost exclusively affects males at a prevalence of 1 in 25 000. Evidence of the disease is usually seen before the age of 5 years as delay in walking, abnormal gait, frequent falling and difficulty in climbing stairs. The important signs on examination are a waddling gait with lordotic posture, abnormal run and hop, difficulty in rising from the floor owing to weakness to pelvic girdle muscles (Gowers' sign) and pseudohypertrophy of the calves (Fig. 7.22A, B) The boy may try to accommodate for proximal weakness by 'toe-walking'. There may be associated cardiomyopathy. As the disease progresses, musculoskeletal deformities such as equinovarus, scoliosis and eventually fixed flexion contractures are seen. There are no sensory or reflex abnormalities until late stage wasting develops. Plantar responses are flexor and the sphincters are not involved. The clinical course is relentless with progressive loss of function and eventual wheelchair existence by 12 years of age. Respiratory infections are common and death generally occurs by the early 20s.[37,68,83–85] A slower progression and continued ambulation after 12 years of age should suggest the milder X-linked recessive Becker muscular dystrophy.[37,68,86]

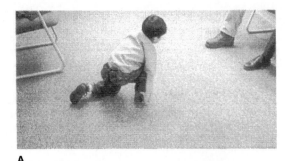

A

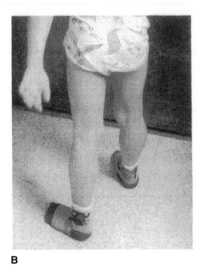

B

Figure 7.22 **(A)** Gower's sign. **(B)** Pseudohypertrophy of the calf muscles in a boy with Duchenne muscular dystrophy.

Investigations demonstrate an elevation in serum creatine phosphokinase levels, increased ultrasound echogenicity of muscle, myopathic electromyography and muscle biopsy showing degeneration of muscle fibers with evidence of regeneration with variation in fiber size, internal nuclei and excessive fat and connective tissue. DNA analysis is also highly reliable in identifying affected children[87] as well as unaffected carriers.

There is no effective treatment for Duchenne muscular dystrophy but it is important to avoid excessive immobilization and to encourage physiotherapy in order to prevent fixed deformities. Physiotherapy and rehabilitation must be individualized for the patient. Timely use of splints or calipers may prolong active gait for years.

Occasionally, surgery for tendon transfer[69] or flexion contractures may be necessary but the benefits must be weighed against the disadvantages of discomfort from several operations and frequent hospital admissions with only transitory benefit. Eventually, the energy expended from walking and the risk of falls and injury make the need for a wheelchair inevitable.

Foot and ankle deformities in muscular dystrophy

Equinus. The progressive form of muscular dystrophy described in boys by Duchenne is extremely well documented and studied, and motor deterioration and subsequent deformities may be accurately predicted. Initial functional loss begins proximally. Hip extensors are involved early in the course of the disease and changes in gait are the first manifestation. Progressive weakness of hip extensors results in an inability to maintain the hip in extension by muscle power alone. To keep upright, the boy must extend the hips by posterior displacement of the center of gravity behind the axis of hip motion by increasing lumbar lordosis so that the center of gravity (located high in the thorax) now comes to lie behind the hip joint axis. Early involvement of the hip abductors results in gait characterized by waddling from side to side as well as forward thrusting of the pelvis caused by hyperlordosis of the lumbar spine and decreased thoracic kyphosis.

As the disease worsens, the knee extensors become involved. In order to continue functioning, the boy preferentially develops a toe-to-toe gait pattern. Equinus gait in patients with Duchenne muscular dystrophy is actually necessary for continued function.[88,89] Without equinus, the boy would have extreme difficulty in balancing the center of gravity posterior to the hip joint and anterior to the knee axis.

As functional equinus persists, over time the gastrocsoleus complex develops myostatic contractures and a fixed ankle equinus results which eventually becomes complicated by subtalar varus when the child ceases walking. Once the child becomes chair-bound, equinus interferes with the ability to position his feet flat on the wheelchair platforms. This destabilization results in pelvic obliquity, progressive knee and hip flexion contractures and hip abduction contractures. Shoes become impossible to fit on the deformed feet. Even the child with advanced muscular dystrophy must occasionally go outdoors in inclement weather.

Therapy. The first goal in children with Duchenne muscular dystrophy is to keep them walking for as long as possible. This requires early aggressive physiotherapy to maintain ranges of motion and prevent the development of disabling contractures. As long as the gait remains efficient, the child can remain walking in hyperlordosis, knee-flexion and ankle equinus while allowing participation in a wide variety of physical activities.

AFOs are used at night in order to prevent the development of early and severe ankle contractures. For boys who have existing contractures, bracing slows down the process.[90]

Bracing the ankle at neutral during ambulation causes problems when the knee extensors become weak. Once this happens, it becomes necessary to design KAFOs which will allow the child to function in some equinus, the knee slightly flexed but stabilized by the orthotic and weightbearing on the ischial tuberosity. Such devices must be kept light in order to allow the weakened boy to function.

Achilles tendon surgery for the ambulating boy should be approached very cautiously. Although the equinus deformity may appear to be a problem, it is actually necessary for continued ambulation once hip and knee extension weakness reaches a certain level. If it is surgically released, the child will go into crouch gait that precludes walking. As the end of ambulation approaches, the equinus makes gait impossible. If this is the case, Achilles tendon lengthening and KAFOs may allow a few more months of semi-independent walking.

Habitual toe-walking

The normal gait pattern for children and adults is characterized by the initiation of stance phase by heel contact followed by full flat in midstance and ending with toe-off. When the infant first begins to walk, the pattern is one of full flat followed by toe-off. This quickly matures to the adult form by 2 years of age. Any other pattern during this time is considered pathological. Toe–heel and toe–toe gait patterns are never normal.

Some children do walk in equinus. They walk persistently up on their toes and the heels do not touch the ground. This gait pattern often has a basis in neurological disease. Many times, equinus gait is the result of static encephalopathy and resulting CP. However, some children have normal neurological examinations. In the absence of a specific neurological diagnosis, these children are diagnosed as having habitual or idiopathic toe-walking syndrome.[91] The role of congenital contracted Achilles tendon is controversial.[92–94]

Work-up includes a careful history to identify risk factors for CP and other neurological causes. Delay in major motor landmarks should be documented. Family history of other toe-walkers should be sought. Physical examination should include a search for contractures and a careful neurological examination. The skin over the spine should be examined for cutaneous signs of underlying cord pathology. X-ray examination is indicated. In suspicious cases, an MRI of the brain and spinal cord may identify CNS lesions that explain the symptoms. In a small percentage of cases, work-up identifies neurosurgically operable lesions. Boy toe-walkers should have a creatinine phosphokinase and aldolase drawn to rule out Duchenne and Becker muscular dystrophies.[91] The diagnosis of habitual (idiopathic) toe-walking becomes one of exclusion after all equinus-producing conditions have been ruled out.[95]

The history of the toe-walking in habitual toe-walkers is typical. They pass all of their major motor landmarks on time. They begin to walk at the appropriate age, but their pattern is equinus from the time they first start walking. They will come down on command if instructed to do so, but will revert to a toe-walking pattern as soon as they are distracted. They function in this pattern in a very coordinated manner. They can walk and run in all directions with ease.

Physical examination. Ankle range of motion is age-dependent. In infancy, there may be as much as 25–30° of dorsiflexion motion at the ankle when the knee is extended and the subtalar joint is neutral or inverted. Fixed ankle equinus is not a clinical issue at this age,[95] but loss of motion does occur with time. By age of 3 years, a certain degree of gastrocnemius equinus will develop. This is recognized by decreased ankle motion when the knee is extended compared to a greater range when the knee is flexed.

By age of 6 years, there is usually clear gastrocsoleus equinus evidenced by significant loss of ankle joint motion with the knee both extended and flexed. During this examination, it is important to control the subtalar joint, since pronatory subtalar motion allows some degree of foot dorsiflexion. This is a frequent compensatory mechanism for equinus, and is the reason why the child can walk heel to toe for short periods of time when commanded to do so.

As a condition for the diagnosis of habitual toe-walking, the neurological and orthopedic examination must be normal. The presence of neurological soft signs rules out this diagnosis. Attention deficit disorder (ADD) and hyperactivity disorder (HD) occur so frequently in idiopathic toe-walkers that the diagnosis should be questioned if ADD/HD is not present. In addition, the development of knee and hip flexion contractures and lumbar lordosis are so uncommon in habitual toe-walking syn-drome that their presence should suggest other etiologies.

Differential diagnosis

Duchenne and Becker muscular dystrophies. This is the most important differential diagnosis in toe-walking boys. They have delay in acquisition of the motor landmarks. Specifically, they do not walk independently until 18 to 24 months. There are often delays in the earlier acquired landmarks.

The gait pattern is also helpful in the differential diagnosis. Toe-walking is usually a later finding in Duchenne and Becker muscular dystrophies. The boys are usually 5 or 6 years of age when they come up on their toes. Earlier gait abnormalities are more likely to be hyperlordotic waddling patterns that result from hip extensor and abductor weakness. Creatinine phosphokinase and aldolase are grossly elevated in Duchenne and Becker muscular dystrophies, but are in the normal range for the boys with habitual toe-walking syndrome. DNA analysis is confirmatory for the muscular dystrophies.

Cerebral palsy. The perinatal history offers clues that point to this diagnosis. Prematurity, meconium aspiration, hypoxia, respiratory distress, other forms of fetal distress and postnatal seizures are risk factors for CP.

Examination will identify movement patterns such as spasticity, ataxia and athetosis. There may be hyperreflexia and upgoing plantar reflexes. Cerebral dominance at an early age is often the first finding of hemiplegia on the nondominant side.

Hereditary equinus deformity. The existence of this condition is controversial.[94] Most neonates have exaggerated ankle dorsiflexion. It is so unusual to identify fixed equinus in newborns that some other diagnosis should be considered. Occasionally, bilateral equinus deformity may be a component of arthrogryposis multiplex congenita.

Talipes equinovarus. Talipes equinovarus is a congenital problem that is immediately recognizable at birth. The four recognized forms are idiopathic, postural/positional, teratological and syndromic. Similar clinical presentations may occur after infancy, but they should not be confused with talipes equinovarus. Most acquired deformities with equinus, adductus and varus have neurological or neuromuscular etiologies. The differential diagnosis between talipes equinovarus and other forms of equinus should not prove to be difficult because talipes equinovarus is a triplane deformity.

Cavus deformity. All cavus deformities produce equinus because the talus becomes maximally dorsiflexed in the ankle mortise resulting in decreased available sagittal motion since there is no additional talar excursion. The talar neck rests on the anterior lip of the tibia.

Treatment. The three goals of treatment are to obtain an adequate range of ankle dorsiflexion, maintain that range once achieved and retrain gait to a heel–toe pattern. Treatment should not be attempted until the likelihood of more specific etiology is excluded. The target is 10–15° of ankle dorsiflexion with the knee extended. This may not be possible if there is a myostatic contracture. A course of physiotherapy is begun followed by serial casting if the response to physiotherapy alone is not satisfactory. Serial casting probably succeeds by a combination of weakening of the muscle and decrease in tone from immobilization disuse.

Once the target range of motion is achieved, bracing is utilized to prevent gradual loss of motion. AFOs are used to control sagittal plane motion at the ankle – for use during the day as gait modifiers and at night to prevent equinus sleeping postures. They can be of the solid or the articulated ankle design. It is found that initially most children tolerate AFOs better if their first braces have solid ankles. Subsequent bracing can be of the articulated ankle type. Articulated AFOs allow unrestricted ankle dorsiflexion with plantarflexion only to ankle neutral. With their use, additional ankle stretching occurs during stair-climbing and squatting. Both ankle designs act to retrain gait because it is very difficult to walk in equinus with the ankle fixed at neutral. it can happen if the child walks in knee and hip flexion. Bracing is continued for a minimum of 6 months before an attempt is made to wean the child out of AFOs.

This therapeutic protocol is best used for children of 5 years of age and younger. Children over the age of 5 usually prove resistant to stretching. If an adequate range of motion cannot be achieved, it becomes necessary to lengthen the Achilles tendon surgically.

Hypotonia

The hypotonic infant or child looks floppy, feels floppy, has an excessive range of joint motion, appears relatively immobile and shows a delay in the acquisition of motor milestones.[68]

Hypotonia is a symptom that may have neuromuscular and non-neuromuscular causes. Hypotonia associated with muscle weakness is most likely to be neuromuscular in origin, while hypotonia with normal or near-normal strength is more likely pathology of the CNS. This form is more likely to be a part of a movement disorder. Non-neuromuscular causes include connective tissue disorders.

Spinal muscular atrophy (SMA)

Spinal muscular atrophy is divided into severe (Werdnig–Hoffmann disease), intermediate, and 'mild' (Kugelberg–Welander disease).[37,68,83,96] They are inherited as autosomal recessive disorders, and the pathology in all three is anterior horn cell loss. In the severe form, infants are unable to develop sitting skills. Such children never stand. The intermediate group develops the ability to sit unaided. However, they are unable to stand or walk unaided. In the mild form, children sit and walk independently.[83]

Werdnig–Hoffmann disease is fetal in onset. The clinical symptoms include severe trunk, neck and extremity muscle weakness and hypotonia with preservation of the facial muscles. The distal parts of the extremities may also maintain some function. Most die in the first year of life and there is no orthopedic treatment indicated.

Clinical signs for the intermediate form of SMA start between 6 months and 1 year with weakness in the proximal lower extremities. One of the earliest symptoms is delay in standing and walking with hypotonia. Severe foot pronation and joint laxity are very common. The clinical course may show some apparent spontaneous improvement, or the child may show progressive worsening over years. Orthopedic issues address extremity contractures and preservation of sitting, standing and walking for as long as possible.

Kugelberg–Welander disease may begin at any time between 2 years and late adolescence. Most sufferers are identified before age 5 when a caregiver notices clumsiness in walking or running. They often have difficulty climbing. Such children demonstrate Gowers' sign as they attempt to rise from the floor. There may be tremor after activity owing to weakness.[68] Long-term walking is a realizable goal. Physical therapy and bracing help to maintain ambulatory potential

Down syndrome

Down syndrome children are hypotonic, have ligamentous laxity and have motor landmark delay. Many do not walk until 2 years or later. They have severe pronation without true ankle valgus. Heel eversion is severe enough to require orthotic management. They are also prone to progressive metatarsus primus varus and severe hallux valgus.

Treatment

Most of these children have difficulty with low profile in-shoe orthotics. This is one of the conditions for which SMOs are clearly indicated.

Many of these children are referred to physiotherapy for assistance in managing the tonal issues and acquiring ambulatory skills. Cognitive dysfunction, muscle weakness, fear of falling and collapsing valgus foot deformity all delay walking. An AFO will keep the heel vertical and the ankle at neutral. Often, this is the only intervention necessary to motivate the child to stand and walk. As walking skill matures, pronation is the major problem. Such pronation is usually very severe, and it is difficult to control these children in a UCBL-type orthotic. An SMO is much better tolerated. It is designed to control rearfoot varus and valgus, but does not control the sagittal plane.[35]

Hallux valgus deformity associated with extreme metatarsus primus varus (greater than 15–18°) begins toward the end of the first decade. It is complicated by hypermobile first ray. These deformities do not respond to orthotic management. Surgical management with fusion level at the first metatarso-cuneiform often is the procedure of choice.

Unilateral foot deformity

Differences in foot size and position are usually caused by a combination of decreased size

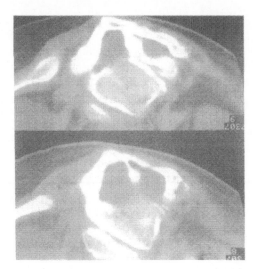

Figure 7.23 Diastematomylelia.

of the bony elements and of abnormality of the muscles of the foot and the leg secondary to paralysis and other forms of decreased muscular innervation. The explanation for this phenomenon very often is based in spinal cord neuroanatomy.

Tethered cord

During normal development of the spinal cord, upward migration of the conus medullaris occurs until it reaches the level of L2. Mechanically impaled cord (diastematomyelia) (Fig. 7.23), entrapped and shortened filum terminale, fibrous adhesions and soft tissue masses (such as lipoma) prevent migration and cause traction on the nerve roots resulting in altered sensory and motor dysfunction. UMN symptoms develop in association with foot deformity, scoliosis and bowel–bladder dysfunction.[97–100] Cutaneous findings include dermal sinus, tufts of hair, subcutaneous lipomas, hemangiomas and pigmented lesions (Fig. 7.24A, B).

Signs of tethered cord can occur at any age from infancy to young adulthood. The three common findings suggestive of tethered cord are small and deformed single foot and leg, gait disturbance (most commonly described by caregivers as 'clumsy') and bladder dysfunction.[101]

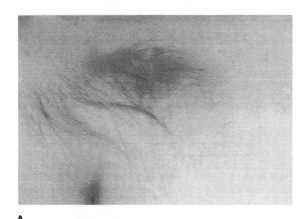

A

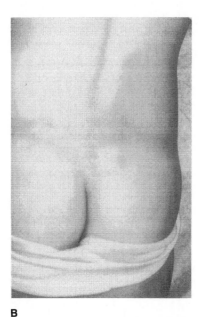

B

Figure 7.24 A & B   Cutaneous findings include tufts of hair, dermal sunuses, subcutaneous lipomas and pigmented lesions.

The foot deformities range from pes cavus to an extremely pronated foot. Calf muscles are usually small and the involved limb may be short. The apparently normal side may also be involved to a lesser extent.

Frequent falling, incoordination, variations from normal gait patterns as well as intoeing and outtoeing are frequently considered evidence of clumsiness to the parents. Incoordination and lack of 'fine motor skill' are more consistent with clumsiness in the context of tethered cord. Associated bowel and bladder dysfunction points strongly to a tether.

Diastematomyelia is a form of failure of proper neural tube closure. It occurs when a bony or cartilaginous spicule impales the cord and prevents its normal migration with growth.

By definition, all patients with myelomeningocele are tethered. The cord is tethered in the scar at the level of surgical closure. This prevents cephalad migration of the lower cord. Additionally, traction is placed on the brain stem as the unaffected thoracic and lumbar spine segments grow.

There has been a renewed interest in spina bifida occulta and tethered cord.[102] Many cases of spina bifida occulta are radiological diagnoses made incidentally when X-rays are taken for other reasons. This may occur in 15% of the population. Hemangiomas, hairy patches, dimples, skin tags and nevi in midline associated with radiographic appearance of occult spina bifida are more likely to be associated with neurological symptoms.

MRI is the definitive imaging technique for diagnosis of tethered cord. This allows imaging of the cord and surrounding structures for soft tissue changes suggestive of tethering and shows the level of the conus. Past the age of 5 years, conus lower than the L2 to L3 interspace is abnormal.

The treatment for tethered cord is surgical repair. This prevents the progression of neurological loss. However, the prognosis for recovery of function lost by tethering is not good. Once neurological dysfunction develops, recovery occurs in only 25% following release of tethering.

REFERENCES

1. Ghosh D, Pradhan S. 'Extensor toe sign' by various methods in spastic children with cerebral palsy. J Child Neurol 1998;13(5):216–220.
2. Brain. Aids to the examination of the peripheral nervous system. London: Baillière Tindall; 1986.
3. Fiorentino M. Reflex testing methods for evaluating C.N.S. development. Springfield: Charles C Thomas; 1963.
4. Willis J, Jay RM. Neuromuscular disorders and reflexes. In Jay RM, ed. Pediatric foot and ankle surgery. Philadelphia: WB Saunders; 1999;50–54.
5. Flett P, Stern L, Waddy H, et al. Botulinum toxin A versus fixed cast stretching for dynamic calf tightness in cerebral palsy. J Pediatr Child Health 1999;35(1):71–77.
6. Bobath K. The neurophysiology of cerebral palsy and its importance in treatment and diagnosis. Cerebral Palsy Bull 1959;1(8):13.
7. Bobath K, Finney N. Re-education of movement patterns in everyday life in the treatment of cerebral palsy. Occupational Therapy 1958;21(6):23.
8. Bleck E. Locomotor prognosis in cerebral palsy. Dev Med Child Neurol 1975;17:18–25.
9. Banks H. The foot and ankle in cerebral palsy. Philadelphia: Lippincott; 1975.
10. Baker L. Triceps surae syndrome in cerebral palsy. Surgery 1954;68:216.
11. Jay RM. Equinus: anterior advancement of the tendo achilles. In: Jay RM, ed. Pediatric foot and ankle surgery. Philadelphia: WB Saunders; 1999;320–321.
12. Silfverskiold N. Reduction of the uncrossed two-joint muscles of the leg to one-joint muscles in spastic conditions. Acta Chir Scand 1923–1924;56:315.
13. Strayer L. Recession of the gastrocnemius, an operation to relieve spastic contracture of the calf muscles. J Bone Joint Surg 1950;32A:671.
14. Vulpius D, Stoffel A. Orthopaedisch Operations-lebre. 2nd ed. Stuttgart: Ferdinand Enke; 1920.
15. White J. Torsion of the achilles tendon: its surgical significance. Arch Surg 1943;46:784.
16. Banta J, Sutherland D, Wyatt M. Anterior tibial transfer to the os calcis with achilles tenodesis for calcaneal deformity in myelomeningocele. J Pediatr Orthop 1981;1:125.
17. Herndon C, Strong J, Heyman C. Transposition of the tibialis anterior in the treatment of paralytic talipes calcaneus. J Bone Joint Surg 1956;38A:751.
18. Turner J, Cooper R. Posterior transposition of the tibialis anterior through the interosseous membrane. Clin Orthop 1971;79:71.
19. Hoffer M, Reiswig J, Garrett A, et al. The split anterior tibial tendon transfer in the treatment of spastic varus hindfoot of childhood. Orthop Clin North Am 1974;5:31.
20. Thomson S. Hallux varus and metatarsus varus. Clin Orthop 1960;16:109.
21. Jones C, McCrea J. Tenotomy of the abductor hallucis for correction of residual metatarsus adductus. J Am Podiatr Med Assoc 1980;70(1).
22. McCrea J. Pediatric orthopaedics of the lower extremity. Mount Kisco: Futura; 1985.
23. Agnew R. Evaluation of the child with ligamentous laxity. Philadelphia: WB Saunders; 1997.
24. Abel M, Juhl G, Vaughan C, et al. Gait assessment of fixed ankle–foot orthoses in children with spastic diplegia. Arch Phys Med Rehabil 1998;79(2): 126–133.
25. Katz D, Haideri N, Song K, et al. Comparative study of conventional hip–knee–ankle–foot orthoses versus reciprocating-gait orthoses for children with high level paraparesis. J Pediatr Orthop 1997;17(3):377–386.
26. Quan A, Adams R, Ekmark E, et al. Bone mineral density in children with myelomeningocele. Pediatrics 1998;102(3):E34.
27. Anshuetz R, Freehafer A, Shaffer J, et al. Severe fracture complications in myelodysplasia. J Pediatr Orthop 1984;4:22.
28. Drennan J, Freehafer A. Fractures of the lower extremities in paralytic children. Clin Orthop 1971;77:211.
29. Kumar S, Cowell H, Townsend P. Physeal, metaphyseal and diaphyseal injuries of the lower extremity in children with myelomeningocele. J Pediatr Orthop 1984;4:25.
30. Rodgers W, Schwend R, Jaramillo D, et al. Chronic physeal fractures in myelodysplasia: magnetic resonance analysis, histologic description, treatment, and outcome. J Pediatr Orthop 1997;17(5):615–621.
31. Dias L, Murali J, Collins P. Rotational deformities of the lower limb in myelomeningocele. J Bone Joint Surg 1984;66A:215.
32. Harding A. The inherited ataxias. Adv Neurol 1988;48:37–46.
33. Ackroyd R, Finnegan J, Green S. Friedreich's ataxia: a clinical review with neurophysiological and echocardiographic findings. Arch Dis Child 1984;59(3):217–221.
34. Nelson K, Ellenberg J. Epidemiology of cerebral palsy. In: Schoenberg B, ed. Advances in neurology. New York: Raven Press; 1978;421.
35. Zelnick N, Giladi N, Goikhman I, et al. The role of botulinum toxin in the treatment of lower limb spasticity in children with cerebral palsy – a pilot study. Isr J Med Sci 1997;33(2):129–133.
36. Hagberg B, Hagberg G, Olow I. The changing panorama of cerebral palsy in Sweden. 1954–70. II Analysis of the various syndromes. Acta Pediatr Scand 1975;64:193–200.
37. Fenichel G. Clinical pediatric neurology. 3rd ed. Philadelphia: WB Saunders; 1996:1103.
38. Papile L, Burstein J, Burstein R. Incidence and evolution of subependymal hemorrhage. A study of infants with birth weights less than 1500 grams. J Pediatr 1978;92:529–543.
39. Kudrjavcer T, Schoenberg B, Kurland L, et al. Cerebral palsy: survival rates, associated handicaps and distribution of clinical subtypes. Neurology 1985;35(6):900–903.
40. Sobel E, Giorgini R. Problems and management of the rearfoot in neuromuscular disease. A report of ten cases. J Am Podiatr Assoc 1999;89(1):24–38.

41. Sparrow S, Zinger F. Evaluation of a patterning treatment for retarded children. Pediatrics 1978;62:137–150.

42. Bobath B. The very early treatment of cerebral palsy. Dev Med Child Neurol 1967;9:373–390.

43. Hainsworth F, Harrison M, Sheldon T, et al. A preliminary evaluation of ankle orthoses in the management of children with cerebral palsy. Dev Med Child Neurol 1997;39(4):243–247.

44. Wilson H, Haideri N, Song K, et al. Ankle–foot orthoses for preambulatory children with spastic diplegia. J Pediatr Orthop 1997;17(3):370–376.

45. Rethlefsen S, Kay R, Dennis S, et al. The effects of fixed and articulated ankle–foot orthoses on gait patterns in subjects with cerebral palsy. J Pediatr Orthop 1999;19(4):470–474.

46. Carmick J. Managing equinus in a child with cerebral palsy: merits of hinged ankle–foot orthoses. Dev Med Child Neurol 1995;37(11):1006–1010.

47. Radtka S, Skinner S, Dixon D, et al. A comparison of gait with solid, dynamic, and no ankle–foot orthoses in children with spastic cerebral palsy [see comments] [published erratum appears in Phys Ther 1998;78(2):222–224]. Phys Ther 1997;77(4):113–118.

48. Sussman M, Cusick B. Tone-reducing casts as an adjunct to physical therapy of patients with cerebral palsy. Johns Hopkins Med J 1970;145:112.

49. Corry I, Cosgrove A, Duffy C, et al. Botulinum toxin A compared with stretching casts in the treatment of spastic equinus: a randomized prospective trial. J Pediatr Orthop 1998;18(3):304–311.

50. Cosgrove A, Corry I, Graham H. Botulinum toxin in the management of the lower limb in cerebral palsy. Dev Med Child Neurol 1994;36(5):386–396.

51. Davids J, Foti T, Dabelstein J, et al. Voluntary (normal) versus obligatory (cerebral palsy) toe-walking in children: a kinematic, kinetic, and electromyographic analysis. J Pediatr Orthop 1999;19(4):461–469.

52. Unnithan V, Dowling J, Frost G, et al. Cocontraction and phasic activity during gait in children with cerebral palsy. Electromyogr Clin Neurophysiol 1996;36(8):487–494.

53. Dyck P, Lambert E. Lower motor and sensory neuron disease with peroneal muscle atrophy. I. Neurologic, genetic and electrophysiologic findings in hereditary polyneuropathies. Arch Neurol 1968;18:603.

54. Dyck P, Lambert E. Lower motor and primary sensory neuron disease with peroneal muscle atrophy. II. Neurologic, genetic and electrophysiologic findings in various neuronal degenerations. Arch Neurol 1968;18:619.

55. Carter G, Abresch R, Fowler W, et al. Profiles of neuromuscular diseases. Hereditary motor and sensory neuropathy, types I and II. Am J Phys Med Rehab 1995;74(5 Suppl):S140–S148.

56. Njegovan M, Leonard E, Joseph F. Rehabilitation medicine approach to Charcot–Marie–Tooth disease. In: Goad RN, Harris EJ, eds. Clinics in podiatric medicine and surgery. Philadelphia: WB Saunders; 1997:99–116.

57. Bird T. Hereditary motor sensory neuropathies. Charcot–Marie–Tooth syndrome. Neurol Clin 1989;7(1):9–23.

58. Miller G, Hsu J, Hoffer M, et al. Posterior tibial tendon transfer: a review of the literature and analysis of 74 procedures. J Pediatr Orthop 1982;2(4):363–370.

59. Siegel I. Cavus versus planus in the neuropathic foot (peroneal muscular atrophy reconsidered) [letter]. Muscle Nerve 1996;19(6):797.

60. Stillwell G, Kilcoyne RF, Sherman JL. Patterns of muscle atrophy in the lower limbs in patients with Charcot–Marie–Tooth disease as measured by magnetic resonance imaging. J Foot Ankle Surg 1995;34(6):583–586.

61. Krampitz D, Wolfe G, Fleckenstein J, et al. Charcot–Marie–Tooth disease type 1A presenting as calf hypertrophy and muscle cramps. Neurology 1998;51(5):1508–1509.

62. Williams P. Restoration of muscle balance of the foot by transfer of the tibialis posterior. J Bone Joint Surg 1976;58B:217.

63. Tachdjian M. Pediatric orthopaedics. 2nd ed. Philadelphia: WB Saunders; 1990.

64. Hibbs R. An operation for 'claw-foot'. JAMA 1919;73(1583).

65. Jones R. The soldier's foot and the treatment of common deformities of the foot. BMJ 1916;1:749.

66. Cole W. The treatment of claw foot. J Bone Joint Surg 1940;22:895–908.

67. Japas L. Surgical treatment of pes cavus by tarsal V-osteotomy. Preliminary report. J Bone Joint Surg 1968;50A:927.

68. Dubowitz V. Muscle disorders in childhood. 2nd ed. London: WB Saunders; 1995.

69. Carroll N. Assessment and management of the lower extremity in myelodysplasia. Orthop Clin North Am 1987;18(4):709–724.

70. Bunch W, Scarff T, Dvonch V. Progressive neurological loss in myelomeningocele patients. Orthop Trans 1981;5:32.

71. Selber P, Dias L. Sacral-level myelomeningocele: a long-term outcome in adults. J Pediatr Orthop 1998;18(4):423–427.

72. Chambers G, Cochrane D, Irwin B, et al. Assessment of the appropriateness of services provided by multidisciplinary myelomeningocele clinic. Pediatr Neurosurg 1996;24(2):92–97.

73. Liptac G, Bloss J, Brisken H, et al. The management of children with spinal dysraphism. J Child Neurol 1988;3(1):3–20.

74. Hoppenfield S. Orthopedic neurology: A diagnostic guide to neurologic levels. Philadelphia: Lippincott; 1977.

75. Greene W. Treatment of hip and knee problems in myelomeningocele. Rosemont, Illinois: American Academy of Orthopaedic Surgeons; 1999.

76. McLone D. Care of the neonate with a myelomeningocele. Neurosurg Clin N Am 1998;9(1):111–120.

77. Drennan J. Current concepts in myelomeningocele. In: Zuckerman J, ed. Instructional course lectures. Rosemont, Illinois: American Academy of Orthopaedic Surgeons; 1999:543–550.

78. de Carvalho Neto J, Dias L, Gabrieli A. Congenital talipes equinovarus in spina bifida: treatment and results. J Pediatr Orthop 1996;16(6):782–785.

79. Thomson J, Ounpuu S, Davis R, et al. The effects of ankle–foot orthoses on the ankle and knee in persons with myelomeningocele: an evaluation using three-dimensional gait analysis. J Pediatr Orthop 1999;19(1):27–33.

80. Sharrard W, Grossfield I. The management of deformity and paralysis of the foot in myelomeningocele. J Bone Joint Surg 1968;50B:457.

81. Bartonek A, Saraste H, Samuelsson L, et al. Ambulation in patients with myelomeningocele: a 12 year follow-up. J Pediatr Orthop 1999;19(2):202–206.

82. Mandell J. Dystrophin. The gene and its product. Nature 1989;339(6226):584–586.

83. Dubowitz V. Color atlas of muscular disorders in childhood. Chicago: Yearbook Medical Publishers;1989.

84. McDonald C, Abresch R, Carter G, et al. Profiles of neuromuscular diseases. Becker's muscular dystrophy. Am J Phys Med Rehab 1995;74(5 Suppl):S93–S103.

85. McDonald C, Abresch R, Carter G, et al. Profiles of neuromuscular diseases. Duchenne muscular dystrophy. Am J Phys Med Rehab 1995;74(5 Suppl):S70–S92.

86. Ishpekova B, Milanov I, Christova L, et al. Comparative analysis between Duchenne and Becker types muscular dystrophy. Electromyogr Clin Neurophysiol 1999;39(5):315–318.

87. Richards S, Iannaccone S. Dystrophin and DNA diagnosis in a large pediatric muscle clinic. J Child Neurol 1994;9(2):162–166.

88. Kelly C, Redford J, Zilber A, et al. Standing balance in healthy boys and children with Duchenne muscular dystrophy. Arch Phys Med Rehabi 1981;62:324.

89. Williams E, Read L, Ellis A et al. The management of equinus deformity in Duchenne muscular dystrophy. J Bone Joint Surg 1984;66B:546.

90. Seeger B, Caudrey D, Little J. Progression of equinus deformity in Duchenne muscular dystrophy. Arch Phys Med Rehabil 1985;66:286.

91. Harris E. An approach to toe-walking: appropriate decision making. In: Jay R, ed. Pediatric foot and ankle surgery. Philadelphia: WB Saunders; 1999;284–302.

92. Burnett C, Johnson E. Development of gait in childhood. Part I: Method. Dev Med Child Neurol 1971;13:196–206.

93. Burnett C, Johnson E. Development of gait in childhood. Part II. Dev Med Child Neurol 1971;13:207–215.

94. Hall J, Salter R, Bhalla S. Congenital short tendo calcaneus. J Bone Joint Surg 1967;49B:695–697.

95. Stricker S, Angulo J. Idiopathic toe walking: A comparison of treatment methods. J Pediatr Orthop 1998;18(3):289–293.

96. Carter G, Abresch R, Fowler W, et al. Profiles of neuromuscular diseases. Spinal muscular atrophy. Am J Phys Med Rehab 1995;74(5 Suppl):S150–S159.

97. Brand N, Haimi-Cohen Y, Weinstock A, et al. Tethered cord syndrome presenting as a nonhealing cutaneous ulcer. Childs Nerv Syst 1996;12(9): 562–563.

98. Cornetre L, Verpoorten C, Lagae L, et al. Tethered cord syndrome in occult spinal dysraphism: timing and outcome of surgical release. Neurology 1998;50(6):1761–1765.

99. Klekamp J, Raimondi A, Samii M. Occult dysraphism in adulthood: clinical course and management. Childs Nerv Syst 1994;10(5):312–320.

100. Shariff S, Allcutt D, Marks C, et al. 'Tethered cord syndrome' – recent clinical experience. Br J Neurosurg 1997;11(1):49–51.

101. Jeelani N, Jaspan T, Punt J. Lesson of the week: tethered cord syndrome after myelomeningocele repair. BMJ 1999;318(7182):516–517.

102. Gregerson D. Clinical consequences of spina bifida occulta. J Manipulative Physiol Ther 1997;20(8):546–550.

8

Cutaneous diseases in childhood

John Thomson

The skin is the largest organ in the body and it can give many clues to the wellbeing of the patient. The skin may show signs of underlying systemic disease, e.g. paleness in anemia or cyanosis in respiratory failure, or of disorders peculiar to it such as psoriasis or eczema. In order to arrive at a diagnosis of a particular skin complaint, the clinician must follow a stepwise logical process through the clinical history, the physical examination and when appropriate by means of further investigations, e.g. biopsy. A correct diagnosis followed by appropriate treatment is satisfying to both patient and podiatrist.

EMBRYOLOGY

Epidermis

The epidermis starts to form around the fourth week of fetal life. A single layer soon divides into two:

1. an outer periderm
2. an inner germinative layer.

The layers of the epidermis develop from the germinative layer. Starting with the basal cells, each layer develops separately, slowly at first, then speeding up until all are complete at about 6 months when the postnatal structure is seen (Fig. 8.1). At this stage the periderm is shed contributing to the fetal greasy coating, the vernix caseosa.

By 8 weeks, the dermis is a thin structure. In 3 months, this resolves separating from the subcutis. The development of the dermis is always delayed compared to the epidermis, especially in

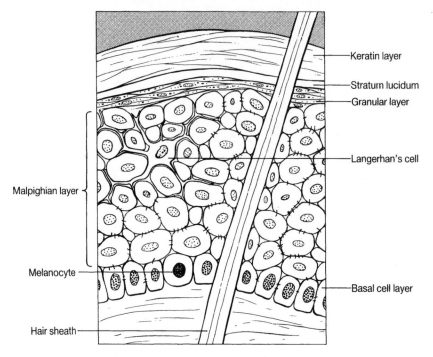

Figure 8.1 The normal epidermis.

relation to its thickness, hence the visible network of dermal blood vessels and 'wasted' appearance of some newborn, especially the premature.

Nails

The nail fold and matrix appear at approximately 3 months. The nail plate develops shortly thereafter.

Hair, sebaceous and eccrine glands

During the third and fourth months, certain germinative cells crowd together growing down to form the primitive hair germ and shaft. Sebaceous glands associate with the hair and become functional around the fourth month; the resulting sebum also contributes to the vernix caseosa. The eccrine glands form first on the palms and on the soles at around the third month. Those in other areas develop more slowly.

ANATOMY

The basic structure of the skin consists of the outer epidermis and the underlying dermis (Fig. 8.1). The epidermis does not contain any blood vessels or specialized structures such as sweat glands or sebaceous glands although parts of these structures traverse through it. All of the above structures are situated in the dermis.

The skin is modified in different parts of the body. The feet exhibit two main skin types:

1. the soles of the feet are hairless and have no sebaceous glands and consist of a thick compact outer layer of keratin with encapsulated sense organs in the dermis. Such non-hairbearing skin (glabrous) also occurs on the palms of the hands.
2. the skin on the dorsa of the feet has hair and sebaceous glands, but there are no encapsulated sense organs.

PHYSIOLOGY AND FUNCTIONS OF THE SKIN

The skin protects against:

- loss of fluids
- absorption of fluids and poisons
- entry of infection
- damage from heat and cold
- damage from ultraviolet radiation
- mechanical damage

The above listed complex mechanisms may be modified under certain conditions or may fail in disease.

The immunological functions of the skin are crucial. Invading organisms and chemicals are gathered in the 'arms' of the dendritic Langerhans cells which are the equivalent of the macrophage cells found in blood. These foreign organisms are then presented to the immune systems in the lymph nodes. The antibodies produced may be beneficial and be used to kill off invaders or they may cause an inappropriate reaction to environmental substances as seen in contact dermatitis. The skin is also an endocrine organ and prevents rickets by synthesizing vitamin D in conjunction with sunshine.

PATHOLOGY

It is usual for pathological changes to occur in both the epidermis and the dermis. Interpretation of these changes is a skilled job for the pathologist and at times requires the services of a specialist dermatopathologist. However, it is the responsibility of the clinician to furnish an accurate history and the site of the biopsy. An adequate specimen as described under the section on further investigations is essential, as histological examination is a logical process working from the keratin layer down. Meetings between clinician and pathologist are very worthwhile.

An abnormally thick keratin layer (hyperkeratosis) may result from increased keratin production or from decreased desquamation. The retention of nuclei in the keratin layer (parakeratosis) is usually seen when there is abnormally rapid cell differentiation such as in psoriasis.

When the epidermal cell turnover slows, thinning or atrophy follows. When the cell turnover increases, thickening or acanthosis results.

The cells of the malpighian or prickle cell layer are attached by anchoring filaments, the tonofibrils. Tonofibrils may be stretched and may partially give way when edema is present giving an appearance similar to a sponge (spongiosis) as in eczema. When tonofibrils are destroyed, e.g. by an antigen–antibody reaction as in certain blistering conditions, the cells round off and lie free. This is known as acantholysis. Changes can also occur at the dermal epidermal junction, which often leads to blister formation.

In the dermis, a variety of changes may occur in the vessels, in the supporting collagen or in the elastic fibers. There may be infiltrates of different cells in a miscellany of patterns.

The subcutaneous fat may also be inflamed leading to panniculitis.

REACHING A DIAGNOSIS

Dermatological diagnosis is reached by a logical progression through the history, the examination and by special investigations. Attempts to diagnose without a history should be avoided; occasionally, the diagnosis may be correct but inevitably vital information such as the patient's drug history will be missed. Similarly, any special investigations should be an adjunct to the history and examination and not a principal means of diagnosis.

In the child, the history may need to be taken from, or augmented by, an adult. Certain vital questions require to be answered. For example, the duration of the condition and its initial site; the initial type of lesion and the subsequent pattern; whether any rash is symptomless, itchy or painful. Are there any fluctuations in severity? Since certain skin conditions are recurrent, is there a past history of previous skin problems? Certain skin conditions are familial; therefore, it is essential to enquire about the family history. An awareness of any general medical problem may help in diagnosing its cutaneous manifestations. It is also essential to obtain a drug history from the patient although specific enquiry may be needed regarding certain preparations such as aspirin, tonics and cough medicines as these may not be regarded as drugs by the patient. Even when the answers to these questions are negative, a 'drug rash' may occur from chemicals in foodstuffs.

Previous treatment may modify the condition, rendering the diagnosis more difficult. When treatment seems to have been adequate and appropriate to the initial diagnosis, but unsuccessful, an alternative diagnosis should be considered. Hobbies and sports may be relevant.

A thorough examination is necessary. The pattern and distribution of a rash may give the vital clue. It may not be possible for the podiatrist to examine completely all the skin but readily available areas should be looked at and a careful history used as a substitute for inaccessible areas. Individual lesions should be carefully assessed.

The initial or primary lesion is the most useful lesion on which to base a diagnosis. A number of skin diseases present with one of the following:

- *macules* are small impalpable lesions, e.g. a freckle
- *papules* are small palpable lesions
- *pustules* are small palpable lesions containing pus, e.g. acne; they may be due to infection but not necessarily so
- *blisters* – small blisters are termed vesicles and large blisters (> 0.2 inches (> 0.5 cm)), bullae.

Secondary skin lesions may evolve from primary lesions by scratching or infection, e.g. excoriation, crusting and ulcers. Diagnostically, these are less useful. Mucous membranes and finger and toe nails should also be examined.

GENODERMATOSES

Many skin diseases are partly determined by genetic make-up but are modified greatly by external or environmental factors. The genodermatoses are essentially unaffected by these factors and are the result of a single gene or chromosomal abnormality.

Down syndrome (mongolism) (1:700 births)

Generalized dryness (xerosis) may affect the lower limbs, which may be short with lax ligaments. Lichen simplex affecting other areas may also involve the ankle.

Neurofibromatosis (1:4000/5000 births)

Abnormalities include nerve and skin tumors, which are usually benign but may become malignant. There are two types: Von Recklinghausen's neurofibromatosis (neurofibromatosis 1; NF1) and another associated with an acoustic neuroma (NF2) which has a different genetic pattern.

The general features of NF1 include soft skin tumors, which may number from a few to hundreds. The tumors may be small, medium or very large. On palpation, it may be possible to herniate them down to the dermis. Multiple axillary freckles are a hallmark of the disease in addition to a number of pigmented, flat spots (café au lait spots). Neurofibromata or the pigmented lesions may affect the skin of the lower limb.

Tuberous sclerosis (1:6000 births)

Tuberous sclerosis is inherited via a single autosomal dominant gene with variable penetration. Mutations may arise and a number of organs may be affected. The skin features predominate. On the face, small reddish brown papules aggregate around the nose (adenoma sebaceum). Periungual fibromata vary in size and may distort the nail plate (Koenen's tumors). Depigmented areas, accentuated by Woods ultraviolet light and with the appearance of ash tree leaves may also be seen. Thickened soft flesh-colored areas are described as shagree patches because of their resemblance to a type of leather. Mental deficiency and/or epilepsy complicate certain cases.

With the exception of the facial lesions all the other features may affect the lower limb.

PHYSICALLY INDUCED SKIN DISORDERS

Although the skin is tough and resilient, certain agents may physically damage it:

- insects
- cold
- heat
- trauma.

Insects: arthropod bites and stings

Insects may be divided into two main groups:

1. those which sting, usually in defense
2. those which bite, often to ingest blood.

The damage may be direct trauma (horsefly); tissue damage from noxious chemicals (bee sting); or an antigen–antibody reaction in the previously sensitized. Secondary superficial infection may be introduced. The symptoms and signs vary considerably. Exposed areas are vulnerable although some arthropods prefer humid, sweaty areas, e.g. under clothing bands. The foot and ankle are especially vulnerable and lesions may be solitary or linear.

The clinical appearance depends on the damage. There may be:

— a central puncture mark
— an urticarial weal occurring within a few moments of the assault, progressing to a papule in 24 to 48 hours, resolving over a few days
— more severe reaction, e.g. blisters or tissue necrosis.

Lymphangitis, lymphadenopathy, cellulitis, malaise or fever are all possible sequelae. Occasionally, collapse owing to anaphylaxis may occur in hypersensitive patients. A current problem, especially in the USA, is Lyme disease resulting from a tic bite, which produces an annular reaction. Joint, cardiac and neurological complications have all been described.

Cold: chilblains (perniosis)

Vasoconstriction is induced by cold. Rapid rewarming opens up arterioles before venules.

Local edema ensues accompanied by a red, swollen, painful itchy area. This appearance subsides to a livid color in 2 to 3 weeks. Warmer houses have so reduced the incidence that the diagnosis may not be considered.

Treatment is symptomatic. However, warmer clothing may prevent their occurrence. Rapid rewarming of cold areas, especially by direct heat should be avoided.

Heat: burns

Burns may be caused by heat (dry or wet), chemicals, friction or electricity. The extent and depth vary tremendously. Any resulting scarring requires lifelong medical attention, therefore prevention is extremely important. The podiatrist should take great care with corrosive chemicals and with diathermy in association with certain flammable materials, e.g. alcoholic skin cleansers.

Trauma

Crushing or sudden blows produce tissue damage to various skin levels with subsequent bruising and edema. The diagnosis is usually apparent. Corns result from long-term pressure and friction. The initial response may be hyperkeratosis or a callosity, which may be protective. When pressure continues, the keratin is compacted so that a central core develops which tends to overly a bony prominence. The main treatment is reduction of the lesion and removal of pressure from the area with suitable padding. A thorough biomechanical examination and advice concerning footwear may also be appropriate.

Sudden unaccustomed frictional forces may lead to blisters rather than callosities. Sweating and new or ill-fitting footwear are predisposing factors. It may be possible to alter the plane of friction by the judicious application of tape. Once blisters develop, they may be drained. However, when the child is to continue with exercise, it is better to avoid debridement. Measures should be taken to prevent secondary infections.

Post-traumatic punctate skin hemorrhage (talon noir) is the result of bleeding into the skin when sudden shearing forces rupture the dermal rete peg capillaries. Such trauma is common in sports where there are sudden acceleration/ deceleration moves, e.g. tennis or badminton. The border of the heel is a common site (hence talon noir) where a black, slightly speckled, area develops. As this discoloration may be mistaken for a malignant melanoma, a careful history is invaluable. Paring the skin demonstrates and sometimes removes the altered blood.

Bizarre, repeated or unexplained trauma raises the possibility of child abuse. In common with other health professionals, the podiatrist must consider this as a possibility in any differential diagnosis. Great care must be taken to be certain of this diagnosis as to diagnose it wrongly or to miss it entirely are both disasters of equal magnitude.

SKIN INFECTIONS

Normal skin is not sterile at birth. Many bacteria and yeasts are present as permanent or transient inhabitants. Such organisms are not spread evenly over the surface; moist surfaces such as toe clefts may harbor greater numbers. Pathogens may invade through breaks in the skin integrity or because of diminished immune defenses. The main aim of treatment is directed towards the infection, but it is also important to seek predisposing factors such as eczema or diabetes mellitus.

The skin may be infected by mites, as well as by bacterial, viral or fungal agents or it may exhibit signs of internal infection.

Scabies

Scabies is due to the human scabies mite. This is one of the suborders of Acarina called *Sarcoptes scabiei* var. *hominis* (Fig. 8.2).

There is usually involvement of other household members or persons with whom the sufferer is closely involved. The predominant symptom is itching, especially at night or when the patient is warm. Such timing may relate to increased activity of the mite. Itching occurs because of an allergic reaction to the *Sarcoptes* or from its degeneration products. This explains the variable latent period before pruritus commences. On subsequent occasions, itching begins

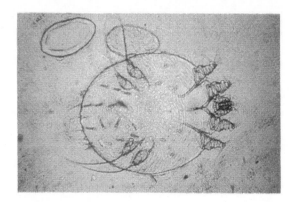

Figure 8.2 Scabies mite.

earlier. The classic sites are the interdigital webs, anterior wrists, axillary folds, the ankles and feet.

The typical lesion is the burrow, usually seen as a small grayish line (Plate 1). Scratching converts these burrows into excoriated papular and/or secondarily infected areas. Usually the diagnosis is easy after the history and examination, but it may be missed. The finding of a mite confirms the diagnosis.

It is essential to explain the condition to the sufferer. Scabies engenders shame and misconceptions about dirt and poor hygiene; thus a sympathetic approach is needed. The entire household (and any other involved households) must be treated simultaneously. Failure to do this will usually lead to recurrences. Gamma benzene hexachloride is effective with one adequate application. However, the itching may take approximately 3 weeks to settle.

BACTERIAL INFECTIONS

The clinical features of bacterial infections depend on the infecting organism, the site of the infection and which layer of the skin is involved. Infection in the keratin layer leads to impetigo; in the prickle cell layer, erysipelas; and in the dermis, cellulitis.

Impetigo contagiosa

Staphylococci or streptococci penetrate the keratin via a minor abrasion. Commonly, this is on the face in a child with a running nose, but it may complicate any skin condition when the skin's integrity is breached. The primary lesion is a blister. On the face, the blister is usually so fragile that it ruptures and secondary 'honey-colored' crusting may be seen. In areas where the keratin is thicker, blisters may remain.

Erysipelas

Erysipelas results from a streptococcal infection (usually group A type) accessing the prickle cell layer through a minor, usually unnoticed breach in the skin. An abrupt onset with malaise and fever occurs. A reddish plaque with a palpable spreading edge commonly occurs on the face but it may affect the limbs. Fungal toe-web infections can allow access to *Streptococcus*. Treatment should be prompt, especially important with facial involvement as the infection may enter the cavernous sinus and then the brain. Penicillin usually settles erysipelas rapidly and should be given for at least 1 week. Recurrence may lead to limb lymphedema. In such cases, the use of long-term antibiotics is justified.

Cellulitis

This dermal infection is usually due to *Streptococcus pyogenes* or *Staphylococcus* penetrating a wound or a macerated area. The characteristic signs of inflammation, redness, heat, swelling and pain usually occur and are soon followed by lymphangitis, lymphadenopathy, fever and extreme malaise. Treatment usually antedates bacteriological identification. Penicillinase-resistant antibiotics such as flucloxacillin or cloxacillin are worth using empirically but penicillin V or phenethicillin may be necessary when *Streptococcus* is proved to be the cause.

VIRAL INFECTIONS

Viruses are very small infective particles that require to harness a host cell in order to replicate. In doing so they may damage or destroy the host cell in a variety of ways. After multiplication, large numbers of the virus may cascade into the blood. Some may be trapped in skin capillaries but are unable to replicate in local cells owing to various defenses. This may explain the transient rash (exanthem) of many systemic viral diseases. Therefore, viruses may affect the skin as transient exanthems in a systemic viral disease or through direct infection.

Common exanthems

Rubella

Malaise and cervical lymphadenopathy precede a pink macular facial rash which then 'runs down' the trunk and the limbs coalescing centrally. The evanescent nature and frequent atypical features may make a diagnosis difficult.

Measles

After an asymptomatic 14-day incubation, fever and malaise are followed by conjunctival suffusion, coughing and a runny nose. A purplish blotchy postauricular rash spreading to the trunk and the limbs succeeds Koplik's spots in the mouth, which have the appearance of grains of salt on a red background. The rash then spreads to the hands and feet where marked desquamation may follow.

Chickenpox (varicella)

A macular rash, followed by tense unilocular blisters, which become pustular and crowded, follows the incubation period of 2 to 3 weeks. Intensely itchy lesions at different stages are mainly confined to the trunk. However, palmoplantar lesions do occur. Fever and constitutional symptoms can be marked. Flat round scars succeed certain lesions.

VIRAL INFECTIONS DIRECTLY INVOLVING THE SKIN

Herpes

Herpes consists of a number of DNA viruses. More associations are being discovered with human disease, e.g. Kaposi's sarcoma. Some have a predilection for nerve and skin tissue.

Herpes simplex

Herpes simplex is a very common infection affecting most people. An undiagnosable viremic illness in childhood is followed by a latent period when the virus remains in a nerve ganglion. Although it usually appears on the face, herpes simplex may occur anywhere including the foot. Ultraviolet light, fevers or the common cold may trigger viral replication. The viruses travel down the nerve root and branches to the skin producing symptoms of tingling, redness, swelling and blister formation. Antibodies would have been produced at the first exposure to the virus and although ineffective during the latent period may attack now. Clearing occurs within approximately 1 week. However, since some virus remains latent in the nerve root, recurrence is common.

Except during the latent stage of the infection, aciclovir is an effective drug; however, it must be started early.

Herpes zoster (shingles)

This DNA virus causes herpes zoster and chickenpox and is therefore called the varicella/zoster virus. Infection in the non-immune causes chickenpox (see above) and in the partially immune, shingles. Usually, the initial childhood infection is eliminated but some virus remains in the nerve tissue, usually the dorsal root ganglia. Later, though rarely in childhood, these viruses are reactivated and pass down the nerve to the skin as grouped blisters. Pain precedes the rash. A unilateral truncal band is commonest but it may affect other areas including the lower limb and the foot. Early treatment with a high dose of aciclovir or similar drug may shorten the course of the attack.

Warts (verrucae)

Deoxyribonucleic acid (DNA)-containing papilloma viruses (PV), a subgroup of the Papova virus family is responsible for viral warts.

The PV is species-specific and the human agent is the humanpapillomavirus (HPV). There are a number of subtypes – currently over 70 and increasing – which may cause infections of specific types or sites. Warts of the hands and feet are usually due to subtypes 1, 2 and 4. HPV can be dormant but remain infectious outside the body for a long time. The virus probably requires an entry portal via an epidermal injury. The finer skin of children is more liable to such minor trauma. Weakening of the normal skin barrier function as in eczema is a predisposing factor. Showers and swimming pools with abrasive non-slip moist surrounds are high-risk areas for contracting plantar warts. Once inoculated, the incubation period is infinitely variable.

After the clinical lesions develop, there is also a variable time before regression; 20–30% of cases clear spontaneously within 6 months. Both humoral antibodies (IgM and IgE) and cell-mediated immunity are involved. Warts can spread rapidly in immunosuppressed patients. The virus may stimulate the basal epidermal cells to divide; however, viral DNA is only found to the depth of the granular layer. Small viral particles in the basal cells may only be able to multiply at a certain stage of cell development in the granular layer.

The diagnosis of the common wart is usually straightforward. Difficulties may occur with plantar warts where there is overlying hyperkeratosis. Partial reduction of the area may reveal petechiae. Skin markings may be seen to be 'pushed aside' by the wart and projecting columns of hyperkeratosis may be interspersed with black dots which represent thrombosed capillaries (Plate 2). Warts vary in number from solitary lesions to hundreds and these may in turn coalesce into masses. Bleeding may occur from trauma or from self-treatment. On weight-bearing areas, warts rarely project to the same extent. A prominent surrounding capsule of hyperkeratosis may mimic a corn. Warts may spread around nail folds giving plate distortion. The patient's main complaint may be the appearance of the wart although pain may occur in pressure areas, especially in plantar warts. The sufferer may be unable to walk or may have a distorted gait. Pain is worse on rising from rest or with direct pressure.

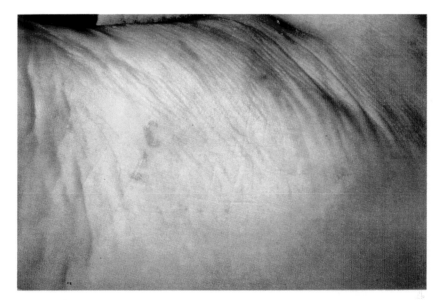

Plate 1 Scabies

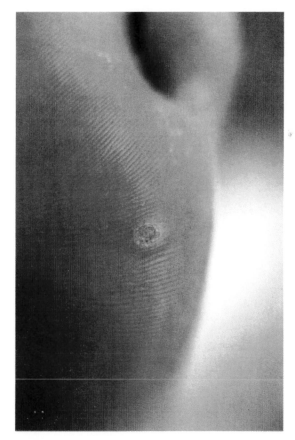

Plate 2 Verruca Plantaris

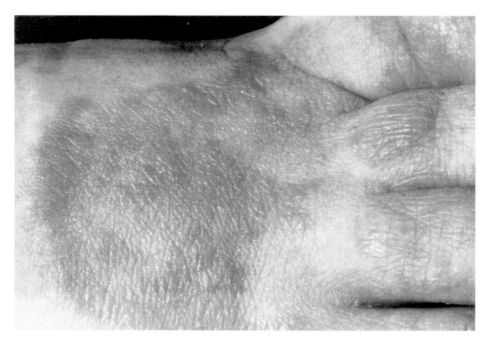

Plate 3 Tinea Pedis

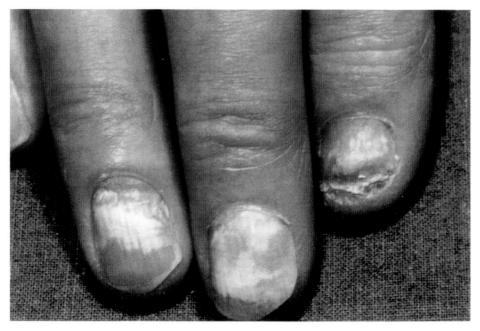

Plate 4 Fungal Leuconychia

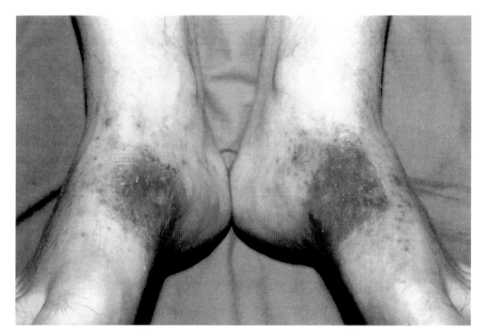

Plate 5 Shoe Contact Dermatitis

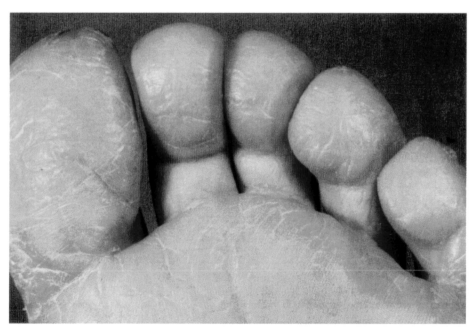

Plate 6 Juvenile Plantar Dermatosis

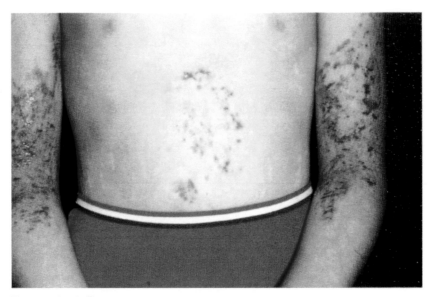

Plate 7   Atopic Eczema

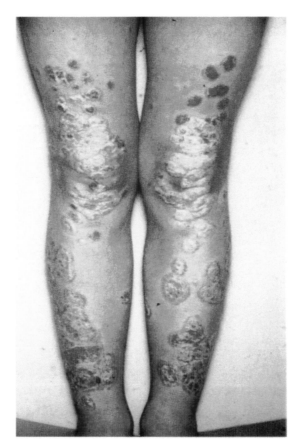

Plate 8   Plaque Psoriasis

Histologically, hyperplasia of the keratin, granular and prickle cell layers occurs. The basal cell layer is intact. The dermal papillae curve under the wart tissue and blood vessels reach high up into it. There may be large keratinocytes with an eccentric nucleus surrounded by a halo (koilocytes or 'bird's eye' cells). These represent viral damage resulting in balloon degeneration to the prickle cells.

There is no specific antiviral drug. Treatment is destructive to the infected area and tends to be painful. Chemically, keratolytic agents such as salicylic acid formulations may be used. Cryotherapy is commonly used, usually in the form of liquid nitrogen. Lasers and electrodessication have their proponents but are still being evaluated.

Hand foot and mouth disease

An uncommon condition reported worldwide, usually caused by Coxsackie A16 although other viruses have been implicated. Young children present with general malaise for 24 hours followed by small painful mouth blisters which rapidly progress to ulcers. Oval vesicles, resembling rice grains, appear on the hands and feet, usually on the dorsa with a periungular predilection. They affect the flexures or hand and feet creases. They usually clear within a week. Contacts may be affected. Histologically, intra-epidermal blisters occur. Specific treatment is unnecessary.

Molluscum contagiosum

Molluscum contagiosum, common in children, is due to a pox virus, and is frequently contracted near swimming pools. After a variable incubation period of 2 to 7 weeks, flesh-colored dome-shaped papules (0.06 inches (1.5 mm)) with a characteristic central depression develop. The papules are usually multiple and are commonly, although not exclusively, found in or around the axillae or groins. Vast numbers may occur in the atopic; in the immunosuppressed; or in those inappropriately treated with topical steroids. From the umbilicated area, caseous material may

be expressed. The appearance may be modified by secondary bacterial infection accompanied by inflammation and pus. Solitary lesions may mimic basal cell carcinoma. When the expressed material is smeared on to a slide and a potassium hydroxide solution added, large balloon cells resembling frog spawn are easily seen.

Normally mollusca resolve in a number of months. Destruction by liquid nitrogen, hyfrecation or squeezing speeds the clearance. Flat scars not related to treatment may be left.

FUNGAL DISEASES

Fungi are a large group numbering many thousands, ranging from small organisms to large mushrooms. Fungi can multiply asexually. Small fragments replicate into whole new organisms whose identical characteristics are good for adaptation. Certain specimens replicate sexually with nuclei fusing and dividing. Such variation makes classification difficult. Microscopically, most fungi appear like a tangled skein of threads. Classifications are made on branching, compartmentalization (by septa), type of replication and from the formation of buds or spores.

Human fungal disease, known as mycoses, may be classified as:

- superficial mycoses which purely affect skin, nails and/or hair
- deep or systemic mycoses affecting deeper structures alone or with secondary skin involvement.

The organisms, which cause superficial mycoses, may be further subdivided into:

1. dermatophytes
   Trichophyton, e.g. *rubrum*
   Epidermophyton, e.g. *floccosum*
   Microsporum, e.g. *canis*
2. yeasts, e.g. *Candida* usually *albicans*.

Dermatophyte infections are designated as tinea (t). The site affected is added as a latinized genitive, e.g. t. pedis, t. capitis, t. corporis or t. unguium. Certain dermatophytes may cause one specific disease while other conditions may be due to one of several fungi. The dermatophytes invade keratin but deeper penetration is prevented by a serum inhibitory factor. In the nail, the entire plate may be affected as far as the growing matrix. In hair, the fungi grow down within or outside the shaft to beneath the skin surface. Therefore, shaving cannot eradicate the infection.

The *Candida* (C) group may also be split into different members. *C. albicans* is the most common but *C. parapsilosis*, *C. tropicalis* and others may be pathogenic. However, this makes little difference to cutaneous therapy. *Candida* may be a normal commensal on the body. It is found near orifices such as the mouth, anus and vagina. The total colony present is kept in balance by the rest of the skin flora. *Candida* is an opportunist and invades when the balance is upset.

Histologically, acute inflammation with pustule formation may be observed. Periodic acid-Schiff (PAS) staining enhances the visualization of small numbers of fungus in the keratin.

Tinea pedis

Tinea pedis is the commonest dermatophyte infection. 10% of the general population (larger in closed communities) may be affected especially when occlusive footwear is worn (Plate 3). Moisture macerates the skin, thereby weakening its defenses and thereby allowing entry of the fungus particularly between the fourth and fifth interdigital webs. The causative fungi may be found around wet areas of showers and swimming pools. Anti-slip surfaces abrade the skin facilitating the infection.

Three dermatophytes predominate – *Trichophyton rubrum*, *Trichophyton mentagrophytes* var. *interdigitale* and *Epidermophyton floccosum*. Certain variations in the clinical picture occur with the different types. The commonest effect is scaling and maceration between the toes, with the fourth and fifth interdigital webs almost invariably affected, either alone or in combination. In many patients, such signs are asymptomatic. However, any dermatophyte may cause this type of clinical picture.

Dry red scaling of the plantar surfaces is usually due to *T. rubrum*. Fine scaling is accentuated by scraping lightly. This occurs spontaneously at skin markings and a network of criss-crossing white lines is seen.

Less commonly, small blisters form usually because of infection by *T. mentagrophytes* var. *interdigitale* and are worse in hot weather. A violent very acute infection together with an associated dermatitis reaction may be crippling and devastating.

The proximity of the toe nails renders them liable to be infected (see below). Recurrent tinea pedis may be due to a reservoir of fungus in the nails. Palmar ringworm (tinea manuum) may be a consequence of a foot infection, particularly with *T. rubrum*. All forms of tinea pedis may lead to a distant sensitization or ide eruption not directly colonized by fungus. Such eruptions are rare in minor infections but are more common when the infection is severe.

When possible, the clinical diagnosis should be confirmed by direct examination with potassium hydroxide or by culture. However, the fungus may be difficult to visualize and may be unpredictable in culture.

Treatment may have limited success. However, the following can help:

- Cleanliness and hosing down communal bathing areas may reduce the incidence.
- Meticulous drying of the feet, especially interdigitally, reduces maceration and the likelihood of penetration by fungus
- Hyperhidrosis is common and should be treated.
- Occlusive footwear should be discouraged.
- Patients with severe infections should be banned from public swimming pools.
- The wearing of plastic socks for swimming may help. However, this may not be popular with children and it is also almost impossible to avoid all foot contact with the wet surfaces.

Topical treatment involves application of an imidazole, e.g. miconazole nitrate cream. Such drugs damage the fungal wall and lead to inhibition of growth and cell death. There are many imidazoles and none would appear to have any significant advantages over the other. The value of antifungal dusting powders for shoes and/or hosiery is difficult to evaluate.

Tinea unguium (onychomycosis)

Most of the predisposing factors for tinea pedis, which may coexist, are pertinent to toe nail fungal infection. *T. rubrum*, *T. mentagrophytes* and *E. floccosum* are again implicated with the emphasis on the first two.

Infection first occurs at the distal nail plate, which may change color. On viewing the nail plate end on, a honeycomb of crumbly nail underlying the smoother upper surface may be seen and is termed distal subungual onychomycosis. Leuconychia (white superficial onychomycosis) may develop due to *T. mentagrophytes* (Plate 4). The fungus may ultimately break through, rendering the upper surface of the nail plate rough and scaly. Onycholysis may be a prominent feature. Onychomycosis, which occurs much more commonly in toe nails, involves one or two nails initially but gradually others may be affected.

The differential diagnosis includes trauma, psoriasis and other nail dystrophies. Traumatic changes usually affect only one or two nails and there may be a history of a particular incident. Changes caused by eczema and other skin diseases are usually identifiable after a history and examination. Changes in the nail as the result of pure nail dystrophies may be more difficult.

In the management of tinea unguium, concomitant tinea pedis (or manuum) should also be treated. Current topical therapies may not cure the affected nail. However, they may be used around all the nails and digits in an effort to prevent further spread. Tioconazole paint has still not yet been fully evaluated and it is expensive. Systemic drugs such as itraconazole and terbinafine show great promise but cannot yet be used in children.

Tinea incognito

Tinea incognito refers to the modification and masking of a fungal infection by the use of inappropriately prescribed strong topical steroids. Initially, the eruption would seem to improve with lessening of symptoms and paling. However, the symptoms never completely clear and when the steroid is withdrawn, the condition may flare. The characteristic scaling edge and clearing center may be lost or diminished making an accurate diagnosis difficult. The area is slightly red and frequently nodules are present. Application of the topical steroid should be stopped and appropriate antifungal preparations given.

Candidiasis (candidosis)

Candidiasis is due to one of the yeast-like fungi of *Candida* with *Candida albicans* the main offender. When present on mucous membranes, the condition is described as thrush. *Candida* is a normal commensal when in small numbers but it is an opportunist.

Supercolonization may occur when the skin flora is disrupted by broad-spectrum antibiotics, diabetes mellitus, systemic steroids, immunosuppression or by drug addiction. When the skin defense is reduced by another rash, *Candida* may colonize such an area. *Candida* infections are more common in the obese.

On mucous membranes, candidiasis causes pain or discomfort. White patches on a red background may be swabbed leaving a raw bleeding area.

Candida is most commonly found in moist skin folds. The interdigital webs of toes are potential sites for invasion. Nail folds may be colonized leading to paronychia with a swollen 'bolstered' area, which may result in cuticle destruction and nail dystrophy.

On the skin, a salmon pink patch extends into the depth of the crevice. Frequently, there is a fine scaly fringed edge with small pustules which rapidly burst and crust. Small outlying satellite lesions with redness and crusting outside this plaque are common.

A diagnosis of candidiasis is made by examining appropriate scrapings. A few *Candida* on a swab may be within normal limits. The underlying cause for the candidal infection must be sought and remedied where possible. Correction of diabetes mellitus, stopping broad-spectrum antibiotics or the use of inappropriate steroids will play a major part. If moist areas can be dried, *Candida* will die out or be loath to recolonize.

Nail folds should be kept dry. Hygroscopic, mildly antiseptic agents may help. Shoes and socks should be of the less occlusive type, thereby reducing sweating. Several different preparations of nystatin are available. However, nystatin is not absorbed from the gut and requires topical application. Nystatin is ineffective against dermatophytes. The imidazoles are active against both dermatophytes and *Candida* and are useful when the clinician does not have access to the diagnostic facilities of a laboratory or is unsure of the offending organism.

ECZEMA/DERMATITIS

Eczema and dermatitis should be considered as synonyms and interchangeable. Both terms refer to inflammation of the skin. The classic features of inflammation are present, i.e. redness, heat, swelling, pain (or itch) and loss of function. The relative degree of each symptom will vary from patient to patient. Eczema or dermatitis is not the final diagnosis; the cause must be sought. This disorder may be divided into two main groups:

1. exogenous, e.g. contact dermatitis
2. endogenous, e.g. atopic eczema, juvenile plantar dermatosis, pompholyx, lichen simplex.

Regardless of the underlying cause, the end result on the skin will be similar. A careful history and assessment of the disease pattern are often more important than the local lesion. The degree of redness and swelling present is proportional to the intensity and the edge of the lesion is not clearly demarcated. Blisters when present range from tiny vesicles to large bullae. These blisters may weep profusely or the affected area may be dry, hard and fissured. Moist raw areas are liable to secondary infection and may be covered with loosely adherent yellowish crusts; an associated lymphadenopathy may follow. No scarring will result from uncomplicated dermatitis.

The symptoms of dermatitis are those of inflammation. The patient may complain of pain, heat or intense itching. Swelling, especially on the face and at the extremities, may be very troublesome. On the foot, swelling may make walking impossible and when it affects the hand, loss of joint mobility is extremely incapacitating. Secondary infection leads to an offensive malodor.

Histologically edema develops in the epidermis and upper dermis (Fig. 8.3). The epidermal cells appear to be pushed apart stretching their intercellular attachments (spongiosis). The edema may collect as epidermal vesicles of variable sizes. The epidermis thickens (acanthosis) and disruption of the normal maturation means that nucleated cells are seen within the keratin layer (parakeratosis). Reddening of the area results from dilatation of the dermal blood vessels and from the presence of inflammatory cells.

General management of eczema/dermatitis

Wherever possible, the cause of the eczema/dermatitis should be identified and treated. In endogenous eczema, no remedial cause may be identifiable. In such cases, the treatment of the dermatitis may be undertaken to get symptomatic relief.

Rest and elevation of swollen areas produce great relief. Firm bandaging may help but should be non-occlusive. Protection from irritants by avoidance or by suitable protective wear is essential. As a general rule, the moister the skin lesion the moister the base of the preparation should be. Therefore, an acute weeping eruption would suggest the use of a lotion in the form of a soak or as a compress. As the area becomes progressively drier, a cream (water miscible), then an ointment, then a paste may be applied. Pastes may be difficult to apply directly on to the skin.

Many topical preparations for the treatment of eczema are available. Topical corticosteroids range from mildly potent to very potent. Certain patients may develop an acute contact dermatitis to the steroid molecule itself. When this occurs, the steroid preparation must be changed. Strong topical steroids should be used on a time-limited basis. Great care should be taken on thin skinned areas since long continued use will lead to atrophy of the skin, marked skin striae and rebound of the condition for which they have been prescribed.

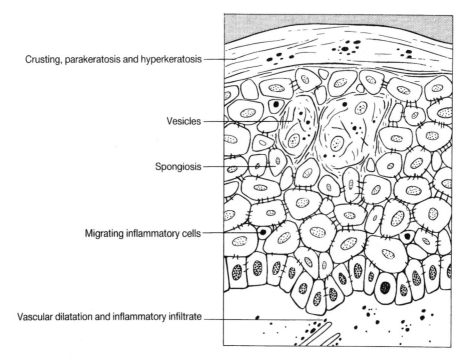

Figure 8.3 Histology of acute eczema.

Secondary infection may well supervene, therefore the incorporation of an antimicrobial agent into the preparation is advantageous, e.g. iodinated quinoline. Likewise, antibiotics such as fusidic acid may also be incorporated into the preparation. However, an allergic contact dermatitis may be caused by the antibiotics themselves. Unfortunately, the strong steroid used in combined preparations may mask such a reaction and may result in a delayed flare thereafter. Therefore, some clinicians prefer to administer antibiotics orally.

Exogenous eczema/dermatitis

Contact dermatitis

Contact dermatitis is a very important condition. When diagnosed, appropriate advice to the patient may have considerable effect on career or lifestyle. The two main types are irritant and allergic.

Irritant contact dermatitis. Normal skin is a highly efficient protective envelope capable of withstanding quite remarkable onslaughts. However, certain substances may overwhelm it, e.g. strong acids and alkalis. Contact with these will provoke an instant caustic burn, which may be described as an acute irritant dermatitis. Such a reaction occurs in all cases and is related to direct cell injury with immunological mechanisms taking no part, at least initially. When these substances are weakened, there will eventually be a stage when the skin can resist them and no reaction occurs. This point will be individual to the particular patient. Most patients with irritant dermatitis have been in contact with subtler substances than caustics. Common causative agents are degreasers, such as soaps, or detergents. Usually, the initial contact does not cause a reaction. However, over time, the skin's protective barriers diminish until the patient's threshold is reached and the disease is manifest. This is termed cumulative insult. The time taken in order to reach the threshold is infinitely variable. As a result, the patient is often confused not realizing the time scale involved. Patients will blame the eruption on a new substance in their environment and will discount the true cause since they have been in contact with this substance for 'a long time'.

The pattern of the dermatitis depends upon the area of contact, e.g. perspiration and occlusive footwear may localize the condition to the feet. The areas of dermatitis are themselves indistinguishable from those resulting from any other cause as is the histology.

Irritant dermatitis is an important diagnosis to make because it should be possible to clear this condition within a reasonably short time. When suitable avoidance can be undertaken, the prognosis should be good. For sufferers, potential irritants should be avoided or a physical barrier interposed. When this is not possible, barrier creams may be tried. Barrier creams can never be absolute and can only complement avoidance and physical protection. Regreasing the skin is advantageous. Simple non-perfumed creams should be used. Prompt treatment for irritant contact dermatitis is highly desirable in order to obviate the development of chronic eczema. In addition, skin damaged by irritants is more liable to allow entry to allergens with the subsequent development of allergic contact dermatitis. Treatment of the dermatitis reaction has been detailed earlier (see above).

Allergic contact dermatitis. Certain individuals are predestined to develop an allergy to a substance should they come into contact with it. Such a reaction may not occur at the first encounter; it may take many such contacts. Therefore, there is no way of predicting such a potential problem. Allergic contact dermatitis is not hereditary. Patch testing may be negative before the clinical problem is manifest. There are concerns that exposure to the allergen by testing may precipitate the condition. The allergens involved in allergic contact dermatitis are usually substances of low molecular weight. In the skin of the vulnerable individual, the allergen combines with normal tissue proteins in order to form antigens. Langerhans cells convey this allergen/antigen complex to the regional lymph node where a specific antibody is produced. The ability to produce this antibody is dependent upon T cells. The specific antibody circulates and when it encounters the original antigen complex, the ensuing reaction provokes allergic contact dermatitis. The entire process takes approximately 14 to 21 days and is therefore termed delayed hypersensitivity. The response relies on cell-mediated rather than humoral immunity. The process is known as **S**kin and **A**ssociated **L**ymphocyte (**T**) system (the SALT system) (Fig. 8.4).

When the reaction is over, a small reserve of memory cells remains and should the original complex, or one similar enough, return, these remaining T cells can multiply rapidly without the fabrication process in the lymphatic tissue and a more rapid clinical response takes place. Therefore, once sensitized, the patient remains so for life. Desensitization is impossible. Although allergic contact dermatitis becomes commoner with advancing age, children can also be affected.

Many factors lead to the unmasking of the innate sensitivity. The more prolonged the contact with the antigen, the more likely sensitivity is to develop. When the normal skin barrier is damaged, e.g. by irritant contact dermatitis, this predisposes to allergic contact dermatitis. It is important to ascertain the area first involved and to what might have been in contact with the skin. Usually, contact dermatitis starts at the area of contact. However, this area may be wider than first thought and in this situation is termed 'wandering contact' (Plate 5). Many substances may cause allergic contact dermatitis and it is good practice to try to identify the agent clinically, before progressing to specific patch testing.

The treatment for allergic contact dermatitis can start when the allergen is suspected as 'best guess' from the clinical history and examination. Treatment will become much more specific once the offending allergens are identified on patch testing. Avoiding contact with certain agents is easy but it may be virtually impossible with others, e.g. nickel. Furthermore, unless contact is prevented by avoidance or by the insertion of a suitable barrier, the problem will not be resolved.

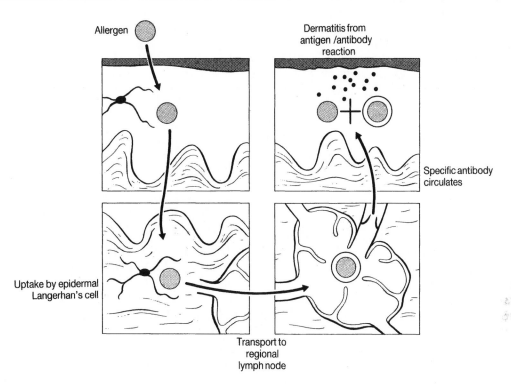

Allergen

Dermatitis from antigen /antibody reaction

Specific antibody circulates

Uptake by epidermal Langerhan's cell

Transport to regional lymph node

Figure 8.4   The skin and associated lymphocyte (T) system (the SALT system).

Endogenous eczema/dermatitis

Atopic eczema

Atopy is a common condition that is increasing in prevalence. Currently, approximately 3% of the population are affected. In many cases, it is more severe in children. The term atopy refers to a complex of problems of which the skin manifestations are only one although often the most prominent feature. A patient with atopy may suffer from asthma, hayfever, allergic conjunctivitis or from food allergies. The etiology of the condition is unknown. Many abnormalities have been uncovered but the whole picture is not yet complete. Food allergy may be a cause or may provoke exacerbations. Immunological abnormalities may be demonstrated in atopic eczema. An elevated level of immunoglobulin E (IgE) is a common finding. However, this may be a nonspecific feature. Cell-mediated immunity is diminished and clinical examples of this are seen in the lessened capacity to cope with many viral skin infections. Encounters with herpes simplex, warts, molluscum contagiosum and other viruses may result in extensive and severe disease.

The small blood vessels in the atopic patient demonstrate a tendency to constrict. This tendency may be secondary to the plethora of vasoactive substances whose proportions are upset in this condition. Firm stroking of normal skin should provoke a red raised line or weal. In the patient with atopic eczema, this line is white and is described as white dermographism. However, white dermographism may also occur in seborrheic eczema or in acute contact dermatitis.

Clinically, atopic eczema may begin at any age but is most common between 2 and 6 months. At this stage, it may be designated infantile eczema. However, there are other causes for dermatitis in infancy. Usually, the first sign is a weeping eczematous facial eruption although many variations are possible. The relative sparing of the napkin area may be helpful diagnostically. As the toddler approaches childhood, the distribution pattern tends to change, exhibiting a pronounced flexural predilection involving the wrists, the elbows, the knees, the ankles and the sides of the neck (Plate 6).

Many patients with atopic eczema have a dry scaly skin elsewhere, known as ichthyosis which spares the flexures which are the areas singled out by the eczema. There are several forms of ichthyosis and some can occur in the absence of atopic eczema. The form seen in atopic eczema resembles an autosomal dominant type. The ichthyosis has a very important bearing on atopic eczema; it is itchy and uncomfortable contributing to the patient's temperature intolerance. In conjunction with the ichthyosis, the child's palm is often dry and hyperlinear. In later life, this may contribute to dermatitis locating there. Similar changes may occur on the sole of the foot. An extra skin crease may be seen under the child's eye (Morgan–Dennie fold). This is due to skin edema. In many patients, the condition gradually settles in late childhood only to go through a spell of increased activity in the teens. Most cases, although certainly not all, clear in the late teens or early 20s. However, in certain patients, the first presentation is at this age.

The skin changes in atopic eczema may resemble those of any other eczema and the diagnosis relies on the history and pattern. However, certain differences do exist, e.g. the pruritus of atopic eczema is usually more intense than in other forms of dermatitis. The skin, especially around the flexures, can become thickened. The skin markings are more pronounced and are similar in appearance to tree bark. This is known as lichenification. Lichenification is highly characteristic of, although not unique to, atopic eczema.

The eczema, the ichthyosis and the pruritus with associated scratching all render the skin liable to secondary infection. Infection may trigger the eczema or vice versa. Although it does not cause the condition, stress plays a considerable part in the development of atopic eczema. Many exacerbations are related to periods of stress.

Management. Cotton clothing is more comfortable. Any aggravating features such as food allergies should be addressed. Liberal use of emollients reduces the need for topical steroids and prompt treatment of secondary infection is essential. Ointments containing preparations of mild tar may help lichenification. Oral histamines have their place in reducing any itch at night. Treatment of the inflamed skin is detailed elsewhere (see above).

Juvenile plantar dermatosis (forefoot eczema; atopic winter feet; glazed feet)

This condition is confined to children and its etiology is unknown. However, there is an increased incidence in patients with atopic eczema. Modern occlusive footwear may be implicated. Patch tests are generally negative for contact factors.

The clinical picture is usually characteristic and the synonyms describe many of the features. Typically, a child of up to 14 years presents with

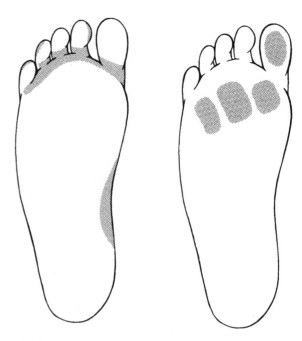

Figure 8.5 Differential diagnosis of tinea pedis and juvenile plantar dermatosis. Left, typical pattern for tinea pedis; right; typical pattern for juvenile plantar dermatosis.

a rash on the weightbearing area of the forefoot, sparing the instep, interdigital webs and the toe arches. The heel or entire sole of the foot may be involved. A pink shiny glazed appearance with scaling may be present. The flexibility of the skin may be lost resulting in fissures, which may bleed and be exquisitely tender. This may make walking impossible (Plate 7).

There may be a seasonal variation with worsening of the condition in winter. However, this finding is inconstant. Usually, the condition resolves spontaneously in the early-to-mid teens.

Many cases are diagnosed as tinea pedis (Fig. 8.5). However, it should be possible to separate these two conditions clinically. When there is doubt, appropriate specimens should be taken. Care should also be taken not to overlook the possibility of genuine allergic contact dermatitis.

Histological changes are unhelpful although there may be sweat gland occlusion. Treatment is unsatisfactory, but less occlusive footwear, thin cotton socks and cork insoles are all helpful. Emollients, when used liberally, may make the skin more supple. Topical steroids have little place in the treatment of juvenile plantar dermatosis.

Pompholyx

Pompholyx refers to eczema of the palms (cheiropompholyx) or soles (podopompholyx). Blisters are a feature of this condition. The exact cause is undefined but it may represent an eczematous reaction that is precipitated by a number of noxious stimuli. Vesicles tend to be prominent because of the hyperkeratosis that is normally found. In certain cases, there would appear to be a fairly good link between pompholyx and distant fungal infections. Associations with irritant contact dermatitis, allergic contact dermatitis, atopy or stress are less obvious. All cases seem to worsen in hot weather.

Clinically, a burning sensation is frequently followed by intensely itchy blisters which are usually small but which may coalesce to form large bullae. Pompholyx is characteristically bilateral and localized to the hyperkeratotic areas of the palms of the hands and the soles of the feet or along the sides of the digits. The vesicles may be deep and may be difficult to see. However, they may be felt deep in the tissue and likened to 'sago grains'. The vesicles progress to the surface, burst, crust and desquamate in approximately 2 weeks. The condition may spread to other areas and secondary infection may occur. Recurrent episodes of pompholyx are common.

Histology shows an eczema with vesicles surmounted by a thick keratin layer. In the management of pompholyx, any convincing precipitating factors should be treated. Dermatitis is dealt with in the conventional manner. Potassium permanganate footbaths may prevent secondary infection. The distressing pain of edematous hands or feet is alleviated by elevation of the appropriate limb.

Lichen simplex chronicus (neurodermatitis)

When lichenification occurs with no apparent initial skin disease, it is termed lichen simplex chronicus or neurodermatitis. Thickening or lichenification of the skin occurs in response to constant rubbing or to scratching. It may be secondary to any, usually itchy, skin condition, of which atopic eczema is a typical example. Rare in childhood, the skin is intensely itchy and the markings stand out like tree bark. Treatment consists of trying to break the itch/scratch cycle.

PSORIASIS

Psoriasis is common, affecting approximately 2% of the world's population. The etiology is unknown. However, the reduction from the normal 28 days progression from basal cell to keratin cell to only 3 to 4 days results in a parakeratotic scaly keratin layer. The thicker acanthotic epidermis is thinner over the rete ridges. The dilated capillaries of these rete ridges impart the red color to the affected skin. Polymorphonuclear leukocytes migrate into the epidermis as Munro microabscesses (Fig. 8.6). These changes may be triggered or modified by heredity, ultraviolet radiation, drugs and/or stress. Many changes are described in cellular immunity and mediators. However, it is yet unclear as to which is cause and which is effect. Psoriasis may first

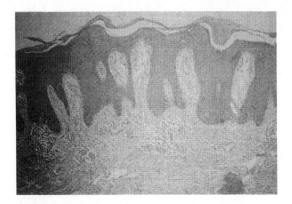

Figure 8.6 Histology of psoriasis.

appear at any age from early infancy to advanced years. The peak incidence is in the late teens or early 20s. The inheritance is autosomal dominant with incomplete penetrance.

Acute guttate psoriasis

Acute guttate psoriasis is the commonest type in the young and often follows a sore throat or other minor infection. Small red drop-like spots spread rapidly over the trunk and limbs. These spots are symptomless and subside in approximately 6 weeks, when they will either disappear or progress to plaque psoriasis.

Plaque psoriasis

Usually, psoriasis takes the form of red, scaly plaques with a predilection for the scalp, the knees, the elbows and/or the sacral region. However, any area may be affected. It occurs mainly on extensor surfaces and it is roughly symmetrical (Plate 8). A variant form affecting the flexor surfaces may be noticed by the podiatrist when nail folds or toe webs are involved. Another type, with a glove and stocking distribution, is more common in children. Psoriasis of palms and soles may be difficult to differentiate from eczema.

The individual psoriatic patches are round or oval, red and scaly. The scaling is silver colored and dry. The prime diagnostic feature is the clear demarcation of the plaque (compare with eczema). Light scraping accentuates the silvery color, the result of an increase of air under the scale, which then acts as a reflector. Surrounding the patches, there may be a white halo known as the 'ring of Woronoff'. Small bleeding points can be seen when the scales are torn off (Auspitz's sign). Such bleeding is the result of damage to the thinner areas of skin overlying the dilated capillaries in the rete ridges. In patients with active psoriasis, injury to the lower epidermis and upper dermis leads to the isomorphic or Koebner phenomenon. This phenomenon will appear in that area within 2 weeks. Diagnostically, such a result may be useful, but it occurs in certain other skin diseases and is therefore not unique to psoriasis.

The mucous membranes and nails of all patients with red scaly eruptions must always be examined. In psoriasis, the mucous membranes are not affected. However, nail changes are observed in about 50% of patients with psoriasis. Such changes may take the form of sharp pits in a linear distribution affecting one or more nails. This presentation is referred to as pepper-pot pitting or thimble nails and is pathognomonic of psoriasis. Another change that may be observed in the psoriatic nail is onycholysis. Commonly, this takes the form of a triangular separation at the distal lateral part of the nail plate. Subungular hyperkeratosis, discoloration or thickened crumbly nails may also be encountered. However, none of these changes is unique to psoriasis and so other conditions must be excluded.

Pustular psoriasis

Pustular psoriasis occurs when the Munro microabscesses are large enough to be seen by the naked eye. There are two forms, both of which are very rare in children:

1. *Localized.* This type mainly occurs on the palms of the hands but more especially on the soles of the feet where the instep is a common site. Crops of deep-seated pustules form on a reddish background, which, with time, mature to a golden brown color and then desquamate. This particular form of psoriasis is often misdiagnosed as a fungal disease.

2. *Generalized pustular psoriasis*. With this form of the disease, the patient is covered in pustules and is gravely ill.

Erythematous/exfoliative psoriasis

This is rare in children. The patient is red and scaly all over. The patient is very unwell and is at risk from infection, from fluid and electrolyte imbalance and from loss of temperature control.

Psoriatic arthritis (arthropathic psoriasis)

Arthritis ranging in severity from mild distal interphalangeal joint involvement to severe mutilating forms occurs in a minority of psoriatics (2%). However all are uncommon in childhood. Psoriatic nail changes in affected digits may help in the clinical diagnosis.

Management of psoriasis

Psoriasis is a disease that often brings misery and embarrassment to its sufferers. Psoriasis is a capricious disease and although chronic in nature, it has phases of inactivity and of flares. Commonly, there is no obvious reason for these. However, stress and infection may unmask or aggravate existing psoriasis. Treatment is tailored to the individual. The vast majority of patients and especially children are treated with topical therapy.

Acute guttate psoriasis. Acute guttate psoriasis tends to clear spontaneously and all that the patient may require is an explanation of the condition and perhaps an emollient such as a simple cream.

Plaque psoriasis. Although crude coal tar 1–10% in soft yellow paraffin for trunk and limbs or wood tar solution such as oil of Cade 6–12% emulsion for the scalp were traditional therapies, they are so messy that the modern patient is reluctant to use them. Cleaner extracted proprietary tars may be employed although these are often less effective. Salicylic acid 5% in white/yellow soft paraffin is keratolytic and therefore reduces patches. However, care must be taken in children in order to ensure that absorption does not lead to salicylism, especially in the smaller child. Anthralin (dithranol in UK) may cause staining when used in paste form. Modern short contact creams are cleaner and as effective and so are better. Calcipotriol is a vitamin D3 analogue, which is very clean and easy to use. However, it is not licenced for use in children.

Topical steroids have only a limited place in therapy where they should be confined to exposed areas and on the flexures. Despite being very effective in their more potent forms, side effects will limit usage.

Erythrodermatous/exfoliative psoriasis; pustular psoriasis. Severe forms require bland emollients and hospitalization. Localized pustular psoriasis is recalcitrant. However, any of the topical preparations already mentioned may be tried.

Nail psoriasis. Psoriatic nail dystrophy is a difficult condition to treat. The severity in the nail changes may fluctuate. Podiatry may help. Topical steroids are rarely effective. Occasionally, steroid injections into the nail matrix may improve the situation.

Systemic or secondline treatment. Since a high proportion of patients with psoriasis find that their condition improves when exposed to sunshine, ultraviolet light may be used for therapy. Natural sunlight has UVA and UVB, i.e. wavelengths of 280–320 nm for B; 320–400 nm for A. The ideal wavelength for psoriatic treatment is approximately 312 nm and this may be administered selectively using TL 01 fluorescent tubes. This form of therapy has largely superseded previous methods where a photosensitizer (Psoralen) was given plus a dose of UVA (PUVA). Long-term concerns regarding skin cancers largely preclude its use in children.

Oral drugs that are prescribed in an attempt to slow down the epidermal cell turnover are by their nature usually toxic. Methotrexate is usually the drug of choice; however, Acetretin, hydroxyurea and cyclosporin A have all been used. The use of such drugs in children would only be ethical in the most dire circumstances owing to potential complications later from immunomodulation such as malignancy.

NAILS

Anatomically, the nail plate is recessed into the lateral and posterior nail folds, the latter being sealed by the cuticle. The nail plate is composed of three layers: the upper layer formed from the dorsal matrix of the proximal end of the nail; the middle layer formed from the intermediate matrix, seen as the half-moon (lunula); and the ventral layer from the nail-bed matrix. Nail growth is affected by many factors; however, the normal toe nail will take approximately 9 months to grow 0.4 inch (1 cm). Finger nails grow three times faster than toe nails and all growth slows with age. Nail growth may be upset after severe illness. This may be seen as transverse indentations across several or all nails (Beau's lines).

Bacteria may invade the nail fold resulting in acute paronychia. The skin overlying the nail fold becomes swollen and 'bolstered' and occasionally beads of pus may be expressed. Ultimately, nail dystrophy with a transverse wavy nail plate develops. Treatment is aimed at drying out the nail fold. Hygroscopic antiseptic preparations are useful. The use of antibiotic/fungal creams is not too successful. However, oral antibiotics with or without surgical drainage may be tried. Elevation of the affected area alleviates pain. In chronic paronychia, the invading organisms change with *Candida* becoming the predominant pathogen.

Ingrown toe nails affecting the lateral nail lead to a paronychia that is especially painful. The abnormal nail plate presses into the fold and damages it, provoking the formation of granulation tissue. Parts of the edge of the nail plate fragment and shards are driven into the area. These shards must be removed and the nail prevented from gouging further by means of reducing its width or by correction of its curvature. Granulation tissue may be cauterized by copper sulfate or silver nitrate and any infection must be treated.

Trauma may also damage the nail. Acute injury that may lead to a subungual hematoma is commonly associated with acceleration or deceleration sports. In such presentations, the differential diagnosis is of a rapidly growing malignant melanoma. The hematoma may be confirmed when altered blood is demonstrated by puncturing the nail plate. Alternatively, it may be possible to gain access to the hematoma from under the distal end of the nail plate. Observation and accurate measurement in order to ascertain if the discoloration is progressing distally may be justified. When there is doubt, it is necessary to remove the nail and biopsy.

Nail biting, habit tics, ill-fitting footwear, certain hobbies or prolonged immersion in water variously lead to nail plate dystrophy, cuticle destruction or onycholysis. Long-standing periungual eczema may lead to cuticle loss. The nails may show pits which mimic those found in psoriasis, but these pits are larger and without the sharp edges found in psoriatic nails. There are many other nail dystrophies, some of which are associated with developmental abnormalities.

CONNECTIVE TISSUE DISEASE

Lupus erythematosus

Lupus erythematosus (LE) is of two types: the purely cutaneous or discoid LE (DLE) and the systemic form (SLE). Both are rare in childhood.

Systemic sclerosis

Systemic sclerosis is rare in childhood. There is usually a history of Raynaud's phenomenon in the hands.

Dermatomyositis

Although there are different causes of dermatomyositis, the cutaneous changes in each type, including the juvenile form, are broadly similar. There is much variation in the degree of skin and muscle involvement. Photosensitivity may be the presenting sign. The classic rash of dermatomyositis affects mainly the face and hands. There is a lilac heliotrope color on the face with edema, particularly of the upper eyelids. Frequently, periungular redness caused by capillary dilatation and ragged nail cuticles may be observed on the hands. Erythema over knuckles gradually extends in a linear pattern to the extensor tendons and over bony prominences. Less commonly, similar changes occur in the feet. A vague erythematous area may be noticed on the 'shawl' area of the trunk. Extruding subcutaneous calcium deposits are a problem, especially in childhood dermatomyositis. The skin histology is not helpful and may mimic that of lupus erythematosus. There is no specific treatment for dermatomyositis. However, symptomatic therapy may be required.

NEVI

A nevus is a developmental abnormality composed of bizarre non-malignant cells. However, certain cells have an increased tendency to transform to cancer. The commonest nevi in the skin affect the vasculature or the pigment-producing melanocyte cells.

Vascular nevi

The medical classification of telangiectasia, capillary and cavernous haemangiomas are used differently by different authors and this results in confusion. Therefore, it seems easier to employ the non-medical terminology.

1. *Salmon patch* relates to a small linear pink area. The occipital area is frequently affected (stork mark) which tends to persist whereas other involved areas tend to fade.
2. *A port-wine nevus* presents as a red area at birth which does not involute. The nevus increases in size proportionally to body size and then darkens to the well-known purplish or port-wine color. Initially, the skin texture is normal but nodules may develop. Very occasionally, there may be deeper angiomatous malformations, e.g. on the meninges, which lead to epilepsy. The histology shows capillary and cavernous vessels. Camouflage is the current best treatment. Modern lasers may be therapeutically helpful.
3. *Strawberry birth marks* are not usually visible at birth. At approximately 2 to 5 weeks, these

marks present and grow rapidly. Rarely do they exceed 2 inches (5 cm) in diameter. Their color varies from red to deep purple and their surface from smooth to puckered. Spontaneous involution after some years is usual and superadded infection and ulceration may hasten this. Histologically, there are thin-walled dilated blood vessels, which gradually obliterate with an increase in connective tissue stroma. Treatment should be expectant with firm reassurance to the parents.

Benign pigmented nevi (melanocytic nevi; moles)

At 12 weeks gestation, pigment-producing cells from the primitive neural crest migrate as melanoblasts, which reach the dermo-epidermal junction at 20 weeks. Certain of these melanoblasts appear to become 'stuck' at various points in this migration and these lead to various pigmented nevi. Certain nevi may develop from epidermal cells 'dropping back' into the dermis. Benign pigmented nevi or moles are common and numerous different classifications exist. It is easier to consider them as congenital or acquired.

Congenital

(1) Congenital pigmented nevi may not be present at birth but should be visible within the first few weeks. They may be subdivided by size into small (< 0.6 inches (1.5 cm)), medium (0.6–7.8 inches (1.5–20 cm)) or large (7.8 inches+ (20 cm+)). Any site may be involved. Mottled pigmentation may be seen with an outer irregular edge. Coarse hair may grow through the nevus. Once developed, congenital nevi persist. Generally the larger the nevus, the more likely there is to be malignant change. Histologically, smaller nevi tend to show aggregations of nevus cells in nests while the cells of larger nevi are more 'cloud-like'. The nevus cells have abundant cytoplasm and may contain melanin. Certain of them possess spindle-like cells and some epithelioid cells. Surgical treatment is not practical for larger nevi. Small nevi may be resectable

depending upon site but such cases are usually left until later childhood as there is little chance of malignancy. However, such lesions should be observed regularly preferably with photographic records.

Acquired

Acquired benign pigmented nevi develop in children, especially in teens and early adult life. Many such nevi disappear slowly with age. These nevus cells may be found in groups at the dermal–epidermal junction, hence the term 'junctional nevus'. When dermal nevus cells are also present, the term 'compound nevus' is used and when they are purely located in the deeper dermis, they are termed 'intradermal nevi'. Junctional nevi may show a uniform scattering of pigmentary stippling which is more easily seen with some magnification after coating the skin with some oil. Although any site may be involved, the soles of the feet, the palms of the hands and the genitalia are common sites. Compound and intradermal nevi show fairly homogenous pigmentation although the color fades in the older intradermal nevi. The edge should not be ragged. The compound and intradermal variety may be dome-shaped but the skin markings are not interrupted. Hair may grow through these, especially in the intradermal type. Histologically, nevus cells of various types are seen in the appropriate site. In the junctional nevi, pockets of cells are observed in this zone. In the deeper varieties, the nests of cells tend to transform into cords and the cells have less cytoplasm. In most cases, surgical removal is only required on account of constant trauma or when there is clinical doubt regarding the benign nature of the lesion.

Malignant melanoma

Very few pigmented lesions become malignant. Even fewer occur in childhood. However, there is an increase in reporting such lesions and to miss one, especially in a child, is a disaster. The increase in incidence may be related to sun exposure abuse, especially episodes of burning. Suspicious symptoms and signs would be complaints of itching, inflammation, bleeding and/or discharge unless there was a convincing history of recent trauma. Increase in size (> 0.39 inches (> 1 cm)) would cause concern as would an alteration in pigmentation with loss of homogeneity. An irregular edge would be ominous as would any abnormality of the skin surface. Malignant melanomas spread by horizontal or vertical paths. The latter have a much worse prognosis in respect of secondary metastases. Histologically, atypical melanocytes with bizarre nuclei and frequent mitoses are seen. The thickness is important in the prognosis and is classified by the pathologist who uses an absolute measurement (Breslow's thickness) or who may relate it to the depth level of other structures (Clark's levels).

Any pigmented lesion suspected of being a malignant melanoma should be assessed by an appropriate doctor as soon as possible.

FURTHER READING

Freedberg IM, Eissen AZ, Wolff K, et al, eds. Fitzpatrick's dermatology in general medicine, 5th ed. New York: McGraw–Hill; 1999.
Hunter JAA, Savin JA, Dahl MV. Clinical dermatology. 2nd ed. Oxford: Blackwell Science; 1995.

MacKie R. Clinical dermatology. 4th ed. Oxford: Oxford University Press; 1997.
Champion RH, Burton DA, Burns DA, et al, eds. Rook/Wilkinson/Ebling textbook of dermatology. 6th ed. Oxford: Blackwell Science; 1998.

SECTION 3

9

Radiological examination of the child's foot

Iain McCall

The standard radiograph has provided an easy and cost-effective method for assessing the foot. Most bone conditions may be diagnosed and the structural alignment and dynamics of the foot easily analyzed with these techniques. In recent years, there has been a number of technological advances which have increased the scope of investigation but which have not replaced the radiograph. Techniques such as computed tomography (CT) and magnetic resonance imaging (MRI) have increased the range of structures that can be imaged and in particular they allow visualization of muscles, tendons, nerves and arteries without the use of contrast agents. The gamma camera with emission computed tomography using [99M]technetium (Tc)-labeled bone-seeking compounds such as methylene diphosphonate (MDP) has provided a means of assessing the dynamics of bone turnover, which is sensitive if non-specific, and enables the identification of early lesions. However, the continued importance of the plain radiograph makes it pertinent that the first consideration should be the radiological investigation of the feet and assessment of the normal development and anatomical variants of development which have no pathological importance save to avoid the mistaken diagnosis of disease.

RADIOLOGICAL TECHNIQUE

The radiological examination of the ankle and foot requires a few standard views in order to demonstrate the major areas of interest, owing to the overlapping structures and multiplicity of normal variants. Routine views of the ankle include an anteroposterior (AP) and a lateral (see Figs 9.4 and 9.5), the former being undertaken with slight dorsiflexion of the ankle and pronation of the foot. In order to evaluate the entire ankle joint space and distal talofibular articulation, the ankle must be internally rotated by 15–20°. The talofibular joint is well demonstrated in this view. Oblique views taken at 45° of external and internal rotation may demonstrate the medial malleolus more clearly but the value is limited. Stress views of the ankle in the AP projection may occasionally demonstrate ligament laxity but comparison with the normal side is essential, as the range of normal is wide. Angulation over 20° or a difference of more than 5° between the two ankles is, however, invariably abnormal and some centers undertake injection of local anesthetic in the ligaments prior to stress views in order to obliterate any guarding effect caused by pain.

The exposure must be adequate to penetrate bone but not too great to blacken out the soft tissues. Demonstration of displacement of the soft tissue outline is of great importance in injury. The pre-Achilles tendon fat pad may be obliterated or displaced by hemorrhage following tears to the ligament or from calcaneal fractures. An ankle effusion is demonstrated by a bulging soft tissue mass displacing the fat line anteriorly and posteriorly.

Routine views of the foot include AP, lateral and oblique projections. The AP view requires two different exposures and centering points for the forefoot and rearfoot. The central beam is perpendicular to the plate for the forefoot but is angled 17° cephalad for the midfoot. The oblique view is performed with the patient supine, the knee flexed and internally rotated and the lateral aspect of the foot elevated 30° from the cassette. The central beam is perpendicular to the cassette and centered over the base of the third metatarsal. The lateral view is usually taken with the lateral aspect of the foot placed against the cassette. Both AP and lateral views may be obtained weightbearing which enhances structural changes that may not be detected on the non-weightbearing films (see Fig. 9.10). Axial views of the calcaneus involve the beam being angled 40° cranially to the cassette with the back of the heel resting on the cassette. This may also be undertaken with the patient weightbearing, standing on the cassette with the tube angled 45° axially, centered on the posterior ankle joint (see Fig. 9.13 A, B). The subtalar joints require specialized views because of their individual angle. The lateral oblique is performed with the limb rotated 60° from the lateral and on a 17° board wedge. The foot is dorsiflexed and the beam is centered 1 inch (2.54 cm) below the medial malleolus and angled 25° to the foot. This view shows the posterior and anterior joints well. The third view is the medial oblique, which has the lower limb rotated medially through 60° and placed on a 30° wedge. The beam is centered on the lateral malleolus and angled 10° cephalad. The sinus tarsus is best demonstrated on these views. The sesamoid bones may be seen on the AP and lateral views but tangential views may also be performed with the patient prone, the toes pushed upwards against the cassette and the beam tangential to the first metatarsal. Weightbearing tangential views of the rearfoot may be obtained with the patient standing in special radiolucent blocks (Coby's views). This demonstrates the line of weightbearing through the talus and calcaneus.

LINEAR TOMOGRAPHY

Linear tomography provides an image in a selected plane, while blurring out structures above and below that plane. Although it has proved highly valuable in the past and has been largely superseded by CT, it remains of value in defining the extent of tethering injury. Injuries and necrosis of the talus may also be well demonstrated and any subtle fracture may be evaluated by this method. Linear tomography is the best method of evaluating bone when metal is present in the foot. Tomograms in both the AP and lateral planes may be required.

COMPUTED TOMOGRAPHY

The anatomy of the foot in the axial plane may be demonstrated in great detail by CT which will also image sagittally and in the frontal plane. The technique involves a rotating X-ray source with an arc of X-ray detectors. The whole system rotates about the foot and the X-ray absorption over multiple projections is measured. The multitude of numbers translated into a gray scale is built up to produce an image which may be manipulated by varying the level and the gray scale, thus allowing both the bone and the soft tissue to be clearly delineated. The acquisition time is now fast and the detail excellent. The angle and position of the slice may be chosen from the scout film and the foot is positioned within the gantry according to the plane of the scan. The technique is particularly good for evaluating the subtalar joint and the rearfoot.[1]

SKELETAL SCINTIGRAPHY

Radioactive isotopes, which are used in imaging, produce gamma rays during their decay process. [99m]Tc is such an isotope and is particularly useful as the energy of the gamma rays is ideal for imaging in a gamma camera. It has a relatively short half-life and is easily produced. It also combines well with phosphonate compounds, e.g. MDP, which act as a transportation system to bone. Following intravenous injection of the [99M]TcMDP, the foot can be imaged immediately to identify the isotope in the blood vessels and within 3 minutes of the injection to demonstrate any increase in activity in the extracellular fluid which may indicate increased vascularity. After 3 hours, the isotope will have cleared from the soft tissue while remaining in bone (see Fig. 9.6). Thus any area that has localized increased blood flow or increased bone activity will show a higher uptake of isotope than the normal surrounding bone. This feature is highly sensitive and a normal bone scan will largely rule out a pathological bone abnormality. However, it does not identify specific disorders. Tumors, fractures, arthritis and infection may all be manifested by increased activity on both phases of the scans. Isotope scanning is particularly valuable in identifying the early lesions shortly after the onset of symptoms but before radiographic changes have manifested themselves. However, normal varia-tions do occur in children and in particular there is increased uptake at the normal growth plates (see Fig. 9.6). Greater specificity for the diagnosis of infection may be achieved using other isotopes such as [67]gallium or by labeling white blood cells with indium III. More recently, techniques to label white cells with [99M]Tc have also been developed. The cell-labeling studies are particularly valuable when infection is superimposed over trauma or after surgery.

ULTRASOUND

When a sonic beam is applied to a structure, the strength of the echo at the boundary of two substances is related to their different acoustic impedance. Bone and soft tissue have widely differing acoustic impedance so that almost all the sound is reflected. However, in the foot, the soft tissues are easily accessible and are superficial to the bone (see Fig. 9.18B). Sonography will therefore demonstrate tendons, muscles and ligaments,[2] and peritendinous fluid accumulation may be detected in cases of tendinitis. Fluid collections in abscesses may also be clearly defined and the ability to visualize structures in real time permits tendon movements to be studied. Its role in relation to MRI has yet to be fully evaluated but it has a major advantage in its low cost, ease of access and rapid examination time.

ARTHROGRAPHY

The cartilage outline in joints cannot be visualized on plain radiographs without the injection of water-soluble contrast medium, air or both. The injections into the joint are simple to perform and have been particularly valuable in assessing the ankle joint. Ligamentous injury around the joint may be demonstrated by leakage of contrast but should be performed as soon after injury as possible.[3] Injury to the lateral complex may also be confirmed by injecting contrast into the peroneal tendon sheath, which will flow into the joint. Connections from the ankle to the posterior subtalar joint and the flexor tendons are a normal variant and occur in 10% and 20% respectively.[4]

Arthrography of the subtalar joints by injecting the talonavicular joint may be valuable in differentiating normal from fibrous or cartilaginous coalition.

MAGNETIC RESONANCE IMAGING

This technique depends upon the intrinsic magnetism of the hydrogen proton and its response when affected by various magnetic fields. The hydrogen proton will alter its magnetic alignment when given energy in the form of a radiowave and will give back this energy in a similar way after removal of the stimulus. This is called relaxation and the density of the hydrogen protons and their differing speeds of relaxation with different tissues enable a detailed tissue image to be produced when analyzed by computer. Two types of relaxation are usually used in imaging. These are the spin-lattice or T1 relaxation and the spin-spin or T2 relaxation. The use of different pulse sequences which vary the time of pulse repetition and echo measurement, i.e. T1 or T2 weighting, will enable differing tissues to be highlighted (Fig. 9.1).

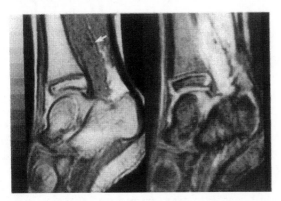

(A)   (B)

Figure 9.1 Hemangioma – MRI scan. (A) T1-weighted image, showing the bright signal of marrow and subcutaneous fat, the slow signal of ligaments, cortical bone and tendons and the intermediate signal of muscle. The low signal of phleboliths are demonstrated (arrow) and there is an accessory soleus in the pre-Achilles triangle. (B) T2-weighted image, showing the intermediate signal of marrow and muscle and the relatively higher signal of articular cartilage, owing to its increased water content. The very bright signal of the hemangioma is seen involving the soleus and accessory muscles.

The advantage of MRI is its ability to demonstrate tissues such as cartilage, ligaments and synovium which are not visible on X-rays and to identify tissue types and fluids more precisely. It is presently used for diagnosis of avascular necrosis and cartilage disorders, particularly of the talus, for tumors and vascular lesions of the foot and for ligament and tendon injuries. However, its role is constantly being evaluated and developed.

DEVELOPMENTAL SKELETAL ANATOMY

The bony skeleton develops from a cartilage template by means of enchondral ossification in primary diaphyseal centers with secondary centers appearing later at the bone ends in the epiphyses. Ossification of the diaphyses occurs early in fetal life but some primary and most secondary epiphyseal centers appear after birth. Fusion of these secondary centers occurs in the second decade.

The only tarsal bones consistently ossified at birth are the talus and calcaneus. The remainder begin to ossify early in the first decade (Fig. 9.2 A, B, C, D). Initially most of the bones are cartilage so that lucent spaces on the radiograph between the ossification centers are wide. The cartilage matrix of the partially ossified bone may, however, be demonstrated on MRI. The development of the ossification centers follows a reasonably predictable format and aging of the skeleton may be achieved by comparing the appearance against standard references (Fig. 9.2).[5]

Growth of the epiphyses and ossification centers in the tarsal bones may not always be sharply defined. Irregularity of the distal tibial and fibular growth plates is common and may contain small areas of ossification. These should not be confused with fractures or areas of infection. The rate of ossification may be irregular and this enhances the appearance of the abnormality.

The epiphysis of the calcaneus can often be irregular, fragmented and sclerotic, despite the fact that this is a normal finding. The calcaneus may develop from two ossification centers, sometimes mimicking a fracture, while overlap of

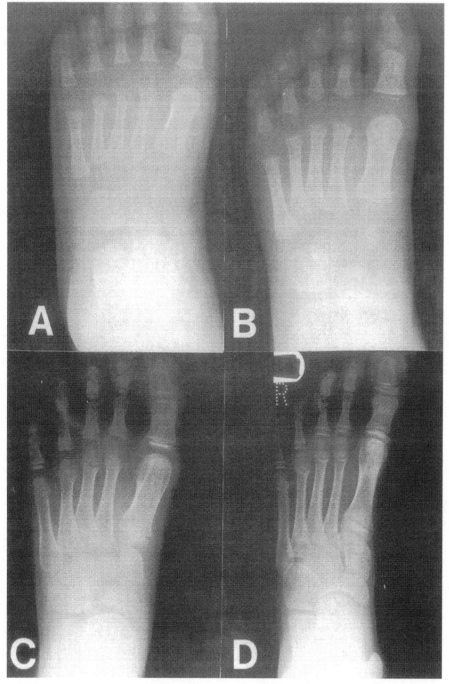

Figure 9.2 Normal development of the ossification centers of the foot at ages (A) 18 months, (B) 3 years, (C) 6 years and (D) 10 years.

epiphyseal lines or other adjacent bones may also cause confusion in cases of trauma. All tarsal bones may ossify in a very irregular fashion and these too may appear rather sclerotic, which in the case of the navicular may mimic osteonecrosis or Kohler's disease.

Conical epiphyseal ossification centers may be seen in the phalanges of asymptomatic children. These changes have been noted in 4–26% of children between 4 and 15 years of age and are usually bilateral and may fuse earlier than the normal epiphysis. Dysplastic splitting of the epiphysis or metaphyseal margin is not uncommon and has been noted more commonly in the distal phalanx of the great toe.[6] The epiphyses at the base of the proximal phalanx of the first toe may divide; it may also be sclerotic and develop as a

single ossification center and then develop a cleft (Fig. 9.3).[7] Incomplete developmental fissures may also be seen through the proximal phalanx of the first toe, distally and laterally. Similar fissures are seen in other toes.

Accessory ossification centers are common in the ankle and foot. Both medial and lateral malleoli may have centers at the distal tip and these must not be confused with avulsion fractures. These centers occur medially in 17–24% of females and up to 47% of males. Most are bilateral and commonly ossify between 6 and 12 years. The well-defined cortical margins and the lack of a sharp line between the two bones should enable an accurate diagnosis (Fig. 9.4).

The secondary ossification center of the talus is located posteriorly. It appears between 8 and

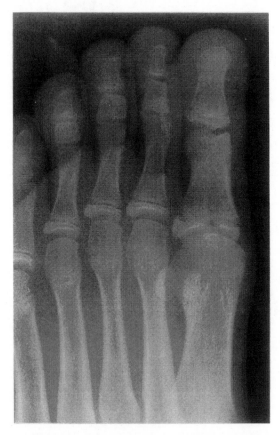

Figure 9.3   The ossification center of the base of the first proximal phalanx of the great toe is divided in the center. This may be misinterpreted as a fracture.

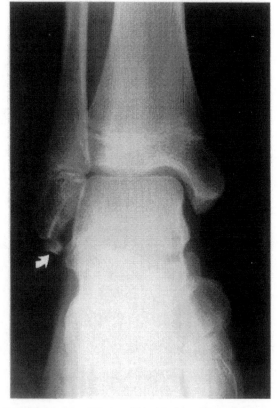

Figure 9.4   Os subfibulare. This AP view of the ankle shows the os subfibulare below the fibula (arrow) and is differentiated from a fracture by its complete cortication.

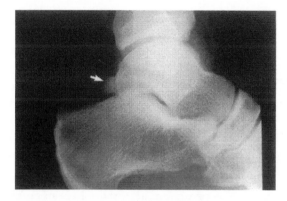

Figure 9.5 Os trigonum. The lateral view of the talus shows the persistent separation of the posterior talar ossification center (arrow).

11 years and normally fuses between 16 and 20 years. It is the posterior part of the talar tubercle and is located lateral to the flexor hallucis longus tendon. When it does not fuse, it is called the os trigonum and may separate in forced plantar flexion (Fig. 9.5). A small anterior os supratalare may also cause confusion with a fracture.

On the medial aspect of the navicular, an accessory ossicle develops in the tendon of tibialis posterior. It is usually situated slightly proximal to the main body of the navicular and may affect tendon function when growth is accelerated during puberty (Fig. 9.6A, B).[8] The os supranaviculare is located on the dorsal margin of the navicular, distal to the joint space; a substantial lump and pain may ensue. On isotope scanning,

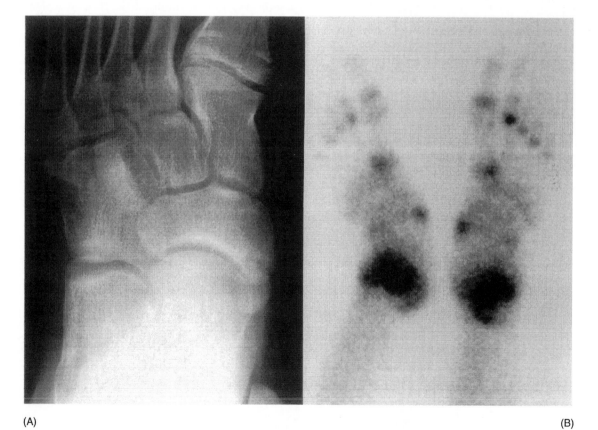

(A)   (B)

Figure 9.6 Accessory naviculi. (A) The well-defined ossicle is situated proximal and medial to the navicular. (B) The increased isotope activity is seen at the site of the accessory navicular. Normal activity is also seen at the ossifying epiphyseal plates. Abnormal activity is seen in the head of the right second metatarsal consistent with Freiberg's disease.

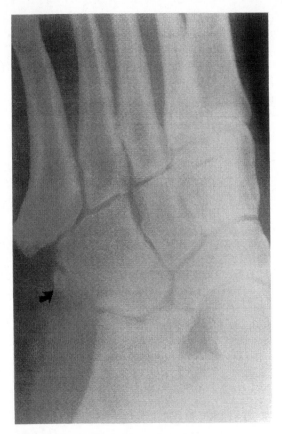

Figure 9.7 Os peroneum. This ossicle lies in the tendon of peroneus longus and is seen on the oblique view of the foot (arrow).

increased activity may be seen in cases of pain. This suggests a stress phenomenon and they must not be confused with an avulsion fracture (Fig. 9.6B). Accessory ossification centers are also found at the distal end of the first metatarsals, while duplication of ossification centers of metatarsal heads may occur. Os intermetatarsum is variable in size and shape, lying between the base of the first and second metatarsal. It may be bilateral, separate or attached.

Multiple sesamoid bones are present in the foot. The os peroneum is commonly seen on the inferolateral aspect of the cuboid, lying in the tendon of the peroneus longus, and may be multicentric and very large (Fig. 9.7). All the metatarsal heads may have sesamoids but the two of the first metatarsals are always present. However, their appearance may vary and bipartite or multipartite bones, some of which are sclerotic, are not uncommon.

The accessory ossification centers and sesamoids are summarized in Figure 9.8.

Other important lesions include the talar beak, which is a developmental variant and may be very large; projections of cortical bone from the surface may be seen in some tarsal bones.

Developmental calcaneal spurs may be seen in infants and will disappear by the age of 1 year.

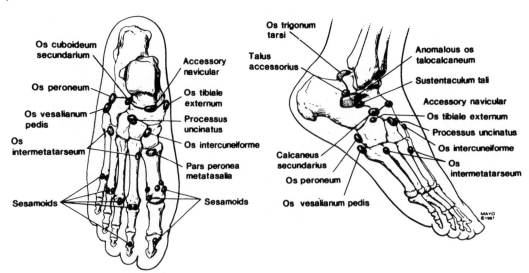

Figure 9.8 The accessory ossicles in the foot are demonstrated. (Reproduced from Berquist TH, Ehman RL, Richardson ML. Magnetic resonance of the musculoskeletal system. New York: Raven Press; 1987.)

Calcaneal cysts may be simulated by the normal arrangement of the trabecular pattern in the body of the calcaneus.

Finally spur-like enlargements of the distal phalanx of the great toe may mimic an osteochondroma but are a normal finding and are of no clinical significance.

ALIGNMENT OF THE FOOT

The talocalcaneal joints are the basis of the alignment of the rearfoot. In young children, the anatomical relationship of the talus and calcaneus is demonstrated on the AP and lateral views. Lines drawn along the longitudinal axis of these bones serve to identify their relationship. The lines are usually constructed through the midaxis of each rearfoot bone but when delineation of the bones is poor on the AP view, the medial cortex of the talus and the lateral cortex of the calcaneus may be utilized. The accuracy of these lines is also lost in the very young when the amount of ossification is limited, giving a different configuration from the mature bone. The normal angle in infants is between 30° and 50°[9] and there is a progressive decrease in the angle until the age of 5 years when it is between 15° and 30°. In the lateral projection, the midtalar–midcalcaneal angle does not change with age and ranges between 25° and 50° and is usually between 37° and 45°.[10]

The normal relationship of the talus and calcaneus may also be assessed by relating it to the metatarsals on the AP view. The midtarsal line passes through or just medial to the first metatarsal and the midcalcaneal line passes through the fourth or fifth metatarsal. Inversion or adduction does not significantly affect such relationships.

On the lateral view, the extension of the midaxial line of the talus aligns closely with the first metatarsal. In certain normal children under the age of 5 years and who have a relative degree of rearfoot valgus, the talar axis may pass medial to and below the first metatarsal on the two respective views.[9] The relationship between the rearfoot could be better made with the midfoot rather than the metatarsals but in infants and small children there is insufficient ossification on the

bones. However, the relationship of the navicular to the talus may be a valuable indication of malalignment in older children. In normal circumstances, it lies immediately anteriorly to the talus in both AP and lateral views.

The forefoot is quite flexible and its appearance may therefore change with weightbearing and non-weightbearing films. However, on the AP films, there is generally convergence and slight overlaps of the base of the metatarsals, while considerable superimposition is the norm for the lateral, where the first metatarsal is superior and the fifth inferiorly positioned.

Owing to the limited ossification of bones and the abundant plantar fat, the arch of the foot is difficult to assess in the infant. However, when pressure is applied, the angle between the calcaneus and fifth metatarsal is usually obtuse on the lateral. In the older child on standing films, an angle of 150–175° is usually seen.

ABNORMAL ALIGNMENT

Pure rearfoot malalignment at the subtalar joint results in altered relationship between the talus and the metatarsals but the relationship of the midfoot and forefoot to the calcaneus is maintained. The ankle mortise limits movement of the talus relative to the tibia and therefore the calcaneus moves relative to the talus.

REARFOOT VALGUS

With a rearfoot valgus, the calcaneus is displaced laterally in the axial plane, and on the AP view, there is an increase in the talocalcaneal angle, with abduction of the calcaneus (Fig. 9.9A, B). The midfoot and forefoot move laterally and as the talus is inhibited in axial movement by the ankle mortise, the longitudinal axis of the talus lies medial to the first metatarsal. If the navicular is ossified, it will lie lateral to the anterior surface of the talus. On the lateral weightbearing view, there is increased talar plantar flexion as the lateral movement of the calcaneus reduces support for the anterior talus. In severe cases, an almost vertical talus may be produced. In these circumstances, the normal longitudinal arch is

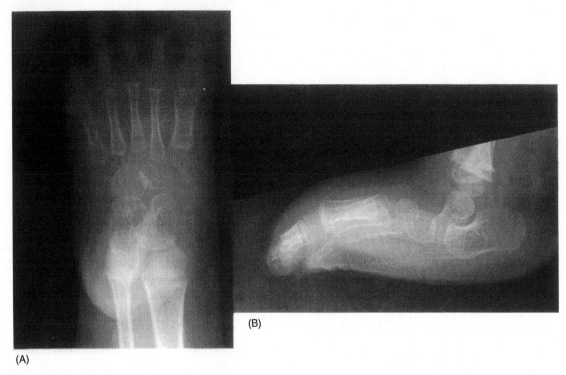

(A)

(B)

Figure 9.9   Congenital vertical talus. (A) On the AP view, the calcaneus is displaced laterally to the talus, although in this case the degree of rearfoot valgus is limited. (B) The lateral view shows the vertical talus. The navicular is not yet ossified.

lost. The navicular may descend with the talus or will dislocate dorsally and relate to the dorsum of the talus (Fig. 9.9B). Rearfoot valgus occurs in planovalgus, congenital vertical talus and neuromuscular abnormalities. Congenital vertical talus may be associated with chromosomal abnormalities, arthrogryposis or myelomeningoceles. It is more common in males and muscle imbalance is a prominent etiological factor.

REARFOOT VARUS

In a rearfoot varus, the calcaneus, the midfoot and the forefoot are displaced medially relative to the talus, in addition to the inversion of the calcaneus. The longitudinal axis of the talus is lateral to the first metatarsal and the talocalcaneal angle is decreased (Fig. 9.10A, B). The navicular projects medially to its normal position. The adduction of the calcaneus leads to dorsal angulation of the talus on the lateral view,

with the longitudinal axes of talus and calcaneus becoming parallel and more horizontal than normal (Fig. 9.9B). Rearfoot varus is commonly seen in congenital equinovarus and certain neuromuscular disorders.

Midfoot equinus is seen when the angle between the calcaneus and the tibia is greater than 90° and occurs in congenital equinovarus and vertical talus.

FOREFOOT ABNORMALITIES

Inversion and adduction of the forefoot combined is referred to as forefoot varus. Inversion is recognized on the lateral as a stepladder effect of the metatarsals and an increase in overlap on the AP views (see Fig. 9.10A, B). Medial deviation of the forefoot alone is seen in metatarsus adductus (Fig. 9.11), and inversion is added in congenital equinovarus. Forefoot valgus is a combination of eversion and forefoot adduction with the radio-

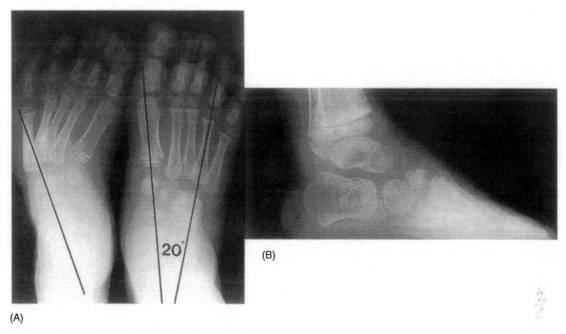

Figure 9.10   (A) Talipes equinovarus of the left foot. The talus and calcaneus are superimposed and the longitudinal axis of the talus is lateral to the first metatarsal. There is inversion and adduction of the forefoot. In comparison, the right foot is normal, with an angle between the talus and calcaneus and the longitudinal axis of each bone passing along the first and fourth metatarsals respectively. (B) The lateral view demonstrates the talus and calcaneus to be parallel to each other.

graphic signs being opposite and may be seen in congenital vertical talus and neuromuscular disorders.

Congenital equinovarus is a combination of forefoot adduction, rearfoot varus and rearfoot equinus. Medial subluxation of the navicular on the talus and a marked degree of inversion are generally present. On an AP radiograph, the talocalcaneal angle is decreased and the midtalar line lies lateral to the base of the first metatarsal. On the lateral view, the calcaneus is plantarflexed and the talus and calcaneus nearly parallel. Medial deviation of the forefoot is present on the AP view with a greater overlap of the metatarsal bases (see Fig. 9.10).

PES PLANUS

When the calcaneus does not maintain its normal dorsiflexion, the longitudinal arch is decreased and the angle between the inferior surface of the calcaneus and the axis of the fifth metatarsal is increased. Pes planus is present in planovalgus foot, tarsal coalition, spastic flatfoot and congenital calcaneovalgus foot. Flexible flatfoot is the most common form of rearfoot valgus. The midtalar line projects medial to the first metatarsal. However, there is normal dorsi- and plantarflexion of the foot.

PES CAVUS

Increased dorsiflexion of the calcaneus and an associated increased plantarflexion of the metatarsals produce an abnormally prominent longitudinal arch. Cavus may be associated with rearfoot valgus or varus and is a prominent feature of some neuromuscular abnormalities, particularly Charcot–Marie–Tooth disease.

TARSAL COALITION

This is a congenital condition in which varying degrees of union occur between two or more

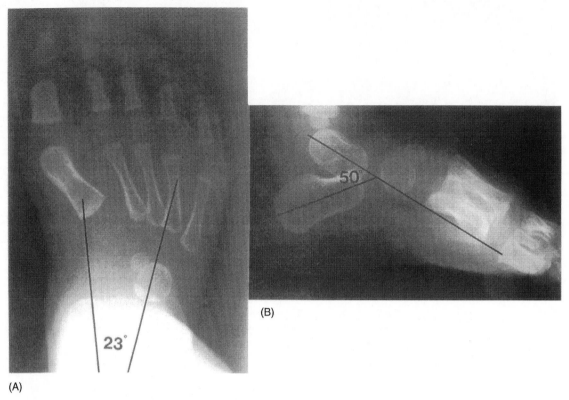

Figure 9.11 Metatarsus adductus. The relationship between the talus and calcaneus is normal, both in the AP (A) and the lateral (B) view. There is medial deviation of the forefoot.

tarsal bones. In the younger child, varying degrees of restriction of motion between involved tarsal bones may become apparent but the condition is not likely to become obvious until pain develops and this usually occurs between 8 and 12 years of age for calcaneonavicular coalition and during adolescence with talocalcaneal coalition. The increase in body weight and strenuous sporting activities may be responsible for the onset or the increase in pain in the subtalar or midtarsal region. Shortening of the peroneal muscles gradually occurs over the course of time resulting in restricted subtalar motion, rearfoot valgus deformity, abduction of the forefoot and tautness of the peroneal tendon, the so-called peroneal spastic flatfoot.

The overall incidence is probably less than 1% and the most common form is the medial talocalcaneal bridge (62%) with the calcaneonavicu-lar (29%) and posterior talocalcaneal bridge (4%) much less frequent.[11] Isolated fusions between other tarsal bones occur in a few cases. There is evidence to suggest that it is an inherited autosomal dominant disorder, with almost full penetration.

The radiological demonstration of tarsal coalition is dependent upon the site and upon whether the bridge is fibrocartilage or bone. Plain radiographs are of little value in the younger child, where much of the cartilage skeleton is unossified. However, in adolescence most lesions may be demonstrated on routine radiographic studies.

Calcaneonavicular coalition is best demonstrated on the 45° oblique views of the foot as there is tarsal bone overlap on the AP and lateral views. When the bridge is ossified, it completely obliterates the gap between the calcaneus and the

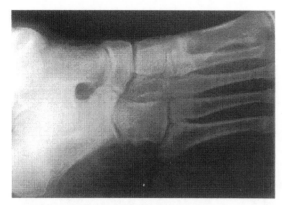

Figure 9.12 Calcaneonavicular coalition. There is a widening sclerosis and irregularity of the adjacent bone ends, with loss of the normal space between the calcaneus and navicular on the 45° oblique view.

navicular but when it is fibrous or cartilaginous, the anterior medial ends of the calcaneus may only be in close proximity to the navicular. In this situation, the contiguous surfaces are flattened and may be sclerotic and irregular, similar to a pseudoarthrosis (Fig. 9.12). Occasionally, the anterior process of the calcaneus may appear as a slender prolongation, owing to the presence of a cartilage bar.

Talocalcaneal coalition is more difficult to diagnose but medial coalition may be suspected from the lateral view when the sustentaculum tali is elongated and prominent because of bony thickening. However, confirmation of bony bridging may be demonstrated on the axial view of the calcaneus taken with good bone penetration (Fig. 9.13A, B). The angle of the axial view may vary between 30° and 45°, depending upon the plane of the sustentaculum tali. When the coalition is fibrous or cartilaginous, a radiolucent line is present along the joint but the margins are irregular and lack cortication. In addition, the plane may be inclined medially and downwards, in contrast to the horizontal position of the normal joint. When there is doubt about the status of the joint, a CT scan in the frontal and axial plane of the ankle and rearfoot will demonstrate the joint clearly (Fig. 9.13C, D).[12] The normal appearance is of well-corticated smooth subarticular bony margins, clearly separated by the normal articular cartilage. Complete bony bridging is well demonstrated and may be sclerotic. Fibrous or cartilage union may be more difficult to diagnose as there is a narrow space between the long surfaces. However, these surfaces will usually be irregular and less sclerotic.

Coalition of the posterior and anterior subtalar joints is uncommon. The former may be demonstrated on medial and lateral oblique axial projections. When doubt occurs, CT in the frontal plane to the ankle will demonstrate the joint clearly. The anterior joint is demonstrated on the oblique lateral dorsiplantar projection of the normal tarsus. In this view, the medial border of the foot is placed on the film with the sole tilted at 45° to the cassette. The tube is centered just below and anterior to the lateral malleolus.[13]

The restriction of movement between the talus, calcaneus, navicular or cuboid may result in other changes on the plain films and such changes may be best shown on the standing lateral. There may be beaking on the dorsal and lateral aspect of the head of the talus adjacent to an otherwise normal talocalcaneal joint (Fig. 9.13A), which may be due to impingement of the dorsal part of the navicular on the films during dorsiflexion. Narrowing of the posterior talocalcaneal joint space and broadening of the lateral process of the talus may also be seen as calcaneonavicular coalition. This may be associated with flattening of the undersurface of the neck of the talus.

When a fibrous coalition is suspected but doubt remains, arthrography of the subtalar joints either with air or contrast may be helpful. This is best combined with the plain films and CT. The contrast is injected into the talonavicular joint on its dorsal aspect and should outline the talocalcaneonavicular joint space. On the lateral view or on the frontal CT, contrast should be seen extending above the sustentaculum tali, which will not be seen in cases of coalition. The posterior and anterior compartments do not communicate but arthrographic demonstration of the former may be achieved through direct puncture from a medial approach although clinically this is rarely warranted.

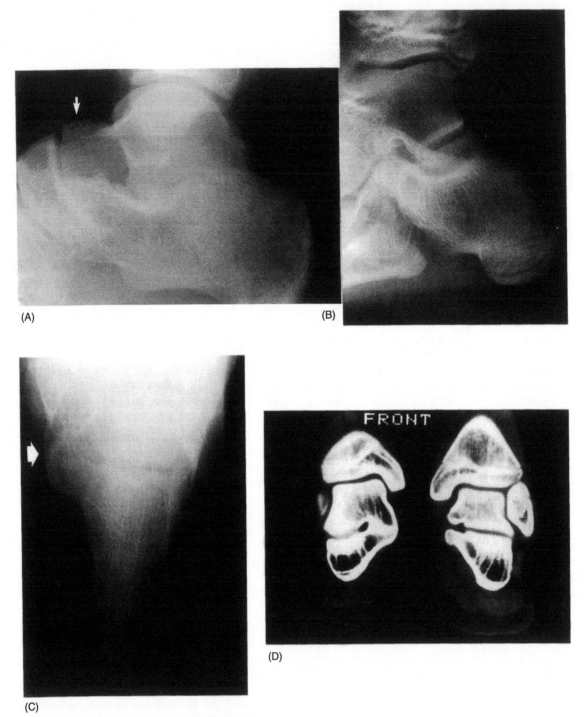

(A)

(B)

(C)

(D)

Figure 9.13   Talocalcaneal bar. The lateral (A) and lateral oblique (B) views show poor differentiation of the middle subtalar joints. Mild beaking is demonstrated in the anterosuperior aspect (arrow). (C) The axial view of the calcaneus shows bony bridging of the middle subtalar joint (arrow). (D) The coalition is confirmed by the CT scan. The normal side demonstrates a clear middle subtalar joint space.

The use of MRI in this condition has not been fully evaluated but the fibrous coalition, which is dark on T1- and T2-weighted images, can be differentiated from a narrow joint or osseous coalition.

INFLAMMATION

The most important inflammatory process to affect children is juvenile rheumatoid arthritis. It is a generalized disease and there are a number of variants, depending upon the extent of involvement and also the presence or absence of systemic manifestations (see Ch. 6). The feet and ankles are commonly involved in juvenile chronic arthritis. The plain radiographs will initially demonstrate increased density of periarticular soft tissues and displacement of the anterior fat lines around the ankle and of the periarticular fat lines around the metatarsophalangeal joints, owing to the presence of joint effusions and synovitis. Osteoporosis in the juxta-articular bone is another important early feature. Joint space narrowing and periarticular erosions are a late feature as the articular and epiphyseal cartilage of children is thick. Periosteal new bone is common in this condition and involves the small tubular bones of the feet. Such new bone is often thick and is seen early in the disease. Bone growth, maturation and epiphyseal fusion are accelerated. The epiphyses may be enlarged but longitudinal bone growth may be retarded because of the premature epiphyseal fusion. The most commonly affected joints are the ankle, proximal interphalangeal, metatarsophalangeal and intertarsal joints. Frequently, joint ankylosis occurs late in the disease and may be asymmetrical.

Ankylosing spondylitis may affect patients in their teens and although involvement is predominantly in the spine and in the sacroiliac joints, calcaneal changes are not uncommon. Fluffy erosive changes in association with osseous proliferation occur at the insertion of the Achilles tendon and plantar fascia on the calcaneus and radiographic changes may be seen around the metatarsal and interphalangeal joints.

INFECTION

Most frequently, pyogenic osteomyelitis occurs in infants and children and is three times more common in males than in females. It may be of hematogenous origin or it may be caused by external inoculation during puncture wounds. Hematogenous osteomyelitis most commonly affects the calcaneus with other tarsal bones less frequently involved. Clinically, there is pain and limp with soft tissue swelling and tenderness. In infants, vessels in the long bones extend through the growth plate into the epiphysis, whereas in children the vessels terminate in sinusoidal lakes in the metaphysis. This accounts for the higher incidence of epiphyseal and joint space involvement in infants with osteomyelitis and the higher susceptibility of the metaphysis in children. Early diagnosis is best achieved using ^{99M}TcMDP bone imaging, which will demonstrate a marked increase in uptake of isotope on both the early blood pool and late bone phase. Comparison with the asymptomatic joints is essential as increased uptake is seen in normal epiphyseal plates. The earliest radiographic change is swelling of the deep soft tissues, which displace the adjacent fat planes, and this is best seen on radiographs accomplished by reducing the kilovoltage across the X-ray tube. Radiographic changes in bone occur late with lytic areas, loss and distortion of trabecular pattern and periosteal new bone formation. The periosteum is more loosely attached in infants and infection therefore elevates and penetrates it more frequently. The degree of response also depends upon the type of bone affected. When adequate treatment regimens are instituted, such changes will resolve leaving a normal bone. When chronic infection develops, there will be areas of sclerosis and lucency in the bone, and sclerosis and distortion of the cortical surface. Areas of necrotic or dead bone (sequestra formation) may be demonstrated, which are more dense than the surrounding osteoporotic or hyperemic bone (Fig. 9.14).

Localized bone abscesses (Brodie's abscess) may occur, which are usually metaphyseal lucencies, with well-marginated dense surrounding

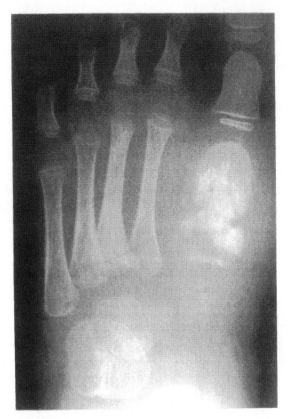

Figure 9.14 Chronic infection. There is considerable soft tissue swelling around the first metatarsal, which is sclerotic with areas of necrosis.

sclerosis. Central sequestra may be present and cortical involvement may produce considerable sclerotic reaction, not unlike an osteoid osteoma. CT will demonstrate the lucency and the central sequestra very effectively. Osteomyelitis, owing to *Salmonella* infection, often affects the diaphysis and may be associated with bone infection, particularly in a patient who has underlying hemopoietic disorders such as sickle cell anemia.

Tuberculous osteomyelitis may involve children of all ages although bone and joint involvement only occurs in 3–5% of patients with tuberculosis. When present, it is usually due to hematogenous spread to the metaphyseal region of the long bones in children.

The shafts of the metatarsals may show obvious layered periostitis, with multiple metatarsals being involved. Soft tissue swelling

of the foot is also a prominent feature. Congenital syphilis may produce similar bone changes but without the soft tissue swelling.[14] Circumscribed cystic lesions may also be demonstrated but these are rare in the foot.

Rubella and cytomegalic inclusion disease in neonates may present mild periosteal changes with mixed lucent and sclerotic changes in the metaphysis.

Infection of bone following fracture may be particularly difficult to appreciate because of the disuse osteoporosis and periosteal callus formation as part of the healing process. Serial radiographs will be necessary in order to identify a failure of the normal healing process and also isotope studies are frequently helpful.

CT is useful in order to demonstrate localized destruction of the tarsal bones and is also the most effective method of demonstrating sequestra in chronic osteomyelitis. MRI demonstrates infection as a dark area on T1-weighted images, while on T2 would be due to edema, contrasting with the bright signal of normal marrow and fat on T1-weighted images. Therefore, MRI demonstrates infection earlier than routine radiographs and identifies the extent of soft tissue involvement.

Differential diagnosis of infection includes Ewing's sarcoma. Differentiation may be difficult as this tumor produces a mixed lytic and sclerotic pattern, especially in the calcaneus and tarsal bones. Cystic lesions with eosinophilic granuloma may be seen and reaction to a foreign body and stress fracture may also cause confusion.

SEPTIC ARTHRITIS

Contamination of the joint may occur from the hematogenous route either by direct spread from soft tissue and adjacent bone or following trauma. Direct spread from adjacent osteomyelitis is more common in infants owing to the vascular supply across the growth plate.

Monoarticular involvement is common and initially the radiograph demonstrates periarticular swelling which is identified as a slight increase in density and by displacement of the pericapsular fat line and muscle planes. Some juxta-articular osteoporosis may be present in the early stages. As the infection progresses, destruction of cartilage occurs, leading to joint space narrowing and finally to bone destruction on either side of the joint. As with osteomyelitis, two-phase Tc bone scans will identify joint infection early. CT scanning is unlikely to add any specific information apart from demonstrating joint destruction in the tarsal bones in the later stages. However MRI will clearly identify the joint effusion as a bright signal within the joint on the T2-weighted images. Cartilage destruction may also be directly visualized. Aspiration of the joint and culture of the fluid is an urgent requirement for the treatment of septic arthritis.

OSTEOCHONDROSIS

Osteochondrosis or osteochondritis are terms that have been used for ischemic disorders of the epiphyses in children. Some of the conditions previously ascribed to this group are normal variations of ossification. This is the case for the changes seen in the calcaneal apophysis in Sever's disease. The apophysis is often sclerotic and fragmented, especially towards the end of the first decade of life and is of no significance as the apophysis develops normally.

Osteochondrosis involving the navicular (Kohler's disease) is more likely to be due to ischemia, although the etiology remains controversial. It is observed between the ages of 3 and 7 years and the appearances are of irregular ossifications and flattening of the bone although the space of the cartilage model is intact (Fig. 9.15A, B). It is difficult to differentiate from normal irregular ossification in the absence of symptoms of local pain, swelling and a decrease in movement, although the frequently unilateral nature of the disorder allows comparison with the normal foot. ^{99M}TcMDP bone scans are often equivocal as activity may vary from a low level to a significant increase over normal epiphyseal activity. The natural history is of bony reconstruction and a normal end result.

Collapse of the metatarsal heads associated with sclerosis is a further form of this condition. Originally described by Freiberg in 1914, it is thought to be due to ischemic necrosis secondary to repetitive trauma. The second metatarsal is most commonly involved, probably because of its greater length, but the changes in the third and fourth metatarsals are also seen. Symptoms occur most commonly in adolescence. Radiographically there is flattening and irregularity of the articular surface of the epiphysis of the

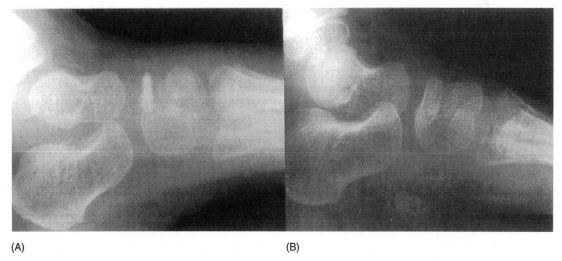

(A)   (B)

Figure 9.15 Kohler's disease. (A) The navicular is flattened and sclerotic and the apparent joint space is increased. (B) 15 months later, the bone growth has returned with the outline of the sclerotic bone still visible inside the new ossification. A small calcaneal spur is seen which is a normal developmental variant.

metatarsal heads and frequently there is a rim of sclerosis on the endosteal margins of the defect. Healing occurs with reconstitution of the sharp subchondral line but flattening of the head persists.

Osteochondrosis of the sesamoids of the first metatarsal may also occur and once more repeated trauma is probably an important etiological factor. Adult females are more commonly affected and sclerosis and irregularity of the sesamoid are seen radiographically. The isotope bone scan may show increased uptake.

DYSPLASIAS

A large number of dysplasias have been described and many will have involvement of the foot. It is inappropriate in this text to give a detailed account of all these conditions. However, there are a few important points that should be stressed.

Deformity and irregularity of a number of epiphyseal centers are most likely to be due to a dysplasia, with multiple epiphyseal dysplasia being the most likely condition, although similar epiphyseal changes may be seen in some of the mucopolysaccharidoses. Multiple epiphyseal dysplasia produces shortened long bones in the feet with irregular frayed metaphyses, small irregular epiphyses and widened epiphyseal plates (Fig. 9.16). The tarsal centers are small and irregular. After fusion, the metatarsals are short and the heads are widened and flattened. In spondyloepiphyseal dysplasia, the peripheral joints are less involved but talipes equinovarus or midfoot valgus may occur. In achondroplasia, the long bones of the foot are short and broad and in Morquio–Brailsford syndrome, the shortening of the metatarsals and phalanges is due to premature epiphyseal fusion but with normal modeling. Rocker-bottom deformity with vertical talus may be seen.

Ossification from multiple centers may be due to dysplastic epiphysealis punctatae but hypothyroidism should also be considered, especially with delayed maturation.

In osteopetrosis, the metaphyses of the metatarsals are expanded and osteosclerotic, without

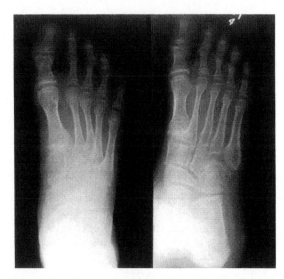

Figure 9.16 The epiphyses are widened, flattened and irregular and the metaphyses are splayed. The outline of the tarsal bone is more irregular than normal.

distinction between cortical and cancellous bone. A bone within a bone appearance may be present in the small bones of the feet and healing stress fracture may occur.

Osteopoikilosis also results in increased sclerosis but the sclerosis has a multiple spotted appearance in the bone ends. It is of no clinical significance and is very rare.

Overgrowth of the foot may be associated with vascular anomalies such as arteriovenous malformations and hemangiomas and also with neurofibromatosis. Hemihypertrophy has been reported in association with Wilms' tumors.

In Marfan syndrome, the feet are unusually long with joint laxity, which may produce pes planus. Talipes equinovarus has also been found.

Acromegaly produces overgrowth of bones and this is both in the length and width of the long bones. Cartilage thickness is also increased, leading to joint space widening, and increased skin thickness of the toes and heel pads is common.

Hypoplasia may be associated with central neurological defects or as a focal peripheral underdevelopment involving one or more sclerotomas. The thalidomide embryopathy is a well-known effect on the extremities.

Microdactyly of the first toe is an associated feature of myositis ossificans progressiva.

Osteogenesis imperfecta is characterized by thin osteoporotic bones with multiple fractures and shortening of bones as a result of healing fractures.

Abnormalities of bone modeling may be due to diaphyseal aclasia, which affects the ankle but rarely the foot. Multiple small exostoses of the distal tibia and fibula may deform the lower ends and may lead to poor formation of the ankle mortise. Ollier's disease produces irregular translucent areas in the metaphyses, with streaks of cartilage alternating with areas of increased density. The diaphysis is not usually extensively involved.

Fibrous dysplasia produces a lack of bone modeling with sclerosis. Bone maturation may be advanced.

In cleidocranial dysostosis, the main feature is short terminal phalanges with cone-shaped epiphysis and pseudoepiphyses.

NEOPLASM

Skeletal tumors of the foot are unusual and constitute only about 3% of primary bone tumors.[15] It is even more unusual for children's feet to be involved. However, all the recognized tumor types that affect children have been reported in feet. All imaging modalities have some value in the diagnosis and evaluation of bone tumors but the plain radiograph is usually the source of initial diagnosis. However, it is important to define the exact site and extent of any lesion and CT and MRI are particularly valuable in this regard. Distant extension and involvement are best assessed with bone-seeking isotopes.

Benign tumors

Osteochondroma is the most common benign tumor but despite this it is still unusual in the foot. It usually manifests in the second decade and may be associated with lesions elsewhere as multiple hereditary exostoses. The radiographic features are those of a peripheral bony projection with flaring or undertubulation of the affected

bone. The trabecular and cortical bone of the lesion is continuous with that of the bone of origin. The periphery of the lesion may be irregular in outline and some cartilaginous calcification may be present. Subungual exostoses are radiologically similar to osteochondroma and arise from the distal phalanx beneath the nail bed and have a predilection for the great toe. This probably represents reactive growth to trauma or pressure.

Osteoid osteoma is a highly cellular tumor of bone containing fibrovascular tissue, immature bone and osteoid, which may generate a vigorous osteoblastic host response. In the diaphysis of long bones, it produces a prominent periosteal reaction but in the bones of the foot it is more often intra-articular and the perifocal sclerotic reaction is not prominent. In these circumstances, there may be osteoporosis or osteosclerosis and the lesion may be more lucent. Epiphyseal enlargement may also occur. The lesions produce increased activity on both the early and late phases of ^{99M}Tc bone scan and may be identified visually with CT.[16]

Aneurysmal bone cyst is rare in the foot but has been found in the tarsals, metatarsals and phalanges. It is composed of cavernous blood-filled spaces with thin fibrous walls. The radiological appearances are of expansion of the bone by the lucent lesion, which has a well-defined endosteal margin and thin shell of bone on the outer

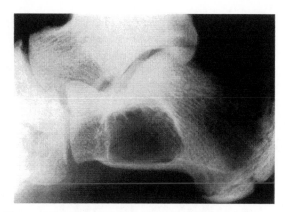

Figure 9.17 Simple bone cyst. A well-defined lucency is seen in the junction of anterior and mid-third of the calcaneus.

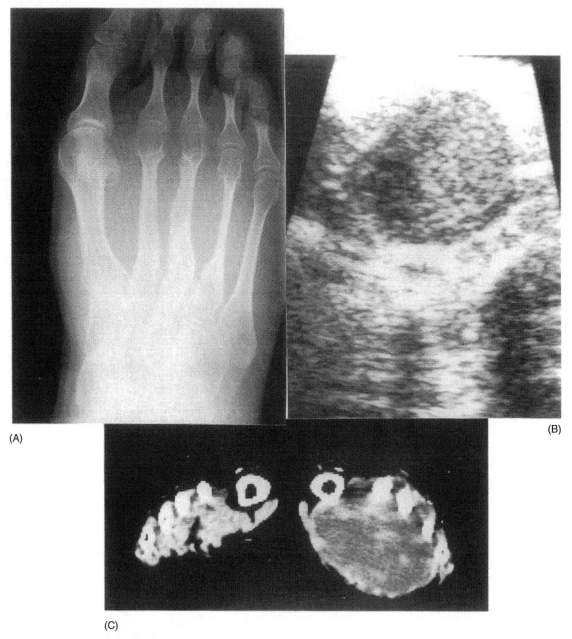

(A)

(B)

(C)

Figure 9.18 Soft tissue tumor. (A) The plain films show splaying of the metatarsals, with bony deformity owing to a soft tissue mass. (B) The ultrasound demonstrates the round mass, which is shown to be solid by the multiple bright echoes within it. (C) The normal and abnormal feet are compared, showing the large, substantially homogenous, soft tissue mass, which was proven to be a fibroma.

margin. Enlargement may lead to a break in the outer shell, with soft tissue extension.

Simple bone cyst occurs in the first two decades and in the foot the most common site is the calcaneus near the junction of the anterior and middle third. There is a well-defined, purely lytic lesion, with mild expansion of the cortex and fine trabeculation (Fig. 9.17). The cyst contains straw-colored fluid.

Enchondroma is a benign hypocellular neoplasm of cartilage, which is most commonly found in the phalanges when affecting the foot. They are intramedullary, expand the cortex and have well-defined margins. Punctate calcification may be seen within the lesion.

Chondroblastoma is a tumor of cartilage, which invariably involves an epiphysis or apophysis. Thus they occur in children but are rare in the foot. The bones affected in the foot are usually the talus and the calcaneus and the appearances are of a sharply marginated lucent expansile mass.

Malignant tumors

Osteosarcoma, although rare, is still the most common malignant tumor to affect the ankle and foot in childhood. It may be either osteolytic,

osteosclerotic or a combination of the two. Destruction of the cortex with an ill-defined endosteal margin is present. In the long bones, periosteal reaction is present and this may be partly destroyed by tumor extruding into the adjacent soft tissue.

Ewing's sarcoma is a highly malignant round cell tumor, which affects children and may affect the foot and ankle, with all bones being potential sites. The tumor produces a motheaten effect in bone, involving the diaphyses. Periosteal reaction may be a prominent feature but this is variable and a soft tissue mass is common.

Soft tissue tumors are often difficult to demonstrate on routine radiographs but soft tissues can be seen on CT and to greater advantage on MRI. Intravenous contrast enhancement may assist the demonstration of lesions in muscle in CT. Benign lesions tend to have sharp margins with a homogenous CT density and MR signal. Malignant lesions often have an ill-defined margin and a variable texture, owing to internal necrosis or hemorrhage. Local invasion or adjacent bone destruction is a feature of malignancy. Tumors that occur in children include lipoma, fibroma and hemangioma (Fig. 9.18).

REFERENCES

1. Solomon MA, Gilala LA, Oloff LM, et al. CT scanning of the foot and ankle 2. Clinical applications and a review of the literature. AJR Am J Roentgenol 1986;146:1204–1214.
2. Fornage BD. Achilles tendon ultrasound examination. Radiology 1986;159:759–764.
3. Olson RW. Ankle arthrography. Radiol Clin North Am 1981;19:255–268.
4. Freiberger RH, Kaye arthrography. New York: Appleton-Century-Crofts; 1979.
5. Hoerr NL, Pyle SJ, Francis CC. Radiographic atlas of skeletal development of foot and ankle. Springfield; Thomas: 1962.
6. Keats TE. An atlas of normal roentgen variants, 3rd ed. Chicago: Year Book Medical Publishers; 1984.
7. Harrison RB, Keats TE. Epiphyseal clefts. Skeletal Radiol J 1980;5:23–27.
8. Caffey J. Pediatric X-ray diagnosis. Chicago: Year Book Medical Publishers; 1978.
9. Templeton AW, McAlister WH, Zim ID. Standardization of terminology and evaluation of osseous relationships

in congenitally abnormal feet. AJR Am J Roentgenol 1965;92:374–381.
10. Vanderwilde R, Staheli LT, Chew DE, et al. Measurements on radiographs of the foot in normal infants and children. J Bone Joint Surg Am 1988;70A:407–415.
11. Harris RI. Retrospect-peroneal spastic flat foot (rigid valgus foot). J Bone Joint Surg 1965;47A:1657.
12. Deutsch AL, Resnick D, Campbell G. Computed tomography and bone scintigraphy in the evaluation of tarsal coalition. Radiology 1982;144:137–140.
13. Isherwood I. A radiological approach to the subtalar joint. J Bone Joint Surg 1961;43B:566.
14. Resnick D, Niwayama G. Diagnosis of bone and joint disorders. Philadelphia: WB Saunders; 1981.
15. Dahlin DC, Unni KK. Bone tumours: general aspects and data on 8,542 cases. Springfield: Thomas; 1986.
16. Cassar-Pullicino VN, McCall IW, Wan S. Intraarticular osteoid osteoma. Clin Radiol 1992;43:153–160.

10

Orthopedic conditions affecting the foot in childhood

Malcolm Macnicol (with a contribution by Peter Thomson)

Children rarely present to an orthopedic clinic with the complaint of deformity or weakness. It is pain, and perhaps problems with footwear, which usually prompt referral. Pain may arise from within the articulations and soft tissue of the foot, or as a result of direct compression, whether over the non-weightbearing areas owing to shoe pressure or from the sole and heel. As a surgeon, there may also be concern about the shape, flexibility and strength of the foot, but the primary clinical problem is pain and any associated tendency to limp.

ABNORMALITIES OF THE FOOT IN INFANCY

Flatfeet (pes planus)

The normal appearance of the foot is flat as the infant usually has appreciable ligament laxity and subcutaneous fat fills the medial arch. Indeed, if the foot does not tend to pronate and flatten when weightbearing during the first year or two of life, there may be an unacceptable degree of rigidity present. At birth, the foot may present with the relatively common calcaneovalgus deformity, which by definition is mobile and therefore correctable passively; or with the, fortunately rare, fixed flattening of convex pes valgus (vertical talus or rockerbottom foot).

Calcaneovalgus

This is considered to be a molding defect, with no underlying structural abnormality. The opposite foot may adopt a similar posture or may be held in a mirror image position (i.e. equinovarus). Many cases of calcaneovalgus resolve spontaneously. As the powerful calf muscles gain tone, the increased ankle dorsiflexion and reduced plantarflexion are reversed and the ankle regains a normal arc of movement in 3 to 6 months.

When the condition is associated with skeletal dysplasia such as the nail–patella syndrome[1] or neuromuscular weakness (including arthrogryposis and polio), the flexible deformity may persist. This is more likely if the peroneal tendons sublux anteriorly over the distal fibula, or if there is any evidence of stiffness.

Traditionally, the parents are encouraged to manipulate calcaneovalgus, stretching the foot into plantar flexion and inversion. When there is doubt about the flexibility of calcaneovalgus, a lateral, plantarflexed (Eyre-Brook/stress lateral) radiograph of the foot may be helpful in deciding which foot will spontaneously resolve and which will possibly require orthopedic care (Fig. 10.1).

Convex pes valgus (vertical talus)

The differentiating features of this deformity are its rigidity and the fact that the hindfoot is held in equinus, producing a 'vertical' talus. The fore-foot is dorsiflexed and the talonavicular joint is dislocated, with the navicular lying dorsal to the head of the talus. The severity of the deformity can be gauged by both the lateral, 'Eyre–Brook' radiograph and the degree of calcaneocuboid separation. Obviously, the more major this midfoot break, the more fixed will be the talar head. The medial arch appears convex because of the prominence of the head of the talus and the ankle and subtalar joints are rigid because of calf muscle contracture.

Etiology

Hamanishi[2] has pointed out that up to two-thirds of these feet are idiopathic, although a positive family history is often present; in the remainder, the baby may be found to have neural tube defects, cerebral palsy, malformation syndromes and chromosomal abnormalities. It is therefore important to investigate fully possible causes of congenital vertical talus, although this medical knowledge may not influence the surgical treatment required.

The surgical correction of convex pes valgus is difficult and the outcome is often disappointing. In milder forms of vertical talus, orthotic support may be all that is indicated. However, the rigid valgus and equinus position of the heel, and the prominence of the talar head medially, lead on to symptoms in later life although not necessarily sufficient to prevent an active career.

Surgical treatment

If surgical correction is considered appropriate, and it may have to be carried out bilaterally, the equinus should be reduced by posterior capsulotomies of the ankle and subtalar joints, coupled with a 0.4–0.8 inch (1–2 cm) step-cut lengthening of the Achilles tendon. The Cincinnati incision allows excellent exposure (see section on clubfoot release and Fig. 10.10) and a concurrent or staged correction of the midfoot dislocation is then undertaken. The dorsally dislocated navicular will need to be reduced between the talar head and the cuneiforms, and the midfoot capsular structures, including the spring liga-

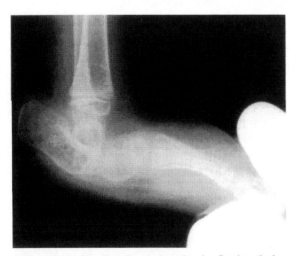

Figure 10.1 The Eyre-Brook view showing fixed vertical talus. (Eyre-Brook A. Congenital vertical talus. J Bone Joint Surg 1967; 49B:618–621.)

ment, carefully tightened. It is wise to stabilize the talonavicular joint with a longitudinal Kirschner (K) wire for 6 weeks, and this joint should be dynamically strengthened by attaching the tibialis anterior tendon to the talar neck and the tibialis posterior tendon to the undersurface of the talonavicular joint. If the peroneal tendons are subluxed, they will need to be realigned behind the distal fibula, or released, as they will otherwise bowstring and encourage the deformity to recur. Similarly, the extensor digitorum tendons often require to be lengthened or released completely. Plaster splintage is necessary for at least 3 months postoperatively, and the medial arch should be supported with an orthosis throughout childhood.

Surgical correction of the foot in the first year of life offers the best prospect of establishing a medial arch and improved foot mobility. However, underlying muscle weakness will militate against a long-term complete correction of the condition.

Structural flatfoot in childhood

When assessing the pronated foot in later childhood, it is useful to classify it as follows:

1. mobile
   a. postural
   b. structural
2. rigid.

Mobile or flexible flatfoot may be differentiated from the rigid type by observing if the medial arch elevates on tiptoe walking or during the Jack test (Fig. 10.2). The mobile flatfoot may be considered postural or structural. The postural flatfoot may be associated with intoeing and knock-knees and is a product of flexibility leading to compensation. The structural flatfoot is often associated with a neurological abnormality. Unlike the rigid foot, the subtalar joint in the structural flatfoot is mobile, at least during childhood.

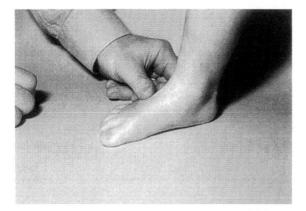 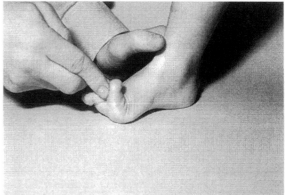

Figure 10.2 The 'Jack test' differentiates postural from mobile, structural flat foot. Dorsiflexion of the big toe creates tension in the plantar fascia which pulls on the calcaneus. The reaction to this tension is compression through the line of the first ray. In the structurally normal foot, these forces effect a rise in medial longitudinal arch because of plantarflexion of the first ray and supination of the subtalar joint. Absence of calcaneal supination may be due to abnormal subtalar joint structure.

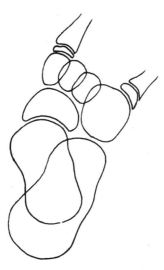

Figure 10.3 Increased talocalcaneal divarication is seen in flatfeet.

Shoe adjustments such as inner flares, medial arch supports or heel cups may offer comfort and improve gait, but will not change the natural history of the developing foot or the eventual height of the medial arch. The non-surgical management of the mobile flatfoot is discussed elsewhere (see Ch. 12).

Surgical management of the mobile flatfoot

In the child with paralytic weakness or congenital hypotonia, pronation becomes severe and the heel valgus leads to significant medial heel wear and distortion of the shoe uppers. The altered subtalar dynamics, with increase in the talocalcaneal divarication (Fig. 10.3), lead to pain and lack of agility so that a subtalar fusion may be required. Classically, this was effected by an extra-articular strut graft, using a segment of the fibula to prop apart the talus and calcaneum in the sinus tarsi laterally. Morbidity from harvesting the fibula has led to the insertion of artificial, inert 'posts' instead, although these have limited application and should certainly not be used before mid- to late childhood.

An alternative procedure uses a screw to support the calcaneum in the correct position under the talus, driving the screw down from the dorsal aspect of the talar neck into the calcaneum with the hindfoot in neutral.[4] Bone grafting is inserted in the older child so that a limited subtalar arthrodesis results. The chronic rigidity of the subtalar joint may produce a 'ball and socket' ankle joint, since an increased degree of accommodative tilting now occurs at the talocrural joint. Midfoot pain and talonavicular sag will also develop with time. Now that well-tailored ankle–foot orthoses (AFOs) are available, surgical intervention for the neurologically deficient foot is less necessary, and associated deformities such as progressive valgus of the hallux and overlapping of the lesser toes can be minimized.

Rigid flatfoot

Rigid flatfoot is fortunately rare. It used to be recognized quite frequently as 'spasmic' or 'spasmodic' flatfoot. The cause of the peroneal spasm is attributed to an irritative lesion of the subtalar joint, such as an intra-articular calcaneal fracture, rheumatoid or infective arthropathy or tumor. Before the days of accurate radiography and computed tomography (CT) or magnetic resonance imaging (MRI), it was often difficult to identify abnormalities, but it is now clear that many of these feet became rigid and painful because a tarsal coalition is present.

Tarsal coalition

The presence of subtalar stiffness should be confirmed by assessing the inversion and eversion of the heel, with the knee flexed and the foot in neutral dorsiflexion, and then the rotation of the forefoot and midfoot upon the hindfoot. The heel should be steadied with one hand and the movement at the talonavicular joint gauged with the other hand, comparing the two feet. The most common coalition is calcaneonavicular (Fig. 10.4), and excision of the bar is usually effective if undertaken in early adolescence before symptoms and adaptive changes become established. It should be remembered that the 'coalition' is due to a failure of the tarsal mesodermal mass to segment properly, and that other abnormalities of the articulations in the hindfoot may be present.

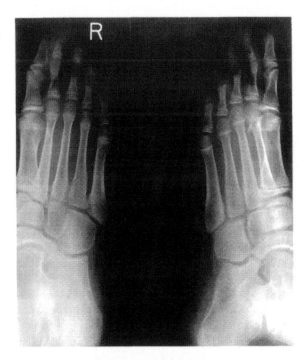

Figure 10.4 The calcaneonavicular coalition is best seen on an oblique radiograph of the foot.

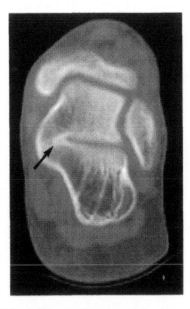

Figure 10.5 A CT scan shows up a talocalcaneal (sustentacular) bar.

The next most common coalition is the talocalcaneal, or sustentacular, bar (Fig. 10.5). If this involves no more than the middle facet of the calcaneum, excision may improve function in two-thirds of cases.[5] However, the principal reason to excise the talocalcaneal bar is to correct fixed valgus or varus of the heel. Since this is a rare deformity, the coalition is best managed conservatively, as are most of the lesser coalitions between other tarsal bones. Mobility is never restored completely after excision, and pain may arise from sites distant to the coalition.

The long-term results following excision of the calcaneonavicular bar are satisfactory, provided that the initial response is good. If excision fails to relieve symptoms, there is no place for a repeated excision as the end result does not improve.[6] A triple arthrodesis in later adolescence may be required in a few cases if pain is persistent, but rigidity of the hindfoot inevitably leads to osteoarthritis of the midtarsal region.

The symptomatic accessory navicular

Another form of structural flatfoot may be encountered when the accessory navicular is symptomatic. In later childhood, either because of pressure from the shoe or due to stress between the accessory and main navicular, pain develops over the instep which is characteristically tender and enlarged medially. Occasionally, a 'foot sprain' is recalled although this is probably coincidental. The type 1 accessory bone is an oval ossicle within the substance of the tibialis posterior tendon whereas the type 2 constitutes a larger, pyramidal or rectangular fragment, joined to the parent navicular by a synchondrosis.

If the pain persists despite orthoses, physical therapy and shoe adjustment, excision of the accessory navicular is indicated.[7] All this seeks to achieve is a recontouring of the prominence medially, and removal of the pseudarthrosis between the two components of the navicular. More elaborate re-routing of the tibialis posterior tendon (the Kidner procedure) is not warranted as the results of simple excision are just as good. As the accessory navicular is hereditary, the parents and the patient's siblings may present with similar lumps, but may be completely asymptomatic.

Os trigonum

The accessory navicular (os tibiale externum) is only one of a number of accessory ossicles of the foot. Most of them remain undetected and are incidental findings when the foot is X-rayed for other reasons. The os trigonum develops at the posteromedial border of the talus in 5–10% of the population. Usually, the ossicle fuses to the talus and forms part of the groove for the tendon of flexor hallucis longus. Fracture of the spur formed by the os trigonum will cause local tenderness and limited plantarflexion. The lesion is relatively common in footballers and usually symptoms after injury settle conservatively.

Os vesalii and fifth metatarsal fracture

The os vesalii is a source of confusion as it is positioned at the tip of the styloid process of the fifth metatarsal where it may be mistaken for a secondary center of ossification at the base of that bone or an avulsion fracture of the insertion of the peroneus brevis tendon (the so-called 'dancer's fracture'). A more distal fracture of the proximal shaft (Jones fracture), between the mobile distal and fixed proximal segments of the fifth metatarsal, is rare in childhood. In the adult, particularly in athletes, the fracture may develop a non-union and require bone grafting and screw fixation.

JUVENILE OSTEOCHONDROSES

Sever's disease

Sever's disease, a traction apophysitis of the calcaneus, is a problem of later childhood and most commonly affects boys between 10 and 12 years. The condition is characterized by posterior and plantar heel pain. Initially, the pain is a low-grade, dull ache which typically occurs on activity after rest (post-static dyskinesia) or after prolonged exercise. The pain may be produced by palpation or by contraction of the calf muscle against resis-

tance. In many instances, the low-grade pain persists for weeks or months before gradually fading. However, in certain patients, it may become severe and disabling and can have a considerable effect on mobility, particularly on high-stress activity such as games, climbing stairs or walking uphill. Here the gait is limping on tiptoe and protective supination is a frequent accompaniment. Limping is often intermittent and its absence may lead to accusations of hypochondria from teachers, peers and family. Therefore, its diagnosis may prove a relief.

Radiologically, the apophysis may appear fragmented and of irregular density but findings in symptomatic and asymptomatic feet may be very similar. Hence the diagnosis is clinical and the cause is probably frequent microtrauma, caused by compression or to traction by a tight Achilles tendon, associated with excessive subtalar joint pronation.

Treatment should aim to relieve Achilles tendon tension and is usually carried out by calf-stretching exercises and the use of a soft (closed-cell rubber or felt) heel raise. Where pronation is a likely cause, antipronatory orthoses should be used. The use of corticosteroids, short-wave diathermy or ultrasound is discouraged as these may influence growth. Complete immobilization with plaster casting is rarely necessary but may be used as a last resort when symptoms are severe.

Osteochondrosis of the navicular

Kohler's disease is a rare, compression osteochondrosis in which the navicular becomes flattened and irregular. Radiological investigation may detect patches of sclerosis and rarefaction.

The peak incidence is among 4-year-old girls and 5-year-old boys. Four out of five cases are found in boys. The problem is symptomatic in approximately one-third of cases with tenderness and possible swelling over the navicular. Inflammation may be noted at the insertion of the posterior tibial tendon. There may be a marked limp but normally there is no loss of motion and passive movement causes little or no discomfort.

The cause is probably compression owing to repeated microtrauma. This compression traumatizes the ossification center of the navicular, restricting the vascular supply and thus producing a crushing aseptic necrosis in the affected area.

Usually pain is exercise-induced so that a supportive in-shoe orthosis is a useful and effective therapy. When the condition is more painful, it may be necessary to immobilize with a walking plaster or to discourage all weightbearing for 2 to 3 weeks. During the healing period (6 to 8 weeks), strenuous activity should be discouraged although this may not prove easy in an active 4- or 5-year-old. Treatment appears to have little bearing on prognosis which is excellent and should therefore be aimed at providing maximum comfort.

Freiberg's infraction

This condition is a relatively common crushing osteochondrosis which is observed mainly in adolescents (peak incidence between 12 and 14 years). Occasionally, active adults may be affected and here the condition is related to trauma. The second metatarsal head is most frequently involved, but the third and fourth may also be affected; 75% of cases are female.

Classically described as an avascular necrosis, recent work using bone scintigraphy[8] supports the idea of an infraction occurring in the early stages of the disease process. The origin of such an infraction is often related to identifiable trauma, but in certain cases it is likely that focal ischemia could result from repeated microtrauma such as stubbing the toe.

Pain is localized to the enlarged second metatarsal head during walking, on tiptoeing and on palpation. The discomfort will frequently fade without treatment, but when there is flattening of the articular surface, it may persist into adulthood as osteoarthritis develops. Radiographs may show thickening, patchy rarefaction and the presence of loose bodies.

Treatment is by means of rest and the provision of a metatarsal bar. Where there is a functional problem, orthoses may help. In persistent cases, the affected metatarsal head is elevated by an extension of the neck of the metatarsal, or by excision of the deformed head. Prognosis is uncertain since many patients with apparently resolved juvenile Freiberg's infraction do not develop osteoarthritis in adulthood. Adults with traumatic Freiberg's infraction tend to develop osteoarthritis as part of the disease process.

Osteochondritis of the talus

Osteochondritis of the talus accounts for around 4% of all cases of osteochondritis. Causation is generally traumatic and is brought about by compression of the talar dome associated with plantarflexion or inversion. Frequently, detection is difficult although modern scanning techniques may help to overcome this. The investigating clinician should ensure that the talar dome is not overlooked in traumatic disruption of the ankle while searching for a more common fracture.

Classification is in four stages of an increasing severity:

- Stage I involves chondral and subchondral damage as the lateral side of the talar dome is compressed against the fibula.
- Stage II involves rupture of the lateral ligaments of the ankle joint, a small degree of subluxation of the ankle and displacement of the osteochondral fragment.
- Stage III involves complete detachment of the fragment.
- Stage IV may see the rotation of the fragment within the joint.

Prognosis is good when the condition is treated early but relatively poor when types II, III and IV are subject to delayed therapy. Arthroscopy makes removal of fragments reasonably straightforward although its long-term effectiveness has yet to be established.

Such fragments should be removed early, particularly when displacement or complete fracture has occurred. Failure to remove fragments may cause further damage and may lead to degeneration of the ankle joint. Generally, treated areas heal well.

Osteochondritis dissecans of the talus

This is a relatively common condition in adolescents. In the foot, trauma may consist of a single major episode, or from a series of microtraumata such as may result from ankle instability or from a change in activity.

Typically, the articular surface or a small area of it becomes avascular. Overlying cartilage becomes softened and there is usually a small fragment of subchondral bone which becomes either fully detached or remains attached by soft tissue. Where complete separation has occurred, this fragment may float around in the joint capsule thus acting as an irritant. Incomplete separation may result in re-adhesion or in detachment. Detachment leaves a roughened, pitted articular surface which eventually remodels. Frequently, the result is a smooth but flattened articular surface and a loss of full movement. Even when this is not apparent in the short term, osteoarthritic changes are common in the long term. In addition to the superior surface of the body of the talus, the first metatarsophalangeal joint may develop a lesion over the metatarsal head, producing hallux rigidus.

The rare forms of osteochondritis are described briefly:

Osteochondritis of the cuneiforms (Buschke's disease) is similar to Kohler's disease. Features include irregular cortical outline and an occasional limp. Duration is around 3 to 4 months.

Osteochondritis of the fifth metatarsal base (Iselin's disease). This condition is a traction apophysitis brought about by repeated trauma and is observed in active children and adolescents, particularly boys. It should be differentiated from fracture (see dancer's fracture) by X-ray. Treatment is by the use of orthoses in order to reduce stress.

DEFORMITIES OF THE TOES

In infancy, the most common toe deformities are bifid toes (particularly the hallux), polydactyly and macrodactyly, and the overlapping fifth toe (digiti quinti varus). A variety of skeletal abnormalities may affect the foot and these are classified as follows:

Terminal transverse
i.   Amelia of the lower limb
ii. Hemimelia of the lower limb
iii. Apodia
iv. Complete adactylia
v.   Complete aphalangia.

Terminal longitudinal
i.   Complete paraxial hemimelia – absence of part of the leg and foot
ii. Incomplete paraxial hemimelia – as above with part of the tibia or fibula present
iii. Partial adactylia – absence of one or more rays of the foot
iv. Partial aphalangia – absence of one or more phalanges of the foot.

Intercalary transverse
i.   Complete phocomelia – in which the foot is attached to the trunk
ii. Proximal phocomelia – in which the foot and lower leg are attached to the trunk
iii. Distal phocomelia – in which the foot is attached directly to the thigh.

Intercalary longitudinal
i.   Complete paraxial hemimelia – as in terminal longitudinal, but the foot is more or less complete
ii. Incomplete paraxial hemimelia – similar also to terminal longitudinal but the foot is also more or less complete
iii. Partial adactylia – absence of proximal or middle digits
iv. Partial aphalangia – absence of proximal or middle phalanges.

Many deformities are functional so that surgical treatment can often be avoided. The principal objective of operations is to ensure that shoe fitment is comfortable and that the toes should flex and extend painlessly. Even extreme deformities such as lobster claw foot, which is often familial, allow normal, asymptomatic walking providing the shoes can be adapted. When predicted shortening of the limb is less than 4 inches (10 cm), leg-lengthening procedures are appropriate, although subsequent ankle and foot function may be compromised. For greater discrepancies, the fitment of an artificial limb (sometimes combined with amputation of the foot) is all that can be offered surgically.

Curly toe

The most common reasons for referring younger children are overlapping (curly) toes, partial or complete syndactyly and the varus little toe. Provided curly toes are mobile with no evidence of skin blistering or nail deformity, the parents should be reassured since the lesser toe overlapping rarely persists into adult life. Occasionally, the affected toe may develop fixed flexion. In such cases, percutaneous flexor tenotomy and splintage with a longitudinal K wire for 4 weeks may be required. Separation of syndactyly is rarely justifiable and is purely cosmetic.

Correction of the overlapping little toe is risky and often the result is disappointment. Moving the toe from a dorsal position over the fourth toe (Fig. 10.6), to a position lateral to the fourth toe may not be enough to relieve pressure over the digit and inevitably function is not improved. In addition to skin and soft tissue releases, a tendon transfer is usually indicated (flexor to the lateral border of the extensor hood). Amputation of the little toe may be the best solution, particularly after failed reconstructive surgery. The fifth toe may also burrow under the fourth toe, forcing the latter dorsally. Wider shoe fitment is all that is necessary.

The lesser toes may also develop three distinct flexion deformities in the child:

1. claw toe (dorsiflexion of the metatarsophalangeal joint, plantar flexion of both interphalangeal joints)
2. hammer toe (dorsiflexion of the metatarsophalangeal with fixed plantarflexion of the proximal interphalangeal joint)
3. mallet toe (plantarflexion of the distal interphalangeal joint).

In all three conditions, the intrinsic muscle control of the toe is deficient, and the toe is often relatively long. In many cases, the exact cause of the deformity is unexplained although it may run in the family.

Once again, treatment by splintage is ineffectual, although an in-shoe device may assist in correcting the hyperextension of the metatarsophalangeal joint which accompanies the flexion deformity distally. Flexor tenotomy with temporary K wire fixation may be sufficient in childhood, but in adolescence and adult life a proximal interphalangeal (for hammer toe) or a distal interphalangeal (for mallet toe) arthrodesis is necessary, thus both correcting the flexion deformity and shortening the toe. A dorsal capsulotomy of the metatarsophalangeal joint is also advisable.

Hallux valgus

Hallux valgus is usually familial and is more common in the flexible, pronated foot subjected to shoe pressure. Metatarsus primus varus (adductus) may promote the valgus deviation of the big toe, as may ligamentous laxity. Pronation of the toe is part of the deformity, and the flexor hallucis longus sesamoids deviate laterally.

The first approach to the management of hallux valgus is conservative, but it may be difficult to ensure compliance when broader shoes are being recommended. If the heel is narrow, it may be appropriate to fit heel cups, allowing a wider shoe fitment. Lower heels are also advisable. Toe spacers of latex rubber or medial border splints are of unproven value and may not be worn much.

If correction of hallux valgus is indicated in childhood or early adolescence, it is best to avoid

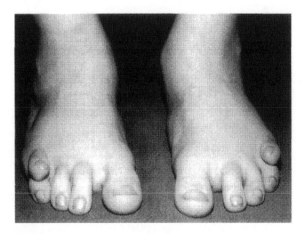

Figure 10.6 Overlapping of the little toe secondary to abnormally dorsal positioning.

skeletal surgery. Release of the adductor from the base of the proximal phalanx, with re-attachment to the neck of the first metatarsal, is combined with medial reefing (capsulorrhaphy) of the deviated joint. After this procedure, particularly with further growth, the valgus alignment is likely to recur. A long first ray and metatarsus primus varus (with an intermetatarsal angle of over 10°) predispose to this recurrence. A first metatarsal osteotomy, either in the distal shaft or at the base of the first metatarsal, will then both shorten and lateralize the affected ray. The medial capsulorrhaphy may need to be repeated, but if it is overtightened it may produce an iatrogenic hallux varus. The Keller's excisional arthroplasty of the first metatarsophalangeal joint is never appropriate in the younger patient as it weakens the foot appreciably.

Hallux rigidus is only post-traumatic in childhood; the classical osteoarthritic form is not seen. An extension osteotomy of the proximal phalanx will increase the range of dorsiflexion at toe-off, thus reducing pain. A metatarsal bar is rarely prescribed and is poorly tolerated. However, a stiff-last shoe may offer some splintage of the joint and thus relieve symptoms.

Pressure over bony prominences

Shoewear produces pressure areas over naturally occurring or abnormal bony prominences. The most common develops over the proximal interphalangeal joint and the thickened skin or corn will only disappear if the flexion deformity is corrected, presuming that shoe adjustment has failed. Callosities may also form under the metatarsal heads in pes cavus, or if a hammer toe causes the associated metatarsal head to be driven into the sole. Callosities or bunions (an adventitial, thickened bursa) form medially in hallux valgus, and laterally when the fifth metatarsal head is prominent (bunionette) (Fig. 10.7). The latter prominence should be managed conservatively and never by shaving off the prominent bone as this will only lead to recurrence. A metatarsal sliding osteotomy (reverse Wilson osteotomy) will relieve pressure by shifting the distal portion medially, and is very occasionally

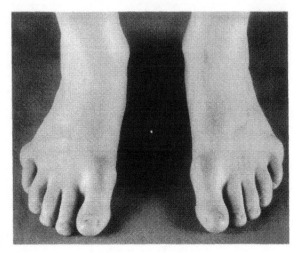

Figure 10.7 A broad forefoot with bunionette (tailor's bunion).

indicated. Excision of the distal third or half of the fifth metatarsal, although described, is too drastic a procedure.

Other prominences such as the overbone (dorsal margin of the tarsometatarsal joints), the heel boss (Hagglund's disease) and the lateral calcaneal lumps in relation to the peroneal tendons should never be excised in children. Pressure over the first metatarsal head in hallux flexus should be treated by correcting the toe deformity – a difficult proposition.

Habitual tiptoe walking

When the child is learning to walk, the calf stretch reflex may be overactive, so instead of walking with some pronation of the foot during stance the child walks on tiptoe. Whereas a short calf may produce a valgus heel and a flattened foot in some neurological conditions, particularly the spasticity of cerebral palsy, the overactive stretch reflex in some, otherwise normal, children induces them to tiptoe. This is more evident when the child is excited or runs, and if asked to concentrate, the heels may drop so that the gait is almost normal.

Tiptoe walking (the ballerina syndrome) may resolve as the child matures and becomes heavier. Shoe heel wear can be monitored to check if this is so. But if the gait remains persistently abnormal, stretching casts, repeated monthly for 12 weeks, may prove effective. In a few children, percutaneous heel cord (Achilles tendon) lengthening is effective although it does not address the true cause, namely the dynamic calf contraction. Although tiptoe walking is sometimes put down to habit, a neurological basis to the condition is more likely, with slight disinhibition of the stretch reflex owing to a nonprogressive upper motor neuron lesion. The use of botulinum toxin to produce partial paralysis at the muscle end-plates is now being established in the management of cerebral palsy, and may have a part to play in this benign condition.

CONGENITAL TALIPES EQUINOVARUS

The other major deformity affecting the infantile foot is congenital talipes equinovarus or clubfoot. The congenital inversion presents with varying degrees of correctability:

1. postural
2. partially correctable (< 20° of fixed equinus and varus)
3. uncorrectable (> 20° of fixed equinus and varus).

The etiology is often obscure, but an association with overt neuromuscular deficit or skeletal dysplasias will make the outcome of surgical treatment unpredictable.

Etiology

There are some pointers towards certain etiological factors. In affected families, the incidence of clubfoot is high and the author has treated one child with five other relatively close family members affected by the condition. The severity of the deformity also varies in families, suggesting variable penetrance or a polygenic trait. In monozygous twins, the likelihood of both babies being affected is 1 in 3, while siblings or children of affected parents have a risk of approximately 1 in 20. Currently, a study is underway in Scotland assessing the national incidence of clubfoot, with both the family inheritance pattern and salivary chromosome analyses.

Intrauterine factors include the 'packing' of the infant, and oligohydramnios has been suggested as a cause of at least the postural deformity. However, the fetus is free-floating at the 0.79–2.4 inch (20–60 mm) stage when the foot is developing, and clubfoot is not more common in twins or the firstborn when there is a presumed increase in intrauterine pressure during the last months of pregnancy.

Intrinsic rather than extrinsic causes are more persuasive, and 'germ plasm defects' have been suggested. Certainly, the dissection of clubfeet often reveals abnormal tendons and altered tarsal relationships, although these may be found in the normal foot. Angiography has revealed deficiency or absence of the dorsal blood supply, with significant attenuation of the dorsalis pedis artery. For this reason, surgical injury to the posterior tibial artery, and dissection around the peroneal vessels when releasing the inferior tibiofibular joint, may have dire consequences. Arrest of the fetal development of the limb may occur at the limb bud stage, secondary to toxic agents, but usually this produces a major deficiency, such as the phocomelia after thalidomide.

The clubfoot deformity is seen in neurological conditions such as myelodysplasia and central core disease. Coupled with the characteristic calf wasting and peroneal muscle weakness, the theory of neurological abnormality is appealing.[9] The literature is now increasingly filled with reports concerning deficits in nerve conduction velocity to the affected limb, altered electromyographic traces and spinal monosynapic reflexes, and, recently, abnormal somatosensory evoked potentials in up to 50% of children studied after clubfoot operations. Microscopic and histochemical studies of muscle biopsies from the affected limb have also revealed alterations. Unfortunately, these results are not consistent and some authors have identified no changes.

It is possible that the neurological imbalance seen in some clubfeet is secondary to viral or bacterial infection in utero. A seasonal variation in the presentation of the condition and spinal cord changes in aborted fetuses with the condition suggest that acquired neurological deficit plays a part, perhaps in those that are genetically susceptible.[10]

Now that screening and immediate splintage of unstable hips have reduced the incidence of hip dislocation and dysplasia, clubfoot represents the most common, severe orthopedic deformity with an incidence of approximately 2 per 1000 live babies. Confusion about the best form of treatment reflects uncertainties about the etiology and prognosis of the condition, the empirical nature of the clinical grading (which represents inadequately a spectrum of deformities) and a lack of convincing long-term reviews of treatment based upon postoperative clinical trials.

Clinical appearance

The clinical appearance is typical, with a small inverted heel and a deep posterior crease above it (Fig. 10.8). The calcaneus is impalpable, so that the ball of the heel is small and soft. The lateral malleolus is posteriorly placed, with loose skin over the sinus tarsi. Supination and adduction of the midfoot and forefoot produce a deep, vertical, medial skin crease where the talonavicular joint is subluxed. The lateral column of the foot is therefore longer than the medial. The equinus masks an underlying varus of the midfoot, and there is a combination of external ankle mortise rotation but internal torsion of the tibia. Calf wasting becomes increasingly obvious as the baby's fat is lost, and, in the poorly corrected case, genu recurvatum and intoeing develop.

Assessment of the deformity relies upon the rigidity of the foot, and other factors such as the size of the foot and calf, and the length of the toes which are often short, flexed and deviated in the type III foot. Initially, twice weekly strapping or fortnightly plasters are employed to correct the mobile element of the deformity. The decision to operate is made from the age of 3 months until walking age, depending upon the response to conservative management or the radiographs (Fig. 10.9). In most cases, it is quite obvious that the foot is structurally deformed, and therefore the need for surgical release can usually be predicted at birth or shortly thereafter. However, it is wise to wait until conservative stretching has been tried for at least 3 to 4 months. Operating at birth has been advocated[11] but brings its own problems; equally, it may be appropriate to release the severely deformed foot later in the first year of life, when the anatomical structures are larger.

Surgical management

The extent of the surgical release varies between surgeons, and may also reflect the severity of the deformity. The Cincinnati lateral–posteromedial incision affords excellent exposure (Fig. 10.10A, B, C) but a combined medial and longitudinal

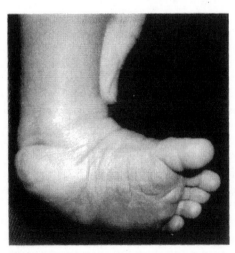

Figure 10.8 Deep transverse posterior and vertical medial creases characterize structural clubfoot.

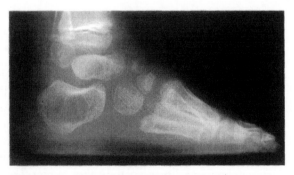

Figure 10.9 The talocalcaneal angle is decreased in clubfoot.

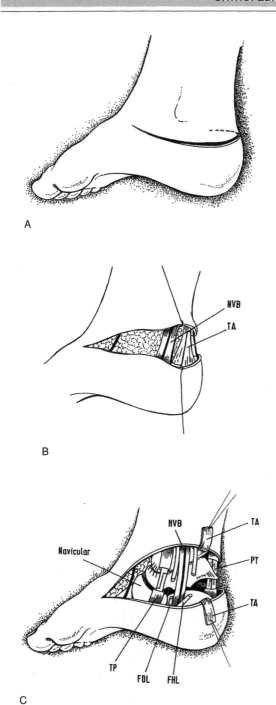

A

B

C

Figure 10.10 The Cincinnati incision affords excellent exposure. (Key: FDL, flexor digitorum longus; FHL, flexor hallucis longus; NVB, neurovascular bundle; PT, peroneal tendons; TA, Achilles tendon; TP, tibialis posterior (tendon).)

posterolateral approach may be preferred. The Achilles and tibialis tendons are lengthened and repaired, the flexor hallucis longus and flexor digitorum tendons often released without repair, and the ankle and subtalar joints opened widely. The talonavicular joint capsule, peroneal tendon sheath and plantar fascia (with the abductor hallucis) are usually released[12] but there is debate about the need to extend the dissection laterally to involve the calcaneocuboid joint.

While some surgeons use K wires to hold the corrected position of the subtalar and talonavicular joints, others feel this to be damaging. The greatest importance attaches to the careful application of padded plasters postoperatively, changing the casts at 2- to 4-weekly intervals. Splintage is recommended for 6 to 12 weeks, and thereafter the foot should be regularly stretched to prevent the tethering effect of surgical scar as the infant doubles its length over the ensuing 12 to 18 months. In the severe (grade III) feet, and when overt neurological deficit or arthrogryposis are present, it is prudent to continue with AFOs until the age of 2 or 3 years. One advantage of operating on the difficult foot later, perhaps at 10 to 15 months, is that the child should then be ready to weightbear on the foot after the operation. However, tarsal deformity becomes more established by the first birthday and therefore most contemporary surgeons prefer to operate earlier, and accept a possibly longer period of splintage.

Relapsed clubfoot

Recurrence ('relapse') of the deformity occurs in 20–40% of feet – most commonly in the bilateral, severe and contracted feet of boys, and least likely in a girl with unilateral, moderate deformity. The soft tissue release can be safely repeated once or twice more, but the dissection becomes much harder and correction more difficult to regain. However, the author considers that soft tissue release can be repeated up to the age of 4 or 5 years. If the foot is mobile but supinates dynamically, a split-anterior tibial tendon transfer (SPLATT) may achieve balance if the lateral lamina of the tendon is inserted into the middle or lateral cuneiform, or to a portion of the peroneus brevis tendon.

In the more rigid foot, bone procedures are an option, but all tend to make the foot smaller. If the heel is inverted, a medial opening wedge[13] or closing wedge osteotomy of the calcaneum may centralize the heel under the ankle. For the bean-shaped foot in the child of $4\frac{1}{2}$ to 6 years of age, wide release of the talonavicular joint is coupled with a calcaneocuboid wedge excision and closure by stapling (Evans procedure[14]). This does not correct supination or hindfoot malrotation, so correction of the midfoot adduction may still leave the child walking on the lateral border of the foot. A number of other orthopaedic procedures have been described to lengthen the medial column of the foot, or to shorten the lateral, but none of them is particularly effective.

Distraction of ligaments

A recent vogue using the Ilizarov distraction external fixator has enjoyed some success.[15] By means of metal rings and half rings, the hindfoot can be distracted from the distal tibia, correcting the equinus and inversion, and concomitant midfoot malalignment can also be straightened. The stretching occurs slowly over 4 to 6 weeks, at approximately 1 mm per day (in small increments), and in theory the soft tissues stretch by 'ligamentotaxis'. Since most feet treated in this way are relatively stiff, the aim is to produce a plantigrade foot which can then be held by plasters in the corrected position for several months. If the deformity is very resistant, distraction may have to be combined with hindfoot and possibly midfoot osteotomies. A number of other fixation devices are in use, but all rely on percutaneous pin fixation which may introduce its own problems of infection, pintrack damage and poor patient tolerance.

By the time the child is 6 or 7 years old, a corrected foot will tend to remain corrected. There may still be a need for occasional later tibialis anterior or tibialis posterior transfers, but any later osteotomy should be delayed until skeletal maturity when a triple arthrodesis or a lesser wedge excisional arthrodesis may be necessary.

These interventions inevitably make the foot smaller and stiffer.

METATARSUS ADDUCTUS

Although this condition, occurring in 2–3 per 1000 live births, is often mistaken for congenital talipes equinovarus, the hindfoot is mobile and the forefoot usually correctable. The function of the foot is perfectly satisfactory although shoe fitment may be difficult in early childhood. Over 90% of these feet correct, so surgical intervention is rarely indicated.[16]

The condition is commonly bilateral and is one of the causes of an intoeing gait. When associated with

a. supination of the midfoot
b. or heel valgus ('skewfoot') (Fig. 10.11)

the deformity may be more troublesome, so these associated deviations should be monitored.

Conservative treatment options for mild to moderate cases are discussed in Chapters 12 and 14.

In the severe case during mid-childhood, there may be a place for distal abductor hallucis tenotomy or proximal muscle slide. The latter procedure may cause hypertrophic skin scarring, and both procedures may disappoint, as they do

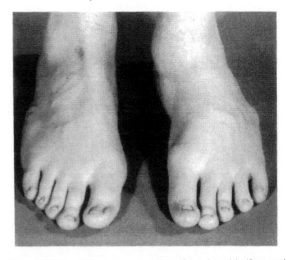

Figure 10.11 Skewfoot, consisting of a valgus hindfoot and an abducted forefoot.

not address the skeletal angulation. Midfoot 'mobilization' by tarsometatarsal capsulotomies or multiple basal metatarsal osteotomies are known to produce midfoot osteoarthritis, so the procedures are best avoided. As with the unnecessary operations carried out on flatfoot in the past, most midfoot releases are not appropriate and may increase symptoms.

PES CAVUS

This is a progressive deformity which is rarely noticeable at birth but becomes increasingly severe during mid- and later childhood. In addition to the heightened medial arch, there may be 'lateral cavus' in the worst cases and the toes become increasingly clawed. This in turn leads to the formation of painful callosities under the metatarsal heads, particularly the first and fifth as a transverse cavus may also develop. In its worst form, the deformity becomes a 'tripod' with skin ulceration and osteitis at the sites of point pressure.

Although some cases of pes cavus seem on questioning to be idiopathic, the deformity is certainly the product of muscle imbalance and subsequent soft tissue contracture, with skeletal deformity later. The condition is seen in hereditary conditions such as the motor and sensory neuropathies (peroneal muscular atrophy or Charcot–Marie–Tooth syndrome), Friedreich's ataxia and other cerebellar or spinal tract diseases. Spinal dysraphism (spina bifida), cerebral palsy, poliomyelitis, the muscular dystrophies and polymyositis are sometimes causative, but in many cases there is no obvious condition. In many families, a high-arched foot is common, representing one end of the spectrum that leads through to familial flatfoot.

Etiology

The muscle imbalance producing pes cavus may be:

1. a weak calf (gastrocnemius–soleus) muscle with overactivity of the long toe flexors
2. a weak tibialis anterior muscle with over-activity of the long toe extensors

3. weak intrinsic muscles of the foot, again leading to overactivity in the long toe flexors and extensors
4. a weak peroneus brevis with overactivity of peroneus longus.

The clinical assessment of the foot should reveal increasing 'dropping' of the first metatarsal into a plantaris position. Not only does this increase the medial arch but it also tilts the forefoot into supination. As a secondary feature, the heel rolls into inversion, although it remains perfectly mobile initially. The heel can therefore be centered under the tibia by a simple procedure known as the 'block test'.[17] The lateral border of the foot, anterior to the calcaneus is supported by a 0.4 inch (1 cm) wooden block while the child is standing. This allows the first metatarsal to drop without tilting the forefoot into supination. As a result, the uninvolved and supple hindfoot straightens up as it is no longer being inverted by the tilting effect of a supinated forefoot.

Stretching or plaster splintage alone has no effect upon the condition. Orthotics and heel cups are sometimes effective in providing comfort, and may be all that is required in the milder deformity. Although plantar fascial release has a time-honored role in the surgical management of pes cavus,[18] it is ineffectual unless combined with some other procedure. This is particularly true of the percutaneous plantar release, which may do more harm than good.

For moderate deformity, step-cut lengthening of the tibialis posterior tendon can be combined with a basal extension osteotomy of the dropped first metatarsal and an open plantar release through the same medial incision. Clawing of the hallux is best corrected by releasing the extensor hallucis longus tendon from its insertion into the base of the proximal phalanx and re-attaching it through a transverse drill hole through the head of the first metatarsal (the Jones procedure[19]). Clawing of the lesser toes is best treated conservatively. However, flexor to extensor tendon transfers are sometimes undertaken as a recognition of the intrinsic muscle weakness.[20] The procedure may leave the toes unnaturally straightened and scarred.

The Jones procedure in the younger child should be accompanied by a tenodesis of the interphalangeal joint to prevent unopposed flexion, and by a K-wire arthrodesis of that joint after the age of 10 or 12 years. The operation may require to be repeated, as may the plantar release. If the deformity recurs, as is very likely in the severely affected foot, a dorsal wedge tarsectomy or calcaneal osteotomy may be indi-cated, although these interventions inevitably stiffen and shorten the foot. A Lambrinudi resec-tion and realignment are of value as a last resort[21] and correct the cavovarus sufficiently to allow the fitment of surgical shoes. A good orthotist has much to offer in this challenging, but fortunately rare, condition. Severe, resistant and bilateral involvement may result in the patient taking to a wheelchair after early adult life.

REFERENCES

1. Högh J, Macnicol MF. Foot deformities associated with onycho-osteodystrophy. Int Orthop (SICOT) 1984;9:135–138.
2. Hamanishi C. Congenital vertical talus: classification with 69 cases and a new measurement system. J Pediatr Orthop 1984; 4:318–326.
3. Wenger DR, Mauldin D, Speck G, et al. Corrective shoes and inserts as treatment for flexible flatfoot in infants and children. J Bone Joint Surg Am 1989;71A:800–810.
4. Dennyson W, Fulford GE. Subtalar arthrodesis by cancellous grafts and metallic internal fixation. J Bone Joint Surg Br 1976;58B: 507–510.
5. Scranton PE. Treatment of symptomatic talocalcaneal coalition. J Bone Joint Surg Am 1987;69A:533–539.
6. Inglis G, Buxton RA, Macnicol MF. Symptomatic calcaneonavicular bars. J Bone Joint Surg Br 1986;68B:128–131.
7. Macnicol MF, Voutsinas S. Surgical treatment of the symptomatic accessory navicular. J Bone Joint Surg Br 1984; 66B:218–226.
8. Mandell GH, Harcke HT. Scintigraphic manifestations of infraction of the second metatarsal (Freiberg's disease). J Nucl Med 1987; 28:249–251.
9. Feldbrin Z, Gilai AN, Ezra E, et al. Muscle imbalance in the aetiology of idiopathic club foot. An electromyographic study. J Bone Joint Surg Br 1995;77B: 596–601.
10. Swart JJ. Clubfoot: a histological study. S Afr J Bone Joint Surg 1993;3:17–23.
11. Ryöppy S, Sairanen H. Neonatal operative treatment of club foot. A preliminary report. J Bone Joint Surg Br 1983;65B: 320–325.
12. Macnicol MF. The surgical management of congenital talipes equinovarus. Curr Orthop 1995;9:71–82.
13. Dwyer FC. The treatment of relapsed club foot by insertion of a wedge into the calcaneum. J Bone Joint Surg Br 1963; 45B:67–71.
14. Evans D. Relapsed club foot. J Bone Joint Surg Br 1961;43B:722–728.
15. Grill F, Franke J. The Ilizarov distractor for the correction of relapsed or neglected club foot. J Bone Joint Surg Br 1987;69B:593–597.
16. Rushforth GF. The natural history of hooked forefoot. J Bone Joint Surg Br 1978;60B:530–532.
17. Coleman SS, Chestnut WJ. A simple test for hindfoot flexibility in the cavovarus foot. Clin Orthop 1977;123:60–63.
18. Steindler A. Stripping of the os calcis. J Orthop Surg 1921;2:8–12.
19. Jones R. Certain operative procedures in the paralysis of children with special reference to poliomyelitis. BMJ 1911;ii:1520–1523.
20. Lambrinudi C. An operation for claw toes. Proc R Soc Med 1927;21:239–243.
21. Lambrinudi CA. Method of correcting equinus and calcaneus deformities at the sub-astragaloid joint. Proc R Soc Med 1933;26:788–793.

FURTHER READING

Coleman SS. Complex foot deformities in children. Philadelphia: Lea & Febiger; 1983.
Fixsen JA, Lloyd-Roberts GC. The foot in childhood. Edinburgh: Churchill Livingstone; 1988.
Helah B, Rowley D, Cracchiolo A, et al, eds. Surgery of disorders of the foot and ankle. London: Martin Dunitz; 1996.

Tachdjian MO. The child's foot. Philadelphia: WB Saunders; 1985.

INTRODUCTION TO FRACTURES AND THEIR MANAGEMENT

Peter Thomson

The treatment of bony injury in children is particularly rewarding as their bones heal quickly and possess a great ability to remodel. Remodeling will occur over an 18-month to 2-year period and angular malunion may correct itself if there is sufficient growth available. In addition, in children post-immobilization joint stiffness is generally not a problem.

Fractures are more common than dislocations in children since their ligaments are relatively very strong. Growing bone is more porous and elastic than in the adult, thus allowing incomplete fractures to occur. In children, the periosteum is strong and thick and rapidly produces abundant callus. Furthermore, the periosteum usually remains intact in pediatric fractures and forms a bridge, which may help in their reduction.

Fractures unique to children include the buckle and greenstick fractures (Fig. 10.12). The bones of children are capable of bending and may reach a point beyond their elastic limit but short of their yield point, thus producing a gentle curve or bowed appearance to the bone.

A buckle or torus fracture (Fig. 10.12A) represents the buckling of the cortex on the compression side of a metaphyseal segment of bone. Typically, such fractures are seen in the distal radius after a fall on the outstretched hand. Greenstick fractures, as their name implies, are incomplete fractures on the tension side of a bone (Fig. 10.12B). The principles of treatment for such fractures are generally as for any fracture.

Buckle fractures require to be protected only until pain free, which may take 2 weeks or less. They have no propensity to displace.

A simple guide to typical healing times of children's fractures is given in Table 10.1. However, all fracture healing must be assessed clinically and radiologically. Clinical union may be said to exist when there is no pain on stressing the fracture. Radiological union, which frequently lags behind clinical union, exists when there is bony continuity of callus across the fracture site.

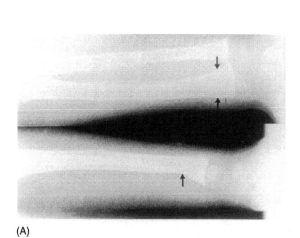

(A)

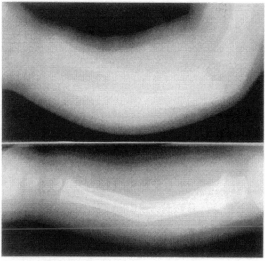

(B)

Figure 10.12   (A) Buckle fracture. (B) Greenstick fracture.

Table 10.1 Approximate healing time (weeks)

Age (years)	Physeal	Diaphyseal
0–3	3	6
4–10	4	8
11–15	5	10

GROWTH PLATE INJURIES

Bone grows in length by endochondral ossification in the growth plates or epiphyseal cartilages.

Two types of epiphysis occur: (i) the pressure epiphysis at the ends of long bones from which longitudinal growth occurs, and (ii) the traction epiphysis at major tendinous insertions.

The weakest area of the epiphyseal plate is the zone of calcifying cartilage and fractures tend to occur through this layer. Thus, the epiphyseal plate always stays attached to the epiphysis. The physis itself is cartilaginous and thus is not visible on radiographs. The classification of epiphyseal fractures most commonly referred to is that proposed by Salter & Harris in 1963[1] (Fig. 10.13). This was later modified by Ogden.[2]

Salter–Harris type I fractures are uncommon and tend to occur in children under 5 years of age. They may also be found in adolescent inversion ankle injuries (Fig. 10.14). Type II fractures are the most common and are frequently found in the child older than 10 years. Type III fractures spare the metaphysis and are usually caused by intra-articular shearing force (Fig. 10.15A, B). Type IV fractures make up about 10% of physeal injuries (Fig. 10.16A, B). Type III and IV injuries are most commonly associated with growth disturbance and must be treated with early anatom-

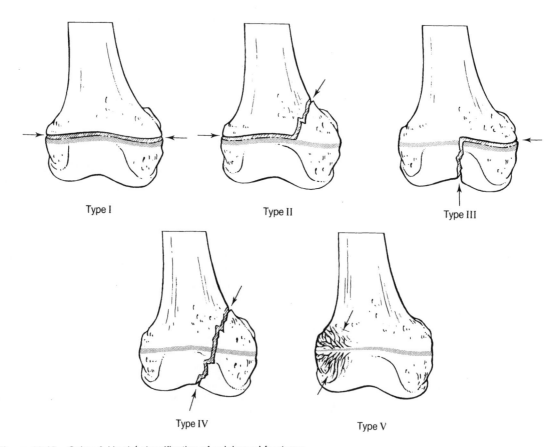

Type I   Type II   Type III

Type IV   Type V

Figure 10.13   Salter & Harris[1] classification of epiphyseal fractures.

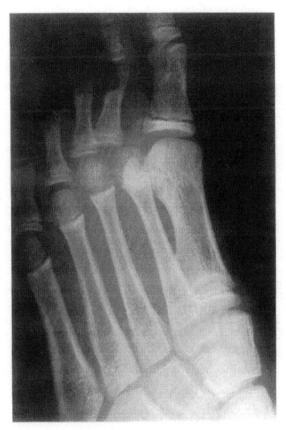

Figure 10.14 Type I fracture. The head of the third metatarsal is rotated following a fracture across the epiphyseal plate. The metaphysis is intact.

ical reduction and usually with internal fixation (type IV always). When at all possible, the internal fixation is not placed across the physis. Screws and wires are restricted to the metaphyseal fragment (types II and IV) and to the epiphysis in type III. If fixation must be used across the plate (unstable type I), unthreaded wires are used, and these are removed as soon as possible. The type V injury is rare and even controversial and may only be diagnosed in retrospect when growth disturbance is noted. Rang expanded the Salter–Harris classification by describing a perichondral ring injury which has been termed Salter–Harris VI.[3] Such an injury may result in angular deformity (Fig. 10.17). Ogden's modification to the Salter–Harris system involved subclassifications to I–IV, which were dependent upon the extent of the fragments that were

visible on X-ray. For example, Ogden classified the type III fracture as either IIIA when the fracture went through the physis or IIIB if it included a small layer of primary spongiosa, thereby raising concern with regard to the vascularization of the fragment. Ogden also added types VII, VIII and IX. However Salter–Harris types I–VI are the forms most commonly referred to.

Most epiphyseal injuries of the ankle may be clearly defined using the routine anteroposterior, lateral and mortise view. Fractures of the fibular physis are the most common and may be subtle. More complex physeal injuries are sometimes best evaluated by CT, which clearly demonstrates the epiphyseal fragmentation and the distal tibiofibular relationship. It is important to define the degree of articular involvement and the degree of separation as displacement of more than 2 mm has significant treatment implications.[4]

The most common complication of growth plate fracture is premature or asymmetrical fusion. Type III and IV tibial fractures with greater than 2 mm displacement, comminuted fractures and type V fractures have the highest risk, occurring in 32% of one series.[5] Growth plate deformity, owing to arrest, will become evident from 6 months to a year after injury and may lead to leg-length discrepancy or angulation deformity (see Fig. 10.16B).

Very careful follow-up of all physeal injuries is indicated in order to ensure that normal growth is proceeding. When arrest of a physis occurs, the anatomy must be carefully defined in order to outline the position of the bar across the plate. This is usually carried out by the use of tomography or CT scanning. Surgery may be performed in order to attempt to resect a bony bridge across the physis and to hold it open with a fatty plug. However, this is technically very difficult and the results are variable.

Angular deformities from physeal injuries may require to be corrected in the older child by osteotomy, which may have to be repeated as the child grows. Complete growth arrest near the end of the growth period may be treated by surgically fusing the contralateral epiphysis (epiphysiodesis).

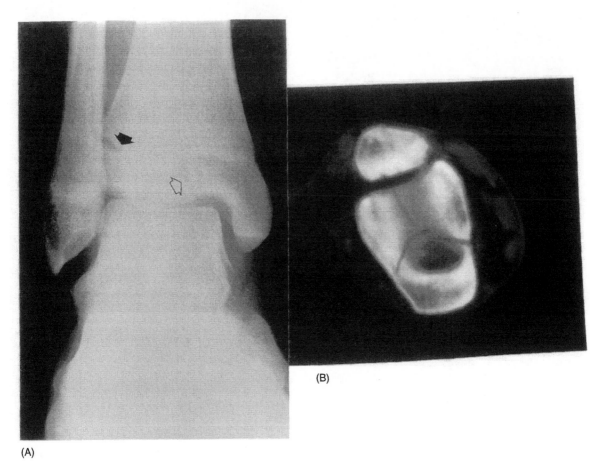

(A)

(B)

Figure 10.15 Type III fracture. (A) There is a vertical fracture through the epiphysis (open arrow) and along the epiphyseal plate, causing slight displacement (solid arrow). (B) The value of CT is clearly demonstrated in evaluating the extent of the fracture.

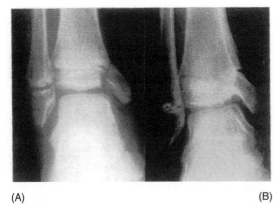

(A)   (B)

Figure 10.16 Type IV fracture. (A) The vertical fracture of the medial aspect of the epiphysis extends through to the metaphysis. (B) Subsequent epiphyseal tethering is leading to further distortion of the joint as growth progresses.

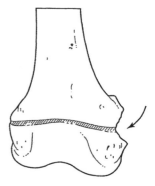

Figure 10.17 Rang's perichondral ring injury, classified as the Salter–Harris type VI fracture.

ANKLE FRACTURES

Fractures of the ankle also have a system of classification. The system upon which most others are based is that of Lauge-Hansen.[6] It is reported that in excess of 90% of all ankle injuries may be classified under this system. However, this method is very detailed and other systems have evolved in an attempt to simplify the classification. In its simplest form, the Lauge-Hansen method describes four main patterns of injury based on the position of the foot (prefix) and direction of the deforming force (suffix) at the time of the injury. Therefore, the Lauge-Hansen method describes:

- supination–adduction
- pronation–abduction
- supination–eversion
- pronation–eversion.

Based on Lauge-Hansen's work, Dias & Tachdjian developed a similar system for the classification of physeal fractures in the young ankle.[7] They too utilized a system whereby the position of the foot and the direction of the deforming force was used. The Salter & Harris classification may also be used to describe the physeal injury.

Distal tibial and fibular epiphyseal fractures are common and are frequently caused by indirect trauma, with the foot being fixed and the body rotating around it. 10% of all physeal injuries occur to the distal tibial epiphysis and are more common in boys between the ages of 11 and 15 years. Towards the end of this period, the growth plate is beginning to close and certain specific fracture patterns occur. The most common distal tibial injury is the type II fracture.

Severely displaced fractures may pull a flap of periosteum from the metaphysis and this flap may slip into the fracture preventing its reduction and therefore surgical treatment may be required. These fractures are usually associated with greenstick fractures of the distal fibula.

Type III and IV fractures of the medial malleolus occur which bring about a far greater incidence of growth arrest and which always require accurate open reduction and internal fixation.

The type I distal fibula fracture is common and is frequently difficult to diagnose as it often slips back to its anatomical position after injury and thus it is not apparent on X-ray. This fracture is usually diagnosed on clinical suspicion. However, a stress inversion X-ray may aid in the diagnosis. Treatment is by rest in plaster until comfortable.

The Tillaux and triplane fractures are complex distal epiphyseal injuries that occur during the period of physiological epiphyseal closure. The Tillaux fracture is a type III injury of the anterolateral part of the distal tibial epiphysis. This is caused by lateral rotation of the foot on the leg and produces a compression torque effect of the talar dome on the distal tibial epiphysis, thus causing shearing. Accurate reduction is essential in order to reconstruct the tibial joint surface. Growth arrest is not a problem as physiological closure is already occurring.

The triplane fracture appears as a type III injury in the anteroposterior plane and as a type II fracture in the lateral plane. It is again an external rotation injury but occurs in a slightly older age group than the Tillaux fracture (average 13 years). The fracture may be two or three part.

Reduction may be by manipulation but it is important to restore the joint surface accurately. A proportion of such fractures will require open reduction.

FRACTURES OF THE FOOT

Accessory bones are frequently misdiagnosed as fractures, particularly during their ossification as they may have a fragmentary appearance on X-ray (Ch. 9).

In children, fractures of the talar neck are uncommon.[8] When they do occur, they are usually the result of an abrupt dorsiflexion of the foot or from direct trauma to the dorsum of the foot. Talar neck fractures may be subtle and may be overlooked, especially as up to 20% of cases may also present with medial malleolar fractures, which are often more obvious. Such fractures are usually undisplaced and may be treated in a non-weightbearing cast. However, complications are particularly frequent following displaced talar neck fractures. Blood supply to the talus is poor since articular cartilage covers a substantial amount of its surface. In addition, there are no direct muscle or tendon attachments. Vascularization is mainly provided by a branch of the posterior tibial artery, which supplies the inferior neck and most of the body. Branches of the dorsalis pedis artery enter the superior aspect of the talar neck and supply the dorsal portion of the neck and the head of the talus. Finally, the peroneal artery supplies part of the lateral wall. Therefore, open reduction risks devascularization of the talar body.

Avascular necrosis is difficult to diagnose on a radiography in the early stages but ^{99M}TcMDP bone scanning has provided a means of early identification. However, MRI is the most specific and sensitive method of diagnosis, with loss of the normal high marrow signal on T1-weighted images. Avascular necrosis becomes evident in the radiographs around 8 weeks with areas of increased density within the bones because of the laying down of new bone on dead trabeculae and the collapse of bone trabecula, which may lead to fragmentation of the articular surface. When displacement has occurred, they can usually be reduced by plantarflexion and can be held either in a plaster or with percutaneous wires.

Inversion and eversion injuries may cause ligamentous 'pull-off' fractures of the medial or lateral side of the talar body. Such fragments are osteochondral in nature and usually heal with rest in plaster, but non-union may occur and excision of the fragment may be necessary. Osteochondral fractures of the talar dome are uncommon in children under 16 years of age and frequently occur with lateral ligament rupture thus allowing varus impingement on the tibial plafond.[9] Medial lesions are deeper and when associated with trauma are due to lateral rotation of the plantarflexed ankle. In such cases, open reduction and internal fixation or excision may be required. Severe fractures and fracture-dislocations are rare. However, all such cases may progress to avascular necrosis of the talar body with possible late collapse and osteoarthrosis.

Calcaneal fractures are relatively rare but are the commonest tarsal fractures in children. Such fractures are caused by falls from a height on to the heels and are always accompanied by extensive soft tissue swelling. Fracture blisters may also occur. Initial treatment is by elevation in order to reduce the swelling and early commencement of active range of movement exercises. 63% of calcaneal fractures in children are extra-articular, rising to 92% in patients less than 7 years of age. Fractures also occur through the anterior or posterior processes.[10] Intra-articular fractures disrupt the subtalar joint and the crushing of the cancellous bone of the calcaneus causes decreased height and increased width of the heel which frequently lead to degenerative changes in the subtalar joint. Routine lateral oblique and axial views will demonstrate most fractures and measurement of the angle of the superior surface of the talocalcaneus (Bohler's angle) may be helpful. Any reduction below 22–48° will indicate a compression fracture. Conventional and computed tomography are the most valuable additional techniques to demonstrate more complex fractures and also avulsion injuries of the calcaneus. CT enables joint alignment to be assessed, detects intra-articular fragments and the integrity of the sustentacular portion of the calcaneus. The talocalcaneal joints are best seen on the frontal scans and the talonavicular and calcaneocuboid articulations are more clearly demonstrated on the axial scans. When tendon and ligament injuries are suspected, MRI may be helpful. Three-dimensional reformatting may be of value in planning treatment of complex fractures.

'Pull-off' fractures of the posterior process by the Achilles tendon require either casting in plantarflexion or open reduction and internal fixation.

Injuries to the other tarsal bones are rare but may be associated with major crushing injuries or Lisfranc fracture dislocations. Soft tissue swelling and possible compartment syndromes must be considered with all major foot injuries. Elevation of the foot and possibly surgical decompression of the interosseous compartments may be required. Such fractures and dislocations are usually easy to reduce and may be held with percutaneous K wires and plaster casts.

Avulsion fractures of the base of the fifth metatarsal by the peroneus brevis tendon are the commonest fractures of the foot. The secondary ossification center at the base of the fifth metatarsal is frequently misdiagnosed as a fracture. However, the growth plate of the fifth metatarsal runs parallel with the shaft whereas the fractures are perpendicular to the shaft (Fig. 10.18A, B). Such fractures may be treated for 4 to 6 weeks in a short leg walking plaster for comfort.

Isolated metatarsal fractures most commonly occur in the shaft of the first or fifth. Direct trauma, such as dropping a heavy weight on to the foot, is the commonest cause. Isolated second metatarsal fractures suggest fatigue fractures.

Most metatarsal fractures are undisplaced because of the presence of strong interosseous membranes. Markedly displaced fractures should be reduced and should be held with wires as the capacity for remodeling, especially of plantar-flexion deformities, is limited. Damage to the growth plate of the metatarsals may interfere with the proper formation of the arches of the foot. There is no association between trauma and Freiberg's infraction.

Fractures through the proximal phalangeal growth plate are more common than metatarso-phalangeal dislocations, which are generally

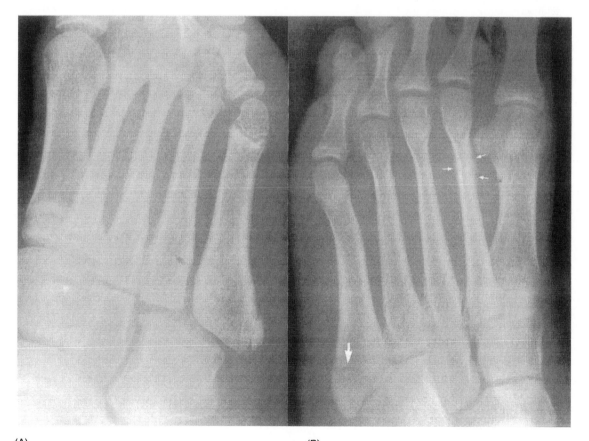

(A)   (B)

Figure 10.18   (A) Normal epiphysis of the base of the fifth metatarsal. (B) The fracture of the base of the fifth metatarsal is perpendicular to the cortex (large arrow). There is also periosteal reaction around the distal shaft of the second metatarsal (see smaller arrows) owing to stress fracture.

encountered in adults. Type III injuries occur here in older children and require accurate reduction and fixation when significantly displaced. Fractures of the lateral toes seldom require much treatment other than symptomatic, but a fracture of a hallux must be well aligned in order to prevent a varus or a valgus deformity.

REFERENCES

1. Salter RB, Harris WR. Injuries involving the epiphyseal plate. J Bone Joint Surg 1963;45A:587–622.
2. Ogden JA. Injury to the growth mechanisms of the immature skeleton. Skeletal Radiol 1981;6:237–253.
3. Rang M. The growth plate and its disorders. London: Churchill Livingstone; 1969.
4. Kling TF, Bright RW, Hensinger RN. Distal tibial physeal fractures in children that may require open reduction. J Bone Joint Surg Am 1984;66: 647–657.
5. Spiegel PG, Cooperman DR, Laros GS. Epiphyseal fractures of the distal ends of the tibia and fibula. J Bone Joint Surg Am 1978;60A:1046–1050.
6. Lauge-Hansen N. Fractures of the ankle II: combines experimental surgical and experimental roentgenologic investigations. Arch Surg 1950;60:957.
7. Dias LS, Tachdjian MO. Physeal injuries of the ankle in children. Clin Orthop 1978;136:230–233.
8. Letts RM, Gibeault D. Fractures of the neck of the talus in children. Foot Ankle 1980;1:74–77.
9. Canale ST, Belding RH. Osteochondral lesions of the talus. J Bone Joint Surg Am; 1980;62A:97–102.
10. McCall I, Cassar-Pullicino V. Radiological examination of the child's foot. In: Thomson P, ed. Introduction to podopaediatrics. London: WB Saunders; 1993:61.

11

Torsional and frontal plane conditions of the lower extremity

Ronald L. Valmassy

The developing child is not merely a small adult. Once the clinician realizes that structural and positional developmental changes occur in a continuous and dynamic fashion, then the satisfactory treatment results which all hope to achieve with a pediatric patient population may be obtained. Knowledge of all the developmental changes that may occur in the growing child's lower extremity should facilitate a successful diagnosis and treatment of a pediatric gait problem. As many have stated, the early years of development represent the golden years of treatment, when the clinician may favorably influence development so that normal gait patterns are achieved by adolescence. Once clinicians understand the continuum of normal development, they will be able to recognize those problems that will require treatment and those that will be outgrown.

Although a clinician will at times be called upon to treat traumatic, dermatological or neurological problems, the vast majority of cases involve a flatfooted condition, associated with either an intoed or an out-toed gait pattern. When a child presents for treatment, the clinician must be aware that often the true etiology of that problem may lie outside the foot. Therefore, it is the purpose of this chapter to present the transverse and frontal plane developmental changes that occur in the leg of the growing child and to discuss how such changes may influence the development of that child's foot and resultant gait pattern. In addition, the ability to evaluate and treat other common pathological conditions such as metatarsus adductus, equinus and talipes calcaneovalgus will also be discussed.

FEMORAL COMPONENT

In reviewing articles dealing with developmental changes occurring in the transverse plane of the femur, antetorsion/anteversion and similarly retrotorsion/retroversion are often used interchangeably. In 1979, the Subcommittee on Torsional Deformity of the Pediatric Orthopedic Society attempted to standardize these definitions. As a result of this, the following definitions were adopted:

- *Version* is the angular difference between the transverse axis of each end of a long bone. This represents the normal angular difference.
- *Torsion* is present when version is increased and occurs when the value for a given measurement falls outside the norm by two standard deviations.
- *Femoral anteversion* is the angle of femoral version made when the femoral head and neck axis are directed forward or anteriorly from the femoral shaft.
- *Femoral retroversion* is the angle of femoral version made when the femoral head and neck axis are directed in a slightly backward direction from the femoral shaft.

Therefore, femoral torsion and antetorsion represent abnormal increases in the femoral version angle. Lateral femoral torsion and retrotorsion represent an abnormal decrease in anteversion or an abnormal increase in retroversion. Although most clinicians understand the concept on which this terminology is based, the interchangeable use of these terms in the literature has led to confusion. In an attempt to clarify and simplify the process of examination, the various causative factors involving rotation of the femoral component are divided into two groups: (1) torsional or bony changes and (2) positional or soft tissue changes. By differentiating between these two groups, the examiner is able to more clearly understand and define the structures involved in the development of the abnormal gait pattern.

At birth, an angle exists between the condyles and the head and neck of femur of approximately 30°. As normal development of this segment occurs, there is a gradual 'unwinding' of this relationship so that by the age of 5 or 6 years a 20° external change has occurred on the transverse plane, thereby leading to an average angle of 8–12°.[1–3] When this change does not occur, or occurs slowly, then an intoed type of gait will be precipitated. The factors that influence this condition include heredity, abnormal sleeping and sitting positions, and ligamentous laxity. Sommerville[4] described how the normally taut ligaments of the hip capsule assist in molding away antetorsion. He reported that when the hip is maintained in its extended position, the anterior capsule tightens, which in turn leads to an external torsional strain on the femoral neck, an area which grows rapidly and is therefore considered extremely malleable. When these ligaments are generally lax, the forces necessary to assist in reduction of the femoral torsion will not be present. It is important to note that there is typically a generalized joint laxity in most cases of persistent internal femoral torsion. In certain cases, this bony unwinding will be delayed up until the age of 13 or 14 years, hence the reason why certain youngsters who appear pigeon-toed for such a long period of time will ultimately appear 'normal' when they become teenagers. Approximately 90% of those youngsters possessing an internal femoral torsion will outgrow the pathology by this age, unless, of course, there was a significant familial tendency towards this deformity. In such cases, there is little likelihood of the torsional component improving spontaneously over time.[5] In addition, it has been reported that youngsters being treated for torsional problems of the femur often demonstrate readily observable angle of gait changes which seem to correspond to overall growth spurts and increases in height.[1] It is postulated that 'growth spurts' not only affect the length of the long bones, but that they may also contribute in part to transverse plane alterations. In other instances, there may be excessive 'unwinding' of the femoral segment, which may result in an external femoral torsion. As this represents an overgrowth, there is generally no treatment that may be easily provided in order to reverse this problem. Such excessive unwinding is often reported as retrotorsion.[2,6] Caution must be exercised when informing parents which problems are most likely to resolve with time. An early external femoral torsion or position may potentially appear worse at age 13 to 14 years depending upon rotational tendencies from the time of diagnosis to adolescence.

The other component of the transverse plane development of the femur is associated with the soft tissue or positional changes which occur over the first few years of life. This soft tissue change involves an internal positioning of this femoral component relative to its position on the acetabulum. As this gradual internal rotation of the entire femoral segment occurs, the long axis of the femur is externally rotating or 'unwinding'. The overall net effect is to have the patella placed on the frontal plane, by approximately the age of 5 to 6 years.[6–8] This positional change is associated with the soft tissue structures affecting the hip joint including the capsule, ligaments and muscles. Such positional adaptation is generally attributed to the child's intrauterine position wherein the fetus was held in an abducted and externally rotated position in utero.[6,9] At birth, the ratio of external to internal rotation is normally 3:1, with a total range of motion approaching 100°.[8–10] As normal development occurs, the overall range of motion, as well as this external position, gradually reduces. Although a tendency towards an external rotation persists throughout the first few years of life, this position should reduce by age 5 to 6 years, at which time the patellae will typically be functioning on the frontal plane in gait. Interestingly, as the child develops into an adult, there is a gradual return to a slightly greater degree of external rotation.

The muscles responsible for externally rotating the femur include: gluteus maximus, obturator externus, obturator internus, gemelli, quadratus femoris, piriformis, sartorius, adductor magnus, adductor longus and adductor brevis. The ischiofemoral ligament will assist in limiting internal rotation.

Internal rotation of the femur is accomplished via contraction of the iliopsoas, tensor fasciae latae, gluteus medius and gluteus minimus. The iliofemoral and pubofemoral ligaments tend to limit lateral rotation.[2,3]

An additional component that may contribute to leg rotation is the position of the acetabulum. Although the normal position of the acetabulum is located in such a manner as to place the head of the femur on the sagittal plane, there may certainly be skeletal variations.[2,8,9,11] The most common variation and certainly a normal variant is one where the acetabulum is more externally rotated, which complements the overall externally rotated position present in the infant. However, when the acetabulum is significantly internally placed, then this would contribute to an internally positioned limb, a factor which some authors feel is significant, yet commonly overlooked, in the overall development of the angle of gait.[2,6,11]

FRONTAL PLANE CONDITIONS OF THE FEMUR

With regard to frontal plane changes associated with the femur, the development of coxa vara or coxa valga is the most clinically significant. Although marked changes associated with frontal plane alterations of the head and neck of the femoral segment are rare, it is still appropriate to discuss them.

The angle of femoral inclination is the angle formed in the frontal plane between the long axis of the head and neck of the femur and the long axis of the femoral shaft. In neonates, this angle is 140–150° and reduces to 120–132° (average 128°) in the first 6 years of development.[3,12]

Coxa valga

When the angle of femoral inclination has not reduced to 128°, the condition of coxa valga is said to exist. The etiology may be due to a lack of development of the head and neck of the femur relative to the shaft of the femur from dysplasia (usually bilateral) or from some type of trauma (usually unilateral). Typically, in this condition there is an awkward gait, and frequently a degree of hip dislocation is present in the varus congenital condition. A clinical result of this may be a concomitant genu varum.

Coxa vara

Coxa vara occurs when the angle of femoral inclination has reduced past 128°. Typically, this represents an overgrowth and may sometimes be seen with a slipped capital femoral epiphysis. It may be caused by trauma or may be developmental in nature. Coxa vara is difficult to evaluate in radiographs of very young infants and is usually first noticed when the child begins to walk. The leg is shorter on the affected side and abduction of the leg is restricted as is internal rotation. Coxa vara may result in genu valgum.

CLINICAL EVALUATION OF THE HIP

Although radiographic studies may be obtained in order to measure some of the torsional parameters previously discussed, this is not common practice when routinely determining the range of motion available at the hip. A combination of off-weightbearing measurements, together with gait analysis, where applicable, is generally sufficient in order to determine whether the problem involves soft tissue or bone. When the primary etiology based on clinical evaluation can be determined, an appropriate treatment plan may more readily be initiated.

Prior to measuring any range of motion, the child should be allowed to walk around the office or clinic, without the hand being held, in order that an overall evaluation of gait may be appreciated. Even in the youngest of children, the position of the head, shoulders and pelvis should be observed in order to determine whether or not a limb length discrepancy is present. Visualization of the patellae will provide the examiner with a general idea as to how the lower limb is functioning. Up until the age of 5 to 6 years, the normal clinical presentation generally places the patellae in an externally located position. This would be expected in a child who had normal torsional and positional development of the femoral segment.

When the child walks in a fairly adducted manner, with each patella on the frontal plane, then the presence of a pseudolack of malleolar torsion, an internal tibial torsion, a metatarsus adductus, a rigid forefoot valgus, or a rigid plantarflexed first ray deformity would be suspected. When one or both patellae function in an internally deflected position, then it may be assumed that at least a portion of the deformity lies within the femoral segment. It is clinically difficult to determine the extent of the involvement from other levels, solely by visualizing the patellar positions. It is also difficult to determine whether an intoed gait associated with internally facing patellae (often reported as the squinting patellae syndrome)[11,13] is due to a soft tissue or osseous anomaly. However, in the case of internal femoral torsion, as the patient walks towards the examiner, it will be noted that the adducted gait pattern is typically consistent in nature, i.e. there is little deviation observed in the angle and base of gait from step to step. However, when the degree of adduction varies with each step, then this inconsistency may be attributed to tight medial musculature. Such tightening during the swing and contact phases of gait initiates the adduction noted. Typically, this motion is caused by a tight medial hamstring. The movement is quite distinct from the marked adduction noted in children with spastic adductors or hamstrings associated with various types of neurological deficits.

Documentation of the angle and base of gait, patellar position and extent of calcaneal eversion should all be recorded at the conclusion of this portion of the examination. Once the gait has been evaluated, the non-weightbearing range of motions should be assessed. Although it is not within the scope of this chapter to present all the diagnostic parameters that are useful in determining the presence of a dislocated or dislocatable hip, no opportunity should be missed to evaluate hip stability and congruency in the developing child. Owing to the dynamics associated with this condition, it is now more appropriately termed 'developmental dysplasia of the hip'. This terminology reflects the potential for this deformity to occur almost spontaneously in a child previously displaying normal hip alignment and stability. The incidence of a frankly dislocated hip is 1 in 1000 live births, with a dislocatable, subluxable hip being present in greater than 1 in 100 live births.[13] The incidence is generally higher in Italy, Israel and Japan.[13] The reason for this is uncertain. There are several etiological factors involved with the development of a dysplastic hip condition:

1. *Heredity*. The first child of normal parents has a risk of about 1 in 1000. When there is one affected child, a male offspring has a risk of 1 in 100, and a female offspring has a risk of 1 in 10. When one parent has a history of congenital dislocation of the hip, a male offspring has a risk of about 6 in 100, and a female offspring has a risk of about 17 in 100. If one parent and one child are affected, the risk to the next child is approximately 40%.
2. *Environmental influences*. These include (a) breech position associated in up to 40% of the cases, (b) first pregnancy and (c) swaddling with the legs in extension.
3. *Hormonal*. Relaxin from the mother during labor may be related to increased frequency in girls. Dislocation is nearly eight times more common in females. Children with metatarsal adductus and torticollis have an increased incidence of a developmental dislocation of the hip.

The importance of this is magnified whenever the opportunity of evaluating the stability of the hips in children under 12 months of age arises. As the status of the hips may change spontaneously, it is essential to evaluate hip stability even when recent examinations by other clinicians have been performed and found to be normal.[13,14]

Clinical signs indicative of a possible dislocated hip include redundant skin folds of the thigh associated with an apparently shortened limb, and a positive anchor sign which is represented by asymmetrical gluteal folds (Fig. 11.1). A Trendelenburg gait with associated mild shoulder and hip drop, along with a unilateral external leg position, are often noted in the ambulatory child with frank hip dislocation. Clinical tests for a dislocatable hip, which may occur in as many as 1 in 100 live births, often become inappropriate after the first few months of life. This is

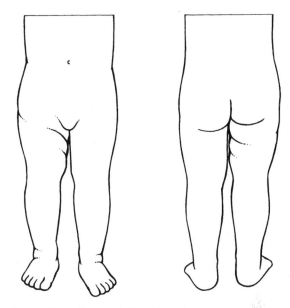

Figure 11.1   Abnormal skin folds and elevated right buttock, indicating positive anchor sign.

due to tightening of soft tissue structures in and around the hip. Spontaneous resolution of this problem is a common phenomenon.[13,14]

Although Barlow's maneuver has been utilized for many years,[15] it has recently been felt to be an ineffective maneuver for eliciting stability of the femoral head within the acetabulum.[14] In addition, there is some concern that the inappropriate application of the manual forces necessary to perform this examination may actually lead to some disruption of normal femoral–acetabular development. Barlow's maneuver as presented in the classical description is most appropriately initiated within the first few months after birth, and is accomplished with the child lying supine with the hips and knees maintained in a flexed position. The middle finger of each hand of the examiner is placed over the greater trochanter, and the thumb of each hand is applied to the inner side of the thigh at the level of the lesser trochanter. The thighs are carried into mid-adduction with the test consisting of the application of pressure backwards and outwards with the thumb.[13]

When the hip is dislocatable, or unstable, this pressure will allow the femoral head to slide backwards over the posterior acetabular rim. Release of the pressure allows re-entry into the acetabulum. The test is limited and becomes less useful as the child becomes older. Although it may be attempted up to the 7th month, the test is most reliable at birth to 4 weeks.

Of greater importance is the ability to actually diagnose the presence of a frankly dislocated hip. Familiarization with the more common and reliable tests for a congenital dislocation of the hip is essential in order that appropriate radiographs may be taken when necessary.

There are three clinical methods that would appear to be reliable in assisting the clinician to determine whether or not a congenitally dislocated hip is actually present. All clinicians involved in the evaluation and treatment of lower extremity disorders in the pediatric population should be capable of effectively performing the following tests:

1. Ortolani's sign (reducing test for congenital dislocation of the hip). With the infant supine, the hips and knees are flexed to 90°. The hips are examined one at a time by grasping the baby's thigh with the middle finger over the greater trochanter and then simultaneously lifting and abducting the thigh to be examined while stabilizing the opposite thigh and pelvis. When the hip is dislocated, the femoral head will move from a posterior dislocated position to a more inferior and distal position within the acetabulum. The examiner can feel the head relocate which is described as a 'palpable click', not an 'audible click'. This test is most reliable in the early months of postnatal life. It must be remembered that there are other structures around the hip such as ligaments that may also cause a clicking and thus although this is a very useful test, it is not pathognomonic for a congenitally dislocated hip.

2. Abduction test. With the child supine and the hips and knees flexed, the hip is gently abducted. There will be restriction of abduction on the dislocated side caused by shortened and contracted hip adductor muscles. This is easily seen in unilateral dislocation.

However, in bilateral dislocations, abduction will be symmetrical but limited. The test is most reliable after 2 months of age. As newborns are generally flexible, it is not uncommon to perceive false negatives.[6,13,16]

3. Galeazzi's sign (Allis' sign). The child is placed supine with the knees and hips flexed and the level of the knees is observed. With a dislocation, the affected side will be lower. This test is most reliable after the age of 18 months. A bilateral dislocated hip deformity will be missed if reliance is placed upon this examination alone.

The last two tests are reliable for quite some time and may be positive even when a dislocated hip has gone undetected for several years. Owing to the ease of performing these tests, they should be carried out immediately prior to the tests preferred in order to determine the status of internal and external hip rotation.

There are numerous methods of determining the ranges of motion of the hips in the transverse plane. The child may be prone or supine, seated or lying down, with the knees either extended or flexed. All the tests are capable of reflecting the information that is necessary in order to reach a correct diagnosis and to fashion an appropriate treatment plan.

One effective method of determining the transverse plane range of motion of the hip involves measuring the internal and external rotation available at the hip, with the child in both a hip-flexed and a hip-extended position. Although it may be necessary to perform the examination on the lap of one of the parents, it is generally preferable to obtain the information with the child directly on the examination table. Initially, the range of motion at the hip should be assessed first externally and then internally in the transverse plane. This may be performed without instrumentation in order to allow the examiner to become correctly oriented with the overall positioning of the limbs. A general impression of the actual available ranges of motion may be achieved if the examiner imagines the face of a clock placed proximal to the patella with an 'hour hand' rising perpendicularly from the center of the patella. When the patella is lying parallel to the supporting surface, the 'hour hand' would reflect a position of 12 o'clock or 0°. Thus each 'hour' position would equate with a 30° change. Therefore, on examining the left extremity of a youngster whose patella approached a '2 o'clock' position with external rotation, this would be documented as an approximate external deviation of 60°. This is only a cursory form of examination and is most useful in screening examinations or at times of initial assessment prior to performing a more complete examination.[2,6,8]

With regard to a specific examination, examiners should utilize whichever of the commonly available measuring devices that they feel are most accurate and reproducible in their hands. Initially, the child is seated in a hip-flexed position with the amount of external and internal hip position recorded for each limb (Fig. 11.2). When measuring external rotation of a limb, care should be taken to ensure that the contralateral buttock does not rise from the couch as this would indicate that excessive force was being generated with the examination technique. In this situation, it would appear that there was a greater degree of external rotation available than was actually present. Conversely, when measuring internal hip rotation, care should be taken not to elevate the buttock of the side being rested as this would erroneously increase the amount of internal rotation present.

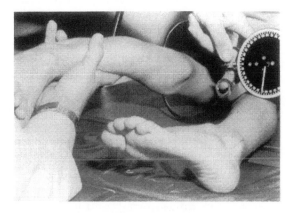

Figure 11.2 Measurement of internal femoral rotation.

The above tests should be repeated with the child's hip in an extended position. Following the recording of the amount of external and internal rotation found at the hip, it must also be noted whether the ends of the ranges of motion were soft and spongy or abrupt and bony in nature.

Children should demonstrate greater external than internal rotation of the femoral segment up until the age of 6 or 7 years. There should exist approximately two to three times the amount of external rotation to internal rotation at that age. The total range of motion available on the transverse plane may be anywhere from 100–120° at birth.[1,3] Over the following years, the general tendency is for internal and external rotations to equalize themselves with the total range of motion generally decreasing to approximately 80°. Any significant alterations relative to these values are generally measured in children with lower extremity gait disturbances.[3,6,8]

When performing the range-of-motion examination of the hips, certain specific clinical observations must be noted. These are extremely useful in establishing a diagnosis for marked internal or external femoral rotation problems.

As mentioned earlier, the quality of the end of the range of hip motion should be recorded. For example, a child whose measurements record 80° of internal hip rotation and 30° of external hip rotation in both hip-extended and hip-flexed positions, and whose 'end of range of motion' was abrupt or 'bony' in nature, would have a clinical presentation consistent with an internal femoral torsion. Conversely, a child who records 90° of external rotation with 10° of internal rotation in both hip-extended and hip-flexed positions, with that same bony feel to the end of the range of motion, would have findings consistent with an external femoral torsion.[3,6]

However, in cases where there was a marked difference in the measured rotations, and the examiner felt that the ends of the range of motion were generally 'spongy' or 'yielding', then the suspected source of the problem would be muscle or ligamentous involvement. For example,[3,6] when the examination reveals 60° of internal rotation and 30° of external rotation with the hip extended, and a similar amount of internal rotation but with 60° of external rotation when the hips are flexed, then soft tissue involvement is likely. Specifically, the pubofemoral ligament, the ileofemoral ligament or the ligamentous teres should be suspected of limiting the external rotation as these structures, when contracted, would limit external rotation with the hip extended. However, once the hip is flexed and these structures become relaxed, an increased available external rotation may be recorded.

When there is the same apparent change elicited in external versus internal rotation produced by examining the child first in the hip-flexed and then in the hip-extended position, the hamstrings should be suspected of being involved in restricting external rotation. In this instance, specific evaluation of the hamstrings would be necessary in order to complete the examination.[8]

With femoral rotation problems, the following clinical possibilities should be noted:

1. An external hip position will be present when the internal rotation available increases with the hip moving from an extended to flexed position, or vice versa. Specifically, when a limited amount of internal rotation is noted only with the hip flexed and knee extended, then there is a tight or shortened lateral hamstring. When the limitation of internal rotation is only present with the hip in an extended position, then a contracture of the iliopsoas must be suspected and this muscle may then be tested on an individual basis.[2,3]

2. A measured range of motion, which remains essentially unchanged regardless of the hip position and which is accompanied by a bony or abrupt feeling at the end of the range of motion, is typically a femoral torsion problem (internal or external). Conversely, a range of motion which is obviously altered in its external or internal measurement, depending upon the flexed or extended nature of the hip, and accompanied by a spongy feel at its end of the range of motion, typically reflects a femoral position problem (internal or external).[3,6,8]

3. Although a soft tissue problem will typically present and remain as a soft tissue problem throughout the child's development and treatment, the same may not hold true for a problem that was originally torsional in nature. An internal or external femoral torsion would most likely lead to a degree of internal or external femoral position as well. As the soft tissue structures crossing the hip joint will most likely contract and adapt to an externally or internally deviated femoral segment, they will often add to the overall deformity.

4. Ranges of motion may vary significantly from individual to individual over a period of years. Therefore, regardless of what is recorded in off-weightbearing measurements, the most important factor is evaluating the overall gait presentation, and any subsequent compensatory changes generated by the alteration of that gait.

Following assessment of the femoral segment, the knee should next be evaluated.

TRANSVERSE PLANE EVALUATION OF THE KNEE

With regard to evaluating the rotations of the knee in the transverse plane, it must be appreciated that the overall available range of motion of this joint is capable of changing a great deal over the first few years of life. As in most major joints of the upper and lower extremity, the rotation present in the knee will be quite large at birth and throughout infancy, with a rapid tightening of the structures noted over the first few years of life. The total range of motion in the transverse plane with the knee extended may be anywhere from 0 to 15–20°.[2,3] As has been pointed out by various authors, it is generally difficult to fully extend the knee in a young infant because of the retention of the in-utero hip-flexed, knee-flexed attitude. As a result of this, the available motion noted is most likely visualized with the knee in a slight degree of flexion. Conversely, evaluation of the transverse plane range of motion with the knee in a fully flexed attitude may exceed 35–45° total range of motion.[3]

When the development of the knee joint together with that of the surrounding ligamentous and muscular attachments proceeds in a normal fashion, there will be no interruption in the development of a normal angle of gait. However, when there is a tightening of the medial structures owing to retention of the in-utero position accompanied by weak lateral musculature or increased intervention of the medial structures, then a developmental and functional asymmetry of the internal versus external range of motion at the knee will exist. In such cases, the tibia will develop and then function in an internally rotated position. Just as it is possible to differentiate between an internal femoral position and an internal femoral torsion, it should be possible to diagnose the presence of an internal tibial position versus an internal tibial torsion. Referred to in the past as a pseudolack of malleolar torsion, and classically described as an increase in the overall range of knee rotation, the deformity should be evaluated and considered in a different clinical perspective.[3] All authors agree that when an intoed gait pattern is present in the early walker and that the child's knee functions in the frontal plane, then the deformity always lies distal to the femoral segment. In cases where there was a measured normal tibial torsion and no other pathology noted in the foot (see previous discussion), then the problem would typically lie within the knee joint itself. As mentioned earlier, this condition was referred to as a pseudomalleolar torsion or pseudolack of malleolar torsion, a rather confusing term at first, but an accurate description of the clinical presentation. That is to say, one in which a child would present with an adducted foot but whose knee functioned on the frontal plane, giving the clinical impression of a low or internal tibial torsion. However, in cases where a normal tibial torsion was present, the resultant deformity was attributed to a hypermobile or loose knee which appeared clinically as being caused by a torsional problem. Such observations led to the description of a pseudolack of tibial torsion.[3,13,14]

Upon clinical examination of a youngster with this presenting problem, the examiner will note that besides the child's gait pattern being adducted, the affected foot will appear to strike in a different position with alternating steps, an effect precipitated via the soft tissue contractures. In addition, there will be a greater tendency towards tripping and instability in gait owing to this gait disturbance.[14]

When performing the non-weightbearing examination for this particular segment of the leg, it is generally unnecessary to use any of the commonly available measuring devices. Clinical interpretation of the amount and extent of rotation will be sufficient, particularly when considered in light of the presenting complaint and initial gait evaluation.

Up to the age of 3 to 4 years, in the child who is developing normally, it would be expected that with the child's knee in full extension, there would be little rotation available as the knee would be 'locked' when in this position. However, upon flexion of the knee, even to a minimal degree, a marked increase in the overall total amount of transverse plane rotation would be noted.

Examination of the knee in this position should normally yield approximately equal amounts of internal and external rotation of the proximal tibia on the distal aspect of the femur. However, if on examination of the tibia in this 'resting' position, a greater amount of external than internal rotation was observed, then it may be assumed that tight medial musculature had placed the resting position of the tibia in an internal position. Any subsequent attempt to produce more internal rotation of the tibia relative to the femur would not yield much movement as the tibia would already be in its abnormal, internally located position.[3,14]

The overall range of motion of the knee would generally remain unaffected, with the actual deformity representing an excessive degree of internal rotation of the tibia. Although the literature cites a variety of effective methods of examining this, the pathology as it should be understood indicates excessive internal rotation of the tibia relative to the femur leading to an adducted gait pattern.[1–3]

Further examination of the child's knee in both hip-flexed and hip-extended position is also beneficial, as is evaluation of hip range of motion in both extended and flexed positions. When the rotation of the tibia changes with hip extension and flexion, the musculature crossing the knee is the primary deforming force. However, when the tibial rotation remains essentially unchanged with hip-extension and hip-flexion, then it may be suspected that the primary etiological problem is ligamentous in nature. Some secondary muscular involvement would also be expected in those instances much in the same manner as there is some musculature contracture at the hip with internal femoral torsion problems.

Appreciation of this fact and an understanding of the biomechanical changes of the knee over the first few years of life will clarify why the deformity is only found in the early walker and is often considered to be a self-limiting process. It should be remembered that the early walker's gait pattern is one of knee-flexion with whole foot contact at 'heel-strike'. Knee-extension occurs much later than at heel contact and for a brief period of time only. Thus, when the knee remains flexed for a prolonged period of time in the early walker, especially at heel contact, and when the medial structures are tight, then it is easily seen why the foot becomes adducted with this specific deformity.[2,6,8]

It is important to remember that as the child matures and develops, a more normal type of gait pattern will develop between 3 and 4 years of age and that more of an actual heel contact with full knee-extension as the foot approaches the supporting surface will be noticed.

DEVELOPMENT OF THE KNEE

Genu varum

The normal amount of bowing at the level of the knee is a result of a lateral curvature of either the tibia or of the tibia and femur and is often found with normal coxa valga. This varus attitude is a normal developmental finding and is typically present in the infant and early walker. Developmental genu varum is present from birth and may be present up until 4 years of age.[6,17]

Normal genu varum may be exaggerated by either an internal rotation of the femoral segment or by an internal tibial torsion, both of which will externally rotate the lateral aspect of the posterior calf musculature. This will tend to emphasize the overall clinical appearance of a normal frontal plane bowing of the knee.[8] The clinical aspect of this condition, which is important to note, is that certain disease processes can mimic or aggravate this deformity, e.g. rickets, Blount's disease or an asymmetrical development of the epiphyses (see discussion under tibial varum, below).[2,6,10] Such conditions must be considered in the differential diagnosis when there is either excessive bowing present or a failure of a varus attitude to reduce significantly by the age of 4.

Genu valgum

A genu valgum or knock-kneed appearance is a normal physiological position noted during a child's development at certain ages. Frequently associated with coxa vara, the position generally develops normally following the normal genu varum position previously discussed. Generally, it is first noticed between 3 and 5 years of age, and will persist for several years before it is eventually outgrown by age 8 years.[6] Certain authors note that a second physiologically normal episode of genu valgum may occur in the 12- to 14-year-old, depending upon other rotational factors influencing the femoral component at that time.[1]

As the child develops, the normal genu valgum attitude may be attributed to the obliquity of the femur, i.e. the medial femoral condyle is lower than the lateral femoral condyle. When this position persists, the lateral femoral condyle will bear more weight than the medial femoral condyle. According to Tax,[6] such a situation, when combined with varying rates of development of the medial and lateral aspects of the tibial epiphyses, will lead to varying degrees of a valgus position, and may be associated with a curvature of the femoral or tibial shaft. Normal epiphyseal plate development, affected by either infection or trauma, may also lead to a significant genu valgum.

In measuring genu varum and genu valgum, the child should lie supine on the examination table.

1. *Genu varum*: the malleoli are brought together and the distance between the medial femoral condyles is measured.
2. *Genu valgum*: the knees are first allowed to come into contact with each other and the distance between the two medial malleoli is then measured.

Based on classic presentation and study of the deformity by Morley,[18] a helpful grading system was introduced for clinical reference.

Grade I: intermalleolar/intercondylar distance = 0.98 inch (2.5 cm).
Grade II: intermalleolar/intercondylar distance = 0.98–1.96 inches (2.5–5.0 cm).
Grade III: intermalleolar/intercondylar distance = 1.96–2.95 inches (5.0–7.5 cm).
Grade IV: intermalleolar/intercondylar distance = 2.95 inches (7.5 cm).

Genu recurvatum

While in the stance position, the child should be examined for pathological genu recurvatum. This posterior deflection of the femur on the tibia may normally be present, measuring approximately 5–10° until the age of 5 years. Any amount greater than that in children under 5 years, or any amount at all after the age of 5 years, may be indicative of some lower extremity pathology.[2,3]

A congenital gastrocnemius equinus may cause this deformity to occur when there is an inability to compensate at the level of the subtalar and midtarsal joints. The genu recurvatum position allows the foot to function in an attitude that is somewhat plantarflexed to the tibia, thereby decreasing the abnormal pull on the posterior musculature. When this type of compensation is allowed to continue, the abnormal deflection of the posterior surface of the knee will become progressively worse and most likely symptomatic. Identification of this condition is essential if future problems are to be avoided.

Consistent monitoring is particularly important when utilizing functional foot orthoses in the treatment of a pes planus deformity associated with a suspected congenital equinus.

When the orthotic device successfully inhibits abnormal subtalar and midtarsal joint compensation, then the Achilles tendon will be placed under constant tension. When there is an accommodative contracture of the posterior musculature, then the Achilles tendon will lengthen and a measurable increase in ankle motion may be appreciated. No change in the original angle of genu recurvatum should be noted during treatment. If, on the other hand, it is observed that the original angle of genu recurvatum is being increased through the use of the functional foot orthoses, then this indicates the likelihood of a congenital equinus. In such instances, the orthotic devices should be discontinued and surgical lengthening considered.[3,7,8]

TIBIA

Transverse plane

Evaluation of the transverse plane rotation of the tibia will allow a full appreciation of all the components leading to the overall development of a patient's angle of gait to be obtained. Along with the previously discussed soft tissue and osseous changes affecting the femur and knee, the twisting or torsion that occurs in the tibia will contribute to the placement of the foot during gait. Most authors agree that there is very little, if any, external rotation noted of the tibia relative to the fibula at birth. However, as the tibia undergoes a gradual 'unwinding' process, in which it will externally rotate relative to the fibula, clinical documentation can be made of the gradual development of this segment and of its effect on the eventual angle of gait.[19,20]

The amount of true tibial torsion, which occurs during development of the tibia on the transverse plane, is between 18 and 23°.[1,3,21,22] This torsion can be measured radiographically, or with computerized axial tomography. However, as it is impossible clinically to measure true tibial torsion, it is the malleolar position that is recorded. Malleolar position is the position of a bisection of the tibial malleolus relative to a bisection of the fibular malleolus.[3] A recent study by Lang & Volpe[22] indicated that the inconsistent values are most likely precipitated by variations in the reference points utilized during examination as opposed to true structural differences.

Malleolar position, or tibiofibular rotation as it has been termed by various authors, changes in a slow, gradual fashion from year to year, with approximately 13–18° of external malleolar position being noted by the age of 7 to 8 years. Whereas external femoral rotation may occur up to 13 to 14 years of age, external rotation of the tibial component is generally completed by this earlier age.[20-23]

In addition, a distinction should be made between a low tibial or malleolar torsion and an internal tibial or malleolar torsion (Fig. 11.3). When the clinical measurement of the tibial position is less than zero, e.g. –8°, then this is a fairly significant deformity which will be difficult to be 'outgrown' as the tibia has not even attained the position which should be present at birth. On the other hand, a less significant deformity would be present if 5° of external malleolar torsion was measured in a 4-year-old who should possess approximately 8° of tibial torsion by this time. A recent study of 281 children between $1\frac{1}{2}$ years and 6 years of age confirmed the views held by other authors, namely that there is a gradual external positioning of the tibia relative to the fibula. The data demonstrated a steady increase in external malleolar position from 5.5° at 18 months to 11.2° at 6 years. The data reported

were consistent with the values reported by other authors that a normal adult position of 13–18° of the transmalleolar position would be achieved by 7 to 8 years.[20]

Measurement of tibial or malleolar torsion is accomplished with the child lying supine or seated, with the knee maintained in as extended a position as is possible. When the measurement is performed with the knee flexed to 90° and when there is an element of internal tibial position present, then the measurement of true tibial or malleolar torsion may be altered. The femoral condyles are placed equidistant from the supporting surface with the patella lying in the frontal plane. By the examiner placing thumbs and index fingers anterior and posterior to each malleolus, the examiner will be able to determine when there is an internal or external tibial torsion present by interpreting the finger position. Each malleolus is then bisected with the position mapped in relationship to the bisection of the fibular malleolus. This examination is carried out with the subtalar joint in its neutral position and the foot held at a 90° angle to the leg. Then, visualizing the angle of the transmalleolar axis relative to the frontal plane, a tractograph or goniometer may be used to document the actual amount of either internal or external tibial torsion which is present (Fig. 11.4).

It is important to remember that when this measurement is obtained, a closed kinetic chain situation is promoted by virtue of the examining technique. Therefore, it is essential to maintain the foot in its neutral position. Inadvertent pronation of the foot will internally rotate the tibial segment and this will cause the examiner to record a lower tibial torsion than is actually present. Conversely, inadvertent supination of the foot may mask an actual low tibial torsion by externally rotating the tibial segment during examination.[23]

Tibial varum

Tibial varum may exist along with genu varum and is often considered as a portion of the overall bowing process of the distal leg. Physiological bowing of the lower extremity is normal from

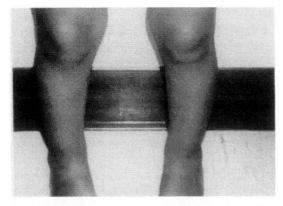

Figure 11.3 Adducted gait secondary to low tibial torsion. Note each patella is on the frontal plane, indicating normal femoral rotation.

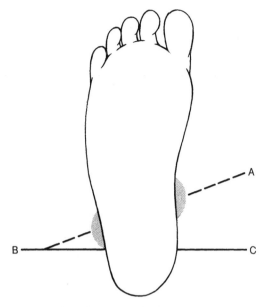

Figure 11.4   Measurement of tibial torsion utilizing bisection of the malleoli.

birth until 2 to 4 years of age, with as much as 5–10° of normal frontal plane bowing present at birth. This bowing gradually reduces to 2–3° at approximately age 2 to 4 years and represents the normal adult value.[3,20] When there is greater than 5° of tibial bowing present, a measure of compensation will be required from the subtalar joint in order to allow the calcaneus to assume a vertical position to the ground. In cases where tibial varum exceeds the subtalar joint range of pronation, the individual will compensate in a varus attitude throughout the gait cycle. Such compensation may lead to chronic lateral instability or to the development of a retrocalcaneal exostosis, or 'pump bump'.

Rickets and Blount's disease must be included in the differential diagnosis of severe bowing of the tibial segment. Although rickets is not commonly seen, the possibility of this process occurring must be borne in mind when evaluating the infant with marked genicular bowing. Causes of rickets can all be associated with a vitamin D deficiency which may be secondary to renal disease, malabsorption problems or to a general lack of the vitamin owing to malnutrition.[6,13] Any

concern regarding the presence of this condition may best be diagnosed via radiographs which will determine an abnormal widening or flaring of the metaphyses.

Blount's disease, on the other hand, is due to a growth disturbance of the medial aspect of the proximal tibial epiphysis and is typically associated with a failure of epiphyseal growth followed by changes in the stress forces affecting the area. This may be manifested in two forms: (i) in the infant and (ii) in the adolescent. The infant form of the disease may be observed in the child aged between 1 and 3 years and is most classically associated with a chubby, active child who was an early walker (prior to 9 months). The adolescent type will be manifested somewhere between 8 and 13 years and is generally not as common as the infant type.

Tibial valgum

This is not a common presentation in the lower extremity. However, when present, tibial valgum is generally the result of an epiphyseal injury or a malunion of a tibial fracture. In evaluating the various etiologies for a flexible flatfoot deformity, an anteroposterior view of the ankle is necessary in order to rule out any abnormal force generated by a valgus ankle joint, with or without tibial valgum.

ANKLE JOINT DORSIFLEXION

At birth, there is unrestricted ankle joint dorsiflexion present so that the dorsum of the foot may approach the anterior aspect of the tibia, an angle of approximately 75°. This amount of dorsiflexion rapidly reduces to approximately 20–25° by age 3 years, 15° by age 10 years and 10° by age 15 years (Fig. 11.5).[3,8] This last value represents the average adult norm. When a congenital tightness is present, there is a consistent lack of dorsiflexion present from birth, with virtually no or minimal measurable dorsiflexion noted. When obtaining this measurement, certain guidelines should be followed in order to ensure accurate and reproducible figures.

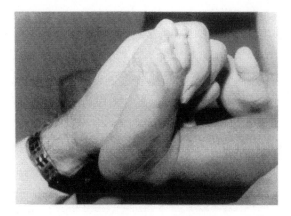

Figure 11.5 Normal ankle joint dorsiflexion in a 2-year-old child.

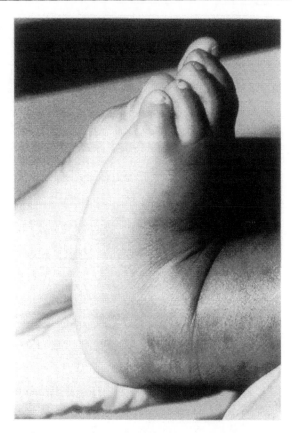

Figure 11.6 Excessive dorsiflexion of the forefoot on the hindfoot during incorrect casting of a congenital equinus has led to a rocker-bottom type flatfoot. Surgical correction was required to effectively increase ankle joint motion.

Generally, it is best to perform this maneuver with the patient supine. The hip may be either flexed or extended. The foot is then maximally dorsiflexed to the leg with the subtalar joint maintained in the neutral position. This is essential as a pronated subtalar joint will cause the midtarsal joint to unlock, thereby introducing additional forefoot dorsiflexion (Fig. 11.6).[3]

Certain children may plantarflex their foot when an attempt is made to passively dorsiflex it. In such cases, the plantar surface of the foot may be stroked and then the foot maximally dorsiflexed as the child is withdrawing. If this strategy is unsuccessful, the problem may be overcome by initially flexing the knee in order to dorsiflex the foot with the gastrocnemius relaxed and then slowly extending the knee again. When recording the actual measurement, care must be taken to place the tractograph so that one arm extends along the lateral aspect of the foot and the other accurately bisects the lower leg. When this measurement is within normal limits for the child's age, it is not necessary to retake the measurement with the knee flexed. However, when there is a marked lack of dorsiflexion, it is necessary to determine to what extent, if at all, the soleus is implicated. When ankle dorsiflexion is limited with the knee extended but greater than 15° with the knee flexed, the child has a gastrocnemius equinus. When the limitation is present in both the knee-flexed and knee-extended posi-

tions, then a gastrocnemius–soleus equinus is most likely responsible; an osseous ankle block would be uncommon in this age group.

When the child's chief complaint is toe-walking, extreme care must be exercised in measuring dorsiflexion. Although most children who exhibit tendencies towards toe-walking have no lower extremity pathology, the clinician must be able to rule out musculoskeletal as well as possible neurological conditions. When there is a true lack of dorsiflexion or brisk reflexes present upon examination, further evaluation is mandatory.[2,6]

The clinician should be aware that an abnormally pronating foot may also cause an apparent equinus condition. In the older child, the pronated foot will unlock the midtarsal joint and initiate dorsiflexion of the forefoot relative to the hindfoot in gait. Over time, foot-to-leg dorsiflexion occurs at the level of the midtarsal joint rather than at the ankle joint.

Subsequently, accommodative contracture of the posterior musculature gives rise to a clinically apparent equinus. It is this type of 'functional' equinus which responds well to orthoses and stretching exercises; a true congenital equinus does not change through the use of either modality.

SUBTALAR JOINT RANGE OF MOTION

A functional orthosis is only appropriate for use in a pediatric patient after the child has initiated a heel–toe type of gait, a situation that generally occurs at age 3 to $3^1/_2$ years. Prior to that time, there is generally full foot contact and the gait is essentially apropulsive. Therefore, an accurate assessment of subtalar joint motion is not an essential part of the examination until functional orthoses are used. At this stage, the calcaneus is bisected and full inversion and eversion of the subtalar joint (in the same fashion employed in the adult foot) are measured. However, one important difference is the range of both inversion and eversion that is present in the developing child's foot. Just as in the other major joints of the lower extremity, the ranges of motion of the subtalar joint are much greater than the standard adult values. Therefore, measurements upward of 45–50° of total subtalar joint motion as compared with 20–30° present in the adolescent or adult foot should be expected.[3,21]

In assessing the subtalar joint range of motion in the child's foot, the borders of the posterior surface of the calcaneus should be established prior to bisecting the calcaneus. The full amount of inversion and eversion of the foot relative to the distal one-third of the leg should then be measured. Care should be taken to maintain the foot in a dorsiflexed position relative to the leg when performing this portion of the examination; a plantarflexed foot will reflect extraneous frontal plane ankle joint motion.

MIDTARSAL JOINT RANGE OF MOTION

A significant varus or valgus deformity, which is often related to the adult foot only, will present in the child's foot as well. Therefore, it is essential for the clinician to fully assess the forefoot to hindfoot relationship in the child's foot.

This portion of the examination is the same as for the adult's foot. The child is placed in the prone position with the calcaneus properly bisected as a reference point. The subtalar joint is placed in the neutral position and the midtarsal joint is locked. This is accomplished by placing a dorsiflexionary force on the plantar surface of the fifth metatarsal, just proximal to the metatarsal head.[24] In this fashion, the two axes of the midtarsal joint (the oblique and the longitudinal) cross each other and limit extraneous midtarsal joint mobility upon examination. In sighting down the hindfoot toward the forefoot, a measurable varus or valgus deformity will become apparent. In no instance should the forefoot be 'loaded' with pressure directed upwards onto the first metatarsal. Such an action would unlock the midtarsal joint and supinate the longitudinal axis of the midtarsal joint, thereby initiating a false degree of forefoot varus. A forefoot varus or valgus deformity present upon examination will generally not be outgrown as the child develops and may require treatment. Any degree of forefoot valgus deformity should be supported to prevent abnormal compensation during development or in later years. It may be appropriate to wait until after the age of 6 years to correct any forefoot varus deformity, as there may be some spontaneous resolution of this deformity up until that age.

METATARSUS ADDUCTUS

One of the most common pediatric abnormalities which responds well to early conservative treatment is metatarsus adductus, a transverse plane deformity occurring at Lisfranc's joint, which is reflected by adduction of the metatarsals toward the midline of the body. There are several factors involved in the etiology of this pathology, the most significant being abnormal intrauterine position with increased uterine wall compression. Other factors are a congenitally tight or malinserted abductor hallucis tendon or a tight malpositioned anterior tibial tendon. Metatarsus adductus occurs in approximately 1 in 1000 births with no sexual distinction; there is a 4–5% transmission rate to the second child regardless of the etiology of the initial problem.[5]

The clinical picture is best visualized by placing the child's foot into a 'V' formed by the second and third fingers. The following signs are then evident:

- concave medial border
- convex lateral border
- prominent styloid process
- increased metatarsus primus adductus.

There is no abnormal subtalar joint range of motion present when non-weightbearing. Clinically, the deformity may be classified into mild (flexible), moderate or severe (rigid). The mild to moderate forms are the most prevalent, and are very amenable to conservative therapy. The clinician must also consider the possibility of a functional type of metatarsus adductus which is commonly associated with a tight or malinserted abductor hallucis tendon. As this form of metatarsus adductus often goes unnoticed until the child bears weight, it is essential for the clinician to pull the infant into a weightbearing attitude in order to determine the presence of such pathology. The resultant loading of the forefoot that occurs is sufficient to cause the tight abductor hallucis to pull the hallux into an adducted position.

Radiography is useful in evaluating this deformity for two reasons. First, it allows the clinician to determine the extent of the metatarsus adductus by measuring the specific amount of adductus present and, second, it provides a baseline radiograph of the pathology. The latter reason is most important as it will allow the clinician to determine if any subluxatory changes are being initiated with overaggressive use of serial plaster immobilization.

The radiographic angle measured is determined by utilizing a bisection of the second metatarsal shaft relative to a perpendicular bisection of the lesser tarsus. The following values are acceptable during normal development:[3]

birth   15–30°
early walker (9–16 months)   20°
4 years   15°
adult   15°.

Positive radiographic findings associated with a metatarsus adductus are:

- an increase in the metatarsus angle
- an apparent decrease of the adductus laterally
- increased metatarsal base superimposition laterally
- hypoplasia of the medial cuneiform
- an associated metatarsus primus adductus.

A metatarsus adductus is a significant lower extremity congenital abnormality. A failure either to arrive at an early diagnosis or to initiate appropriate treatment may result in any of the following in the older child:

1. painful styloid process
2. difficulty with shoe-fitting in the more rigid deformity
3. retrograde pronatory influences into the hindfoot as the flexible type accommodates itself to footwear
4. early bunion formation.[2,3]

The first line of defense in the mild to moderate forms of metatarsus adductus, which is diagnosed within the first few months of life, is passive stretching by the parents. This form of treatment serves two purposes. It may correct a very mild metatarsus adductus, or, minimally, it will increase flexibility prior to the initiation of serial plaster immobilization (see Ch. **14**).

In the moderate to severe deformity, serial plaster immobilization is the most effective method for treating a metatarsus adductus. Whenever serial plaster immobilization is utilized, it is best to initiate it prior to ambulation as the deformity will generally be less rigid and the casts will not hamper the child's initial attempts at walking.

A below-knee cast is most appropriate in treating the non-ambulatory child. However, when the child is ambulating, it is usual to use an above-knee cast for the last two applications. This is recommended as the ambulatory child will otherwise tend to circumduct the below-knee cast, leading to excessive transverse plane motion at the knee which will later cause an internally deviated limb position in gait.

Serial plaster immobilization becomes less appropriate as the child becomes older, with only minimal positive results obtained in the child aged between 24 and 36 months. When correction becomes clinically apparent, serial plaster immobilization should be continued for half as many times again in order to decrease the likelihood of recurrence. When too much motion is achieved too quickly, a radiograph should be taken to rule out midtarsal or subtalar joint subluxation. These are common problems created by overzealous abduction of the forefoot during casting and are to be avoided. This type of subluxation will persist into later life and actually present the patient with more potential pathology than the original complaint.

Following successful treatment with plaster, the clinician must maintain the correction with night splints. The Ganley splint is most appropriate for this as it maintains the forefoot in a corrected position relative to the hindfoot. The splint should be utilized for approximately twice as long as the casting period in order to provide the best possible results (see Ch. **15**).

In conjunction with the splint, the child will have to wear straight last shoes for 2 to 3 years post-casting. Reverse last shoes, or tarsopronator shoes, should generally be avoided at any stage as these may place a constant subluxing force on the developing child's foot. Although they provide apparent cosmetic changes, these types of shoes are not acceptable from a functional point of view. In cases where there is a residual amount of metatarsus adductus present after treatment, and the child's foot exhibits some excessive pronation, rigid functional orthoses should be employed.

In cases where the child's problem is resistant to the preceding conservative therapy or initially diagnosed at a later age, surgical correction is the treatment of choice. Surgical considerations may range from soft tissue release to osteotomies depending upon the child's age and the severity of the condition.

TALIPES CALCANEOVALGUS

This condition is a positional deformity, which clinically presents in a dorsiflexed, abducted and everted position of the forefoot and heel relative to the leg. In many respects, this condition represents a deformity that is the clinical antithesis of a talipes equinovarus. Talipes calcaneovalgus may be either flexible or rigid in nature and is specifically attributed to abnormal intrauterine position and compression. Typically, this positional deformity is found in the firstborn child of a young mother who would be most likely to demonstrate tight uterine musculature thereby decreasing available space for the developing fetus.[2,24]

Although this apparent valgus attitude of the foot relative to the leg is a common positional variation noted at birth, it generally reduces spontaneously. However, when there is a marked tightening of the peroneal musculature combined with prolonged positioning of the forefoot in an abducted and dorsiflexed position, this may require treatment. On those occasions when the deformity does not resolve spontaneously in the first 3 to 4 months, certain characteristic clinical findings may become evident, e.g. a marked redundancy of the lateral skin folds of the foot and ankle; an apparent tightening of the peroneal musculature; and a decreased ability to move the foot into a corrected adducted, inverted and plantarflexed position. A hallmark of a more severe deformity is that when the examiner moves the foot into a corrected position, and then allows the foot to hang freely, it immediately returns to its abnormal position. However, when the foot remains for several seconds in the corrected position, and then slowly moves back into the valgus attitude, then a more flexible, less severe problem exists. In addition, if the child is noted to intermittently and actively adduct and plantarflex the foot, then this also indicates a more flexible deformity which may reduce spontaneously or following minimal treatment.

When the deformity is left untreated, the child will typically be a late walker. When accompanied by an external position of the femoral or tibial component, this combination makes the initial attempts at ambulation an extremely difficult undertaking. When the child finally is able to stand and walk, often as late as 16 to 20 months, the deformity generally will not spontaneously resolve owing to the abducted positioning of the foot. The child's foot then proceeds to develop in a markedly pronated and abducted fashion.

It is for this reason that early treatment ranging from parental manipulative exercises and shoe therapy in the more flexible cases to serial plaster immobilization in the more significant cases is warranted.

Even when a more severe presentation is successfully treated by means of serial plaster immobilization, night splints and shoes, further, prolonged treatment with functional foot orthoses, often for life, becomes an appropriate adjunctive treatment.[25]

TREATMENT CONSIDERATIONS

The most common sequelae of abnormal transverse and frontal plane development of the lower extremities will generally be reflected in the function of the child's foot. Any significant frontal or transverse plane deviation from the norm will place an abnormal pronatory effect on the developing foot and will either precipitate or aggravate any existing abnormal pronation. It must be remembered that the child's foot undergoes constant developmental changes over the first 7 to 8 years. When a child first stands and initiates ambulation, the feet are 'fat, flat and floppy', with no discernible arch and an apropulsive type of gait. This appearance and function are the result of an everted calcaneus and an increased medial fat pad, along with a prerequisite to place the entire foot on to the supporting surface with each step in order to attain some degree of stability. The developing child's foot may be everted by as much as 5–10° with the initiation of weight-bearing, with an average of approximately 7–8° being the norm. Generally, the everted position

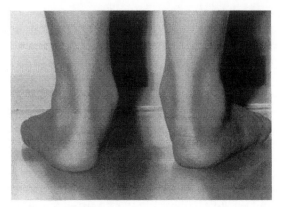

Figure 11.7 Abnormal degree of calcaneal eversion.

of the calcaneus reduces to a perpendicular attitude by the age of 7 to 8 years. However, if the child demonstrates calcaneal eversion in excess of this degree, then it should be suspected that there is an abnormal pronatory force present which is maintaining the foot in this abnormal position (Fig. 11.7). In addition, the fat pad will generally disappear and the foot will take on the overall anatomical characteristics of the adult foot. At approximately 3 to 4 years, the child's proprioceptive capabilities will have improved to the point where the child will develop a heel-to-toe type of gait, as opposed to the full foot contact type of gait associated with the early walker.[8,21] This stage in the child's development is best visualized by noting when the child can maneuver safely up and down stairs without having to stand on a single step with both feet prior to moving on to the next step.

When a frontal or transverse plane deformity is diagnosed in an older child, then some form of treatment must be directed to the foot in order to minimize the pronatory effects of the leg. An internal femoral torsion or position, and an internal or low tibial torsion, will generally lead to adduction of the talus. The internal position of the leg and talus precipitates a closed chain pronatory effect on the child's foot which will maintain or aggravate the already pronated and everted attitude. This pronated foot position and function are typically increased when the child reaches the age of self-awareness at 4 to 5 years.

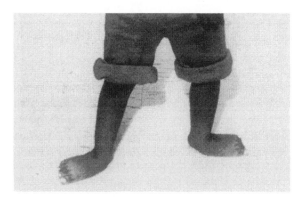

Figure 11.8   Marked external femoral and tibial torsion aggravating a bilateral talipes calcaneovalgus.

At this age, the child will attempt to improve the cosmetic appearance of the feet by actively abducting and pronating them to a greater extent.[1,2]

Conversely, an external femoral torsion or position, or external tibial torsion, may also aggravate or precipitate a significant pes planus (Fig. 11.8) since a markedly abducted gait will maintain the center of gravity in an exaggerated position medial to the subtalar joint axis. In this situation, the foot is constantly maintained in an abducted and everted position with little ability for normal development. A significant genu valgum will also lead to the same type of abnormal pronatory forces being generated into the child's foot. However, in such cases, the valgus forces are transmitted through the frontal plane displacement of the tibia. Once again, the center of gravity becomes shifted to a more medial position relative to the axis of the subtalar joint, which in turn maintains the foot in its pronated and everted attitude.[24]

TYPE AND LEVEL OF DEFORMITY

Night splints and braces may be appropriate methods of treatment for a host of lower extremity soft tissue and osseous malalignment problems (see Ch. **15**). Although the splints are considered to be more effective in correcting deformities attributable to soft tissue contractural involvement, they may also be utilized in the treatment of certain bony conditions. Before undertaking the use of any of these devices, the clinician should be aware of any significant family history for a similar type of problem because this may result in a less than successful conclusion to the treatment regimen. Generally, internal and external femoral torsions do not specifically respond well to the various splinting techniques. Since the majority of the devices are fixed to the feet or in some cases at the knee, it is difficult for appropriate pressure to be placed proximal enough to precipitate any measurable osseous changes.

Infants and children presenting with internal femoral torsion or internal femoral position are commonly found to sleep on their stomachs with their legs and feet rotated in an internal position. Conversely, infants and children with an external femoral torsion or external femoral position generally assume a position wherein their feet and legs are rotated in an external fashion, i.e. they adopt 'positions of comfort' while sleeping. Since sleep represents approximately one-half to two-thirds of the child's early life, significant soft tissue contracture affecting the capsular, ligamentous and surrounding musculature may occur, thereby reinforcing the abnormal position.

Children who have either a marked internal or external femoral torsion will in addition possess some degree of soft tissue contracture. Those youngsters with a primary internal femoral position or external femoral position will also possess increased soft tissue adaptation because of the same type of sleeping positions mentioned above.

Therefore, congenital soft tissue contracture may occur primarily in some children or it may occur secondary to an osseous deformity as described previously. Arguably night splints may be effectively used in either condition primarily to alter the sleeping position and thereby secondarily stretch associated contracted soft tissue structures. Internal or external tibial position and torsion problems may be addressed by splinting and bracing. It should be noted that in certain cases these techniques may be used as the primary method of treatment or they may be used as an adjunctive procedure in more severe examples. In cases in which serial plaster immobilization is used initially, splints and braces may then be used to maintain the correction. Since soft tissue contractures are the cause of tibial position problems, improvements may be expected with such modalities.

True internal tibial torsion may be affected by a variety of the splints in that constant traction on the distal tibial epiphysis is capable of introducing an increased amount of external tibial torsion. External tibial torsion generally represents an overdevelopment or over-twisting of the segment. Bracing techniques may prove unsuccessful in dealing with this condition, since it is difficult to determine to what extent the torsion may ultimately develop. However, splints may be used to inhibit additional outward deflection of this segment of the leg. Although splints that are attached to shoes may appear to correct tibial torsion problems, the level of correction is often attained at the child's knee owing to the large range of transverse plane rotation that exists there. This range of motion may be influenced by any constant internal or external rotatory force, e.g. via a night splint.

Specific foot conditions such as metatarsus adductus, talipes equinovarus and talipes calcaneovalgus may all be addressed via specific splinting techniques. However, it is essential that the clinician is able to determine the extent and severity of the deformity in order to ensure that more aggressive treatment may not be initially required. Although mild cases of any of the aforementioned may improve via regular stretching, shoe therapy and splinting techniques, moderate to severe cases unquestionably require more aggressive treatment.

TYPE OF SPLINT

Over the years, a host of splints and braces have been developed to assist in the development of a normal lower extremity (Figs 11.9, 11.10, 11.11). When selecting a splint, a series of variables must be considered. Certain devices are designed to address specific foot and/or leg deformities. Therefore, the clinician must determine whether the device is to correct one deformity or a combination of deformities. It should be noted that it is common for multiple deformities to be present in the same child. For example, a metatarsus adductus foot type may be exacerbated by the presence of an internal femoral torsion or position or possibly by an internal tibial torsion or position. Conversely, a talipes calcaneovalgus foot type may be exacerbated by the presence of an external femoral torsion or external femoral position or possibly an external tibial torsion or position.

In addition, there also exists the so-called 'windswept' foot deformity wherein the structures of one extremity will be internally rotated while the same structures of the other limb will be externally rotated. For example, a child may demonstrate a metatarsus adductus deformity on one foot, whereas the other foot demonstrates a talipes calcaneovalgus. In cases of multiple deformities, one should employ splints and braces that are capable of affecting each of the involved areas. Therefore, initial selection of the splint or brace should be made in relationship to the type of deformity that is being treated. In cases where the clinician has chosen to use a device that is affixed to the patient's shoe, selection may be based on a number of factors, which may include the materials used; the fabrication of the device; the overall flexibility or rigidity of the device; the ease of application of the device; and finally the cost of the device (see Ch. 15).

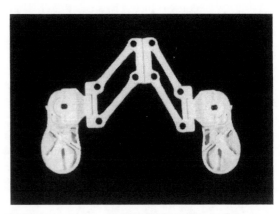

Figure 11.9 Langer counter rotation system splint.

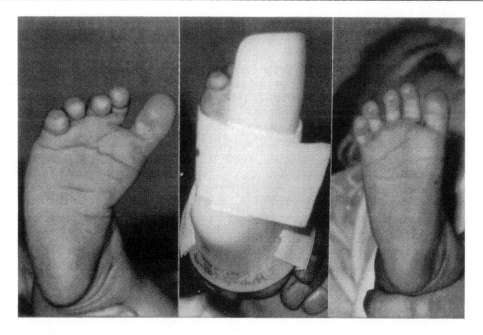

Figure 11.10 Wheaton brace demonstrating correction of metatarsus adductus (courtesy of Wheaton Brace Company, Carol Stream, Illinois, USA).

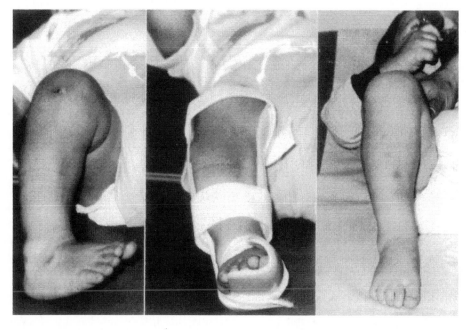

Figure 11.11 Wheaton bracing system demonstrating correction of tibial torsion (courtesy of Wheaton Brace Company, Carol Stream, Illinois, USA)

AGE OF THE CHILD

It is generally considered that the 'golden age' for treatment of pediatric rotational and torsional abnormalities is under 1 year of age; the most successful treatment results are obtained between the ages of 3 and 12 months.[26] Unfortunately, as many of the more common rotational deformities are evidenced only after a child has initiated ambulation, most treatment plans are not implemented until this time. Most of the various splinting techniques are well tolerated by the pediatric patient up to the age of 2 or 3 years, at which time the child may become uncomfortable or agitated by the restrictive nature of some of the splints or braces. After the age of 4 years, certain children may understand that the modality being used is for their benefit and may therefore adapt to the splinting. With regard to specific deformities, the effectiveness of splints and braces on femoral torsion and position problems may prove effective for a few years. Although developmental changes in this segment may occur up to the age of 13 or 14 years, successful alterations of femoral rotation problems are best achieved under the age of 5 years. Position problems affecting the tibia are generally problematical up to the age of 3 or 4 years. At that age, the conditions generally resolve as a result of the normal tightening effect of the developing knee joint.

Since an internal tibial position is responsible for precipitating a significant amount of instability with associated tripping and falling in the 1-, 2- or 3-year-old child, treatment may be initiated on an individual basis. In terms of true tibial torsion problems, it must be noted that the majority of external transverse plane rotation of the tibia is completed by the age of 7 or 8 years, which precludes any attempt at treatment beyond that age. Although significant external tibial torsion problems do not occur as frequently, the same developmental and treatment considerations exist for that condition as well.[2,6,26]

As mentioned earlier in treating specific foot pathology, splinting and bracing techniques are best initiated at an early age. For example, in cases where a talipes equinovarus deformity is untreated prior to the age of 1, splinting techniques are generally ineffective. In cases of a metatarsus adductus or talipes calcaneovalgus, splints and braces may prove effective up to the age of 2 or 3 years, but only in their milder forms. In all the aforementioned cases, the most successful utilization of splints generally follows the implementation of other treatment modalities, such as serial plaster immobilization or surgical intervention.

LENGTH OF TREATMENT

The parents of the child should be presented with the rationale regarding splinting therapy as well as with an idea of the approximate time involvement. The deformity being evaluated must be treated for a period long enough to (a) clinically alter positional torsional changes and (b) to maintain the foot in that corrected position.

When there is no appreciable change elicited over a period of 6 to 10 months, it is likely that the child's problem will not respond even with continued treatment. At this stage, a decision may be taken to terminate treatment. However, regardless of treatment, approximately 10% of these deformities persist into adult life.

In cases involving an internal or external tibial position, the period of treatment depends on whether or not serial plaster immobilization was used. In cases in which this was employed as an initial measure, the casting sequence generally encompasses a period of time extending from 4 to 6 weeks. Following this, a splint or brace is utilized for approximately twice as long as a plaster immobilization, i.e. 8 to 12 weeks. In cases in which serial plaster immobilization was not employed, the overall treatment encompasses approximately 3 to 6 months. Tibial torsion problems, when treated successfully via serial plaster immobilization, may not require additional splinting after correction has been achieved. In cases in which the splint or braces represent the primary form of therapy, the treatment regimen extends for approximately the same length of time as femoral rotation problems, i.e. from 12 to 18 months.[27,28]

Talipes equinovarus, metatarsus adductus, or talipes calcaneovalgus conditions require varying degrees of splinting or bracing, depending on their severity (see Ch. **15**).

EXTENT OF CORRECTION

The child's ability to tolerate a splint often is dependent on a number of variables. The most significant involves the angle of correction of the splint or brace. Over the years, a common prescription provided for any internal leg, knee or foot pathology was for a Denis Browne bar set at 45° abducted bilaterally with reverse last shoes. In certain instances, the bar was initially set at 60° abducted bilaterally. Although this type of bar and shoe modification was tolerated by some children, many did not wear the bar, generally because they could not tolerate the degree of correction. If a child is initially unable to wear a splint or brace because of excessive correction and subsequent discomfort, further efforts, even with the reduced degree of correction, are generally unsuccessful.

Therefore, the clinician should calculate the total degree of external leg rotation available when attempting to use a splint or brace for any internally deviated limb segment. For example, available external femoral rotation should be added to available external knee rotation and this number then added to the degree of external tibial torsion. This number then represents the total available external motion present in this child. If the total range of motion is 30° (hip) plus 15° (knee) plus –10° tibial torsion, the maximum available external rotation for this limb is 35°. If this child were placed in a bar initially set at 45° externally rotated, it is unlikely that the child will tolerate the correction. This measurement should be calculated for both limbs and used appropriately. One method of dealing with the correction is to set the splint or bar initially at a minimum degree of external rotation. This allows the child to become accustomed to the bar as well as to the introduction of a new force or pressure on the affected limb. The child is seen in 2 weeks, then monthly to increase the external correction to a tolerable position. If at any point the child is

unable to adapt to the corrected position, some reduction of that position is required.

Care must be taken not to be overly aggressive while implementing this form of therapy because of avascular necrosis of the femoral head that has been reported in such instances.[13] In cases of unilateral tibial rotation problems, the clinician should be aware that unilateral bracing systems are available and that these eliminate any concern about the preceding discussion. In cases in which a splint or brace is being used to alter an external femoral or tibial rotation problem, the device is most appropriate in altering the child's sleeping position. In these cases, care must be taken to avoid aggressive rotation of the limb into an adducted position. It is essential that the clinician be aware of the possibility of a night splint or brace causing an unstable or dislocatable hip to dislocate. It should be remembered that a dislocatable hip cannot be accurately diagnosed either clinically or radiographically beyond 4 months of age. Therefore, a child with an externally deviated limb may potentially possess this condition and it may not have been detected. Because the motion of hip adduction and internal rotation is what is responsible for dislocating a dislocatable hip, caution must be exercised not to adduct the child's limbs excessively. Because the goal of this treatment is to alter the sleeping position of the child, a corrected position of approximately 25–45° abducted may be sufficient to effect such a change. It is inappropriate to set the correction to a negative or internal value because this has the greatest potential for subluxing the child's hip.[28]

FOOT STABILITY

One of the long-standing concerns regarding any of the splinting and bracing techniques involves the potential for the device to precipitate subluxatory changes of the developing child's foot. Normal structural and functional alterations of the lower extremity should not be achieved at the expense of midtarsal and subtalar joint stability. It is essential to note that the majority of splints and braces act initially at the point of least resistance, which is the foot. Therefore, before the initiation of any force being directed into the tibia, knee, femur or hip, the midtarsal and subtalar joints of the foot are necessarily affected first. In order to eliminate the possibility of this occurring, several modifications may be introduced into the more static or stationary devices to minimize this possibility. Placing a 15–20° varus bend in the bar portion of specific splints (e.g. Ganley, Denis Browne, Fillauer) and placing a triplane or varus wedge in the heel seat of each shoe is advisable. The combination of these two antipronation measures maintains the subtalar joint in an inverted position, which results in a locking of the midtarsal joint.

Therefore, when an external force is directed against the internally rotated limb, the foot moves as a unit, thereby maintaining its structural stability and integrity. In cases in which the splint or brace is available in a variety of widths, the clinician should measure the distances across the child's shoulders or the distance from one anterosuperior iliac spine to the other and add 1 inch (2.54 cm) Either measurement may be utilized to select the appropriately sized bar.

SHOES FOR SPLINTS

As a rule, a stiff-countered, leather-soled shoe is advisable for mounting to any of the splinting or bracing systems necessitating a shoe. Although some of the splints and braces may be used in conjunction with an existing shoe, the clinician should evaluate the shoe for any evidence that it may have adapted to the deformity. For example, children with a metatarsus adductus deformity may have broken down their existing shoes to a point at which they could potentially exacerbate the deformity. When this is the case, the shoe should not be used. When possible, open-toed shoes should be used for adequate ventilation and to provide room for growth. If a closed-toe shoe is selected, the toe box of the shoe should be cut away for the same purpose. In cases in which the shoes are to be utilized for a prolonged period of time, they can be cut along the vamp and into the tongue to allow for expansion of the width of the foot.

When the child is adducted, yet relatively stable and not demonstrating any signs consistent with abnormal pronation of the foot, treatment may not be necessary at all. However, when signs of moderate to severe compensation are present, treatment combining both night splints and custom foot orthoses should be employed in order to provide the child with the best chance of eventually developing a normal gait pattern.

SUMMARY

Early recognition and treatment of the common transverse and frontal plane deformities outlined in this chapter will hopefully lead to a child whose lower extremities are mechanically sound and efficient and capable of carrying the child into adolescence and then adulthood in a comfortable and efficient fashion. The ability to identify those children who require treatment, as well as the ability to identify the type and the extent of the treatment eventually employed, is dependent upon the individual clinician's ability to accurately assess the lower limb development of the young child and to appropriately identify those children requiring treatment.

REFERENCES

1. LaPorta G. Torsional abnormalities. Arch Podiatr Med Foot Surg 1973;1:47–61.
2. McCrea JD. Pediatric orthopedics of the lower extremity. Mount Kisco, NY: Futura; 1985.
3. Sgarlato TE. A compendium of podiatric biomechanics. San Francisco: California College of Podiatric Medicine; 1971.
4. Sommerville EW. Persistent frontal alignment of the hip. J Bone Joint Surg Br 1957;39:106–113.
5. Crane L. Femoral torsion and its relation to toeing-in and toeing-out. J Bone Joint Surg 1959; 41A:255.
6. Tax H. Podopediatrics. Baltimore: Williams and Wilkins;1980.

7. Elffman H. Torsion of the lower extremity. Am J Phys Anthropol 1945;3:255.
8. Valmassy RL. Biomechanical evaluation of the child. Clin Podiatry, Podopediatr 1984;1(3):563–579.
9. Shands AR, Steele MK. Torsion of the femur. J Bone Joint Surg 1958;40A:47–61.
10. Staheli LT, Engel GM. Tibial torsion, a new method of assessment and a survey of normal children. Clin Orthop 1977;86:183–186.
11. Weseley MS, Berenfeld PA, Einstein AL. Thoughts on in-toeing and out-toeing: Twenty years experience with over 5,000 cases and a review of the literature. Foot Ankle 1981;2(1):41–46.
12. Schuster RD. In-toe and out-toe and its implications. Arch Podiatr Med Foot Surg 1976;3(4).
13. Tachdjian MO. Pediatric orthopedics. Philadelphia: WB Saunders; 1972.
14. Valmassy RL, Day S. Congenital dislocation of the hip. J Am Podiatr Med Assoc 1985;75(9):466–471.
15. Barlow TG. Early diagnosis and treatment of congenital dislocation of the hip. J Bone Joint Surg 1967;44B:292.
16. VonRosen, S. Treatment of congenital dislocation of the hip in the newborn. Proc R Soc Med 1963;56:801.
17. Kite J. Torsion of the legs in young children. Clin Orthop 1960;16.
18. Morley AJM. Knock knee in children. BMJ 1957;ii:976.
19. Hutter CG Jr, Scott W. Tibial torsion. J Bone Joint Surg 1949;31:511.
20. Rosen H, Sandwick H. The measurement of tibiofibular torsion. J Bone Joint Surg 1955;37A:847.
21. Root ML. A discussion of biomechanical considerations for treatment of the infant foot. Arch Podiatr Med Foot Surg 1973;1:41–46.
22. Lang MG, Volpe G. Measurement of tibial torsion. J Am Podiatr Med Assoc 1998;88(4):160–165.
23. Swanson AB, Greene PW, Allis HD. Rotational deformities of the lower extremity in children and their significance. Clin Orthop 1963;27.
24. Valmassy RL, Stanton B. Tibial torsion, normal values in children. J Am Podiatr Med Assoc 1989;79(9):432–435.
25. Root ML, Orien WD, Weed JH. Normal and abnormal function of the foot. Los Angeles: Clinical Biomechanics Corporation; 1977.
26. Ganley JV. Calcaneovalgus deformity in infants. J Am Podiatr Med Assoc 1975;65:407.
27. Schoenhaus HD, Poss KD. The clinical and practical aspects in treating torsional problems in children. J Am Podiatr Assoc 1977;67(9):620–627.
28. Valmassy RL. Lower extremity treatment modalities for the pediatric patient. In: Valmassy RL, ed. Clinical biomechanics of the lower extremities. St Louis: Mosby–Year Book; 1996.

12

Developmental flatfoot

Joseph C. D'Amico

Most children's feet are flat, they are not visibly deformed and they are pain-free. Therefore, such feet are assumed to be 'normal'. However, the developmental flatfoot is a poorly functioning, posturally deficient foot that has the potential to cause future deformity and disability. There is an ill-advised tendency for this foot to be ignored or treated with benign neglect. Such attitudes may be the result of disinterest, misinformation or a true belief that the condition is a normal developmental finding and as such causes no problems. Unfortunately, the developmental flatfoot is not normal and the majority of children do not completely outgrow it.

It has been documented that 80% of the population will suffer from foot problems at one time in their lives.[1] The vast majority of these inherent problems are musculoskeletal in nature and are established in childhood. While it is true that symptomatology and deformity may not be evident until the third or fourth decade, the groundwork has been set at birth before the child ever takes the first step. It is the manner in which pediatric foot and limb development takes place that determines whether or not these deficiencies are capable of being outgrown or if they will be retained and allowed to create additional deformity, dysfunction and disability later in life.

PEDIATRIC FLATFOOT

The etiology for most types of pediatric flatfoot is well documented in the medical literature (Box 12.1). There is a great wealth of information available for conditions such as calcaneovalgus,

---

Box 12.1 Selected conditions capable of producing pediatric flatfoot

Calcaneovalgus
Convex pes valgus (vertical talus)
Os tibiale externum
Tarsal coalitions
Neurological disorders
   cerebral palsy
   acute anterior poliomyelitis
Syndromes
   Morquio
   occulocerebrorenal
   Seckel
   Ehlers–Danlos
   Down
   Marfan
Iatrogenic
   post-serial plaster immobilization for talipes equino-
     varus
   post-serial plaster immobilization for metatarsus
     adductus
Mechanical
   genu valgum
   equinus – metatarsal, forefoot, ankle, gastrocsoleus,
     hamstring, iliopsoas
   transverse plane deficiencies – internal tibial torsion,
     internal or external femoral position or torsion
   Morton's syndrome
   limb length discrepancy
   forefoot varus
Developmental

---

convex pes valgus, os tibiale externum, neurological and syndrome disorders, tarsal coalitions, talipes equinus, iatrogenic flatfoot and, to a lesser extent, the mechanically induced flatfoot.[2-5] Of this group of pediatric disorders, by far the largest number of cases are represented by the developmental flatfoot category. The sum total of all flatfoot disorders in each of the other categories would not equal the number of cases in the developmental flatfoot group. Interestingly, many of the major pediatric and pediatric orthopaedic reference texts either do not ascribe any clinical significance to it or fail to mention this type of pediatric flatfoot at all.[2-5]

Definition and occurrence

Developmental flatfoot may be defined as an excessively pronated flexible flatfoot in the weightbearing pediatric population under 6 years of age. Other terms that have been used to describe this type of pediatric flatfoot include pes planus, pes valgoplanus, pes planovalgus, idiopathic hypermobile flatfoot, hyperpronated feet and floppy feet.[6-9] It is the most common condition affecting the musculoskeletal system in a child of this age group. Because this condition is so prevalent it has been equated with 'normalcy'. However, a condition that is normal implies that it is non-pathological. While it is true that the developmental flatfoot is a common finding, it should not be considered normal and it is certainly not the ideal foot type.

Many of the adult musculoskeletal parameters of the lower extremity are achieved by 6 years of age. However, a complete musculoskeletal evaluation of any 6-year-old child will reveal that individual values deviate significantly from the ideal.[10] Should these asymptomatic, undeformed feet be considered 'normal' because they possess commonly occurring, customarily anticipated structural imperfections that cause them to deviate from the ideal but not from the 'norm'?

In theory, if the foundations of a building deviated by the same proportional number of degrees as the 'average' foot, then the building would neither stand straight nor be capable of supporting heavy loads. In addition, the human 'foundations' must be capable of balanced movement, therefore the imperfections present in the 'average' foot become increasingly significant. The structural morphology of the human foot is dictated by the alignment and quality of the osseous structures, the binding ability of the ligaments, and the reinforcing and the secondary stabilizing ability of the muscles and tendons. The developing foot of the pediatric patient is flexible, flat and excessively pronated owing to an immaturity in each of these areas.

The newborn

No child is born with a perfect foot. The structure of the newborn foot contains inherited evolutionary imperfections, which, if they persist, may produce disability in the adult foot. The foot of the neonate is ill adapted for weightbearing. The newborn is not a bipedal human organism. Man is one of the few mammals whose young are incapable of standing erect at or shortly after birth. The human newborn must undergo considerable additional developmental 'unwinding' outside the womb before the organism possesses all the requisites necessary for bipedal locomotion. This critical developmental 'unwinding' takes place on hard, flat, unyielding surfaces in a malleable foot, encased in a shoe and subject to the deforming effects of gravity. A full description of lower limb intrauterine growth and development may be found in Chapter 2.

The average infant begins to stand at 7 to 9 months of age and is walking by 1 year with a range of 9 to 15 months.[11] A heel-contact gait occurs at 2 years of age and a mature, adult-like gait pattern emerges by 3 years of age.[12–17] Up to 6 years of age, skeletal alignment and development of the foot are dictated by the nature and severity of the deforming forces directed through it as well as by its ability to resist these forces. When allowed to continue, these compensatory deforming forces retard ideal development while at the same time encouraging the retention of neonatal deficiencies. According to Wolf's law of bone adaptation, structure will occur in direct response to function, i.e. form follows function. The consequence of poor function is that development will be impaired.

Osseous malalignment

The limbs of the newborn are bent and bowed to such a degree that at birth even the normal newborn possesses significant structural imperfections on all three body planes (Fig. 12.1). It is said that 'Just as the twig is bent so the tree inclined' which is an apt way to highlight the significance that these newborn imperfections may have on the growing lower extremity.[18] On the frontal plane alone, one would note the following: genu varum, 15–20° of tibial varum, 8–10° of subtalar varus and 10–15° of forefoot varus.[11] Therefore, the total amount of 'normal' varus (the sum of all the varus influences into the foot) could reach as high as 45°. All of these must be developmentally reduced before ideal foot function can take place. Most skeletal deficiencies reduce in magnitude by 6 years of age at which point their development is essentially complete.

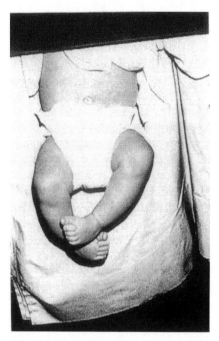

Figure 12.1 The 'normal' newborn exhibiting inherited structural imperfections, which must at least in part be outgrown before efficient weightbearing can occur. Note the crossed-over left limb position.

By 6 years of age, genu varum should have disappeared, tibial varum reduced to 0–2°, subtalar varus reduced to 2–4° and forefoot varus reduced to 0–2°. The total varus component at this point in the ideally developed foot is from 2–8°. However, musculoskeletal evaluation of the 6-year-old child will usually reveal significant unreduced structural deficiencies that are the basis for pathomechanical foot function.

The mechanism of compensation for these congenital structural imperfections in the developing or mature foot is pathological subtalar and midtarsal joint pronation. Of the frontal plane deficiencies present at birth, the most destructive is forefoot varus. Compensation for forefoot varus requires calcaneal eversion beyond the vertical to allow the forefoot to come down to the weightbearing surface. Hence, forefoot varus is capable of producing severe subtalar and midtarsal joint pronation resulting in the development of a flexible flatfoot condition.

On the transverse plane, the range of motion of the hip joint at birth is between 120° and 150°. External rotation exceeds internal rotation in a 2:1 ratio. The range of hip rotation gradually decreases until approximately 4 years of age at which time the range of motion has reduced to 90–120° and is equal internally and externally. In the child under 4 years of age, this developmental externally rotated limb position maintains the foot in an abducted attitude thereby promoting pedal pronation. In addition, there is a concomitant medial displacement of the line of gravity, which further increases the pronatory forces into the foot, encouraging the development and retention of a flexible flatfoot. The medial displacement of the line of gravity also has negative superstructural implications on the developing lower extremity articulations as well as on posture.

Osseous immaturity

Osseous immaturity is another factor which predisposes the developing foot to retain its flexible, excessively pronated, flattened morphology. Osseous maturity in the lower extremity does not occur until epiphyseal–diaphyseal fusion has taken place. The osseous nature and concomitant ability to withstand stress increases directly with age. The osseous framework of a 2-year-old child is distinctly less developed than that of a 6-year-old.

The ossification sequence in the foot occurs for the most part from the rearfoot to the forefoot. The first bones to undergo ossification are the calcaneus and the talus, which are already radiographically visible at birth. The last bone in the foot to undergo ossification is the navicular with an average age of onset of ossification of 33.8 months in males and 23.3 months in females.[19] The last site to ossify in the foot is the calcaneal epiphysis. This area does not undergo fusion until 16 to 20 years of age.[19] It is generally agreed that ontogenic development in regard to basic bone form and position is complete by 7 to 8 years of age; however, overall bone growth continues up to 20 years of age.[11,20] Complete skeletal maturity occurs at 13 years in girls and 15 years in boys.[19,21]

It is interesting to note that at 7 months of age, when the average child begins to stand unassisted, the ossification process for the navicular and for the medial and intermediate cuneiforms has not even begun.[19] These cartilaginous structures are extremely vulnerable to deforming gravitational forces directed from the limb above. At 12 months of age when the average child is already walking, the navicular and the medial and intermediate cuneiforms are still not ossified. In addition, at 12 months, the talus, the calcaneus, the cuboid and the lateral cuneiform are all markedly immature and underdeveloped structures.

The 3-year-old child is already an established mature walker with an adult-like gait pattern. At this stage, the foot is skeletally immature and not ideally suited for its static and dynamic functions of support and locomotion (Fig. 12.2). Once more, this extremely malleable foot is particularly susceptible to deforming forces directed through it from the superstructure above.

The navicular is especially significant in evaluating foot function; it is the keystone of the longitudinal arch. However, although the navicular undergoes relatively rapid ossification and growth from this onset, it is not until 6 years of age that it loses its appearance as a 'bone island' in a large space of lesser density[22] (Fig. 12.3). During this same period, the child is actively developing and refining a well-coordinated,

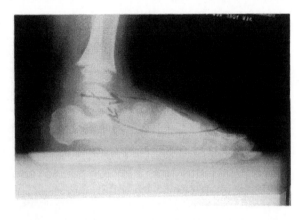

Figure 12.2 Absence of the navicular ossification center in a 2-year-old boy. Note the plantarflexed position of the talus in this established walker with developmental flatfoot.

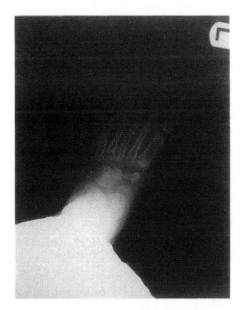

Figure 12.3 Appearance of the navicular as a 'bone island in a sea of lesser density' in a 3-year-old girl.

adult, propulsive, gait pattern. In other words, the navicular is still developing and is therefore vulnerable to forces from the superstructure above and from pathological forces from within the foot at a time when the child is now capable of bearing weight.

Ligamentous laxity

The function of the ligamentous system in the foot is to secure the osseous framework. The ligaments are the 'living' cement that help to prevent the osseous segments from becoming displaced. A developmental inability to accomplish this function results in foot instability and deficiency.

At birth, all children are loose-jointed. Such laxity peaks at 2 to 3 years of age and then begins to diminish,[23] thereafter 70–80% of all toddlers outgrow these lax ligaments.[24] At this early age, it is impossible to determine which children will outgrow this laxity and which children will be left with a significant musculoskeletal system deficiency. Ligamentous laxity should have sufficiently diminished to be clinically insignificant by 6 to 8 years of age in females and 8 to 10 years

of age in males although continued reduction occurs throughout adolescence.[24] Beyond this point, only individuals with severe degrees of ligamentous laxity retain essentially unrestricted ranges of motion.[4,23] When there is a history of familial ligamentous laxity, then it is likely the child will be similarly affected. This is especially true when both parents demonstrate lax ligaments. Schuster & Port[25] hypothesized that individuals with high degrees of ligamentous laxity and accompanying severe pronation suffer from defects in hormonal metabolism.

Ligamentous laxity is the most commonly ascribed etiology for flexible flatfoot in the developing child.[23,24,26,27] Schuster qualifies this by stating that only the generalized familial ligamentous laxity with its associated hyperextensible knees, elbows and wrists is the responsible etiology for 'unusually' flatfeet in children.[28] According to Trott, when ligaments are lax, especially in the case of the calcaneonavicular or 'spring' ligament, there is nothing to prevent medial, anterior and plantarward displacement of the talar head with resultant flatfoot deformity.[11] While this is true, it is the strength and alignment of the osseous structures that primarily and predominantly determine foot morphology.[29–31] Ligaments serve to restrict and maintain this osseous framework along with the additional reinforcement and stabilization provided by the musculotendinous apparatus. In the developing child, the inability of the ligaments to secure the osseous framework and restrict excessive motion results in instability. Since ligaments are expansile and not contractile in nature, prolonged tension, e.g. in an excessively pronated foot, will permanently deform and elongate these structures. Subsequently, abnormal foot function in the form of excessive pronation and medial displacement of body weight will be encouraged at the expense of normal osseous development.

Neuromuscular immaturity

The nervous system of the newborn is immature and does not achieve the initial stages of maturity until 1 to 2 years after birth.[10] The myelinization process begins in the 4th to 6th fetal month. However, the nerve fibers in the lower extremities are the last to receive their myelin coating.[32] Functional maturity and resultant coordination are directly related to the degree of myelinization that has taken place at any point in the continuum. Usually, it is not until 6 years of age that most organ systems of the motor mechanism are completely developed and adult coordination demonstrated.[32]

It is this neuromotor immaturity that characterizes the gait of the early walker. Observation of the gait of a 9- to 15-month-old child will reveal a wide base of gait with short bursts of forward progression. This wide base of stance and gait increases lateral and postural stability. The typical flexed positions of the knee and hip of the early walker serve to lower the center of gravity, thereby further providing stability. The feet are markedly pronated, i.e. more of the plantar aspect is in contact with the ground. This pronated foot position increases the number of plantar proprioceptors in contact with the weightbearing surface, logically improving proprioceptive feedback for balance and stability.

The function of the lower extremity musculature is to reinforce skeletal integrity and to relax ligamentous tension during locomotion and stance. This function is achieved by exerting sufficient tension to resist undesirable motions that would either disrupt joint integrity or promote hypermobility. In an excessively pronated foot, the first body system to exhibit excessive activity is the musculotendinous apparatus. The efficiency of this functional unit is dependent upon (a) proper muscle strength and length, (b) precisely sequenced phasic activity, (c) balanced synergistic and antagonistic muscle function, (d) the innate mechanical efficiency of the tendon and (e) proprioceptor activity.[33] In a pronated foot, proprioceptors respond to the stimulus of ligament stretch by innervating muscle contractions by reflex action to the extent necessary to relieve the tension.

It has been mentioned earlier that the structural morphology of the human foot is dictated by the structural alignment and quality of the osseous framework, the binding ability of the ligaments, and the reinforcing and stabilizing ability of the musculotendinous apparatus. In the developmental flatfoot, the osseous framework is significantly malaligned and immature; the ligamentous binding network is non-existent; and the musculotendinous stabilization apparatus is immature and unable to maintain optimum foot structure and function. It is because of these deficiencies that the foot of the developing child is pathologically flat and excessively pronated. However, it also represents the model from which the adult foot structure and function are derived.

Identification

By definition, the developmental flatfoot is an excessively pronated flexible type of flatfoot in which the calcaneus is markedly everted upon weightbearing (Figs 12.4, 12.5). It is a commonly occurring condition affecting the musculoskeletal system of weightbearing children under 6 years of age. The lateral column of the foot is short relative to the medial column which is lengthened owing to protrusion of the talar head medially.[31] The navicular is abducted and dorsiflexed on the head of the plantarflexed talus. The developmental flatfoot deformity is unique in that it encompasses several major pedal articulations with triplanar axes of motion. Furthermore, add to this the fact that these articulations, namely the subtalar and midtarsal joint complexes, are those responsible for connection of the foot to the leg and the foot to the ground as

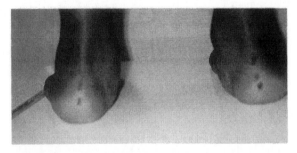

Figure 12.4 Developmental flatfoot in a 3-year-old. Note the convexity of the medial and concavity of the lateral borders of the foot formed by the extension of the medial and contraction of the lateral columns.

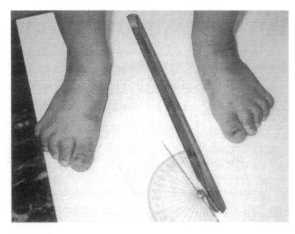

Figure 12.5 Marked calcaneal eversion and medial talar bulging in a 3-year-old child with developmental flatfoot.

well as for translating motions from the super-structure to the supporting surface and vice versa. The combined pathological relationships present in the developmental flatfoot deformity create a midfoot sag with lowering of the longitudinal arch. Therefore, the medial border of the foot is abnormally convex rather than concave (Figs 12.4, 12.5).

Identification of the developmental flatfoot is primarily achieved by elimination. It is a diagnosis of exclusion determined by ruling out other pathological flatfoot disorders (see Box 12.1). Identification proceeds first by determining whether the foot in question is flexible or rigid. The flexible pediatric flatfoot is distinguished from the rigid type by the presence of an arch off-weightbearing and none on weightbearing (Fig. 12.6). In addition, radiographs are normal off-weightbearing but exhibit an increased talometatarsal, increased talocalcaneal and lowered calcaneal inclination angles upon weightbearing (see Fig. 12.2). Finally, owing to the windlass effect of the plantar fascia, the calcaneus will invert from its present everted posi-

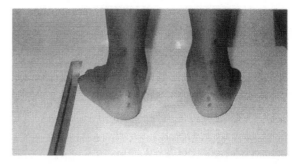

Figure 12.7 Weightbearing developmental flatfoot exhibiting marked calcaneal eversion.

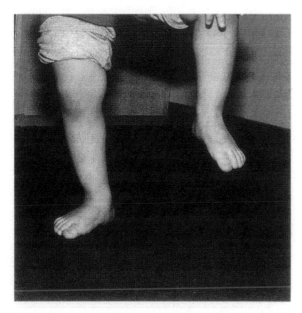

Figure 12.6 Identification of developmental flatfoot in a 2-year-old reveals an arch present off-weightbearing and none present upon weightbearing.

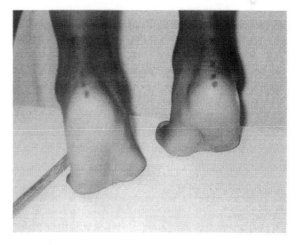

Figure 12.8 Calcaneal inversion in a case of developmental flatfoot as a result of activation of the windlass mechanism by rising up on the toes (Hubshire maneuver).

tion when the patient stands on the toes in a flexible-type flatfoot (Figs 12.7, 12.8). In a rigid-type flatfoot, when performing this maneuver, the calcaneus would remain everted. This test is known as the Hubshire maneuver. Another test that will corroborate the viability of the windlass mechanism is known as Jack's test.[34] This test is performed while the patient is weightbearing by manually dorsiflexing the hallux in order to ascertain whether or not a longitudinal arch may be recreated. The recreation of the longitudinal arch is possible if the flatfoot is flexible but not if it is rigid.

If the flatfoot is considered to be of the flexible type, then it is possible to exclude rigid flatfoot conditions such as convex pes valgus (vertical talus) and, in the older child, peroneal spastic flatfoot. However, if the deformity is of the flexible type, then it must be further differentiated from conditions such as calcaneovalgus, neurological and syndrome disorders, mechanical causes and iatrogenic flatfoot. This can be achieved through clinical and radiographic evaluation. For example, the flexible deformity of calcaneovalgus is easily distinguishable from the developmental flatfoot by the presence of a dorsiflexed and abducted attitude of the foot off-weightbearing. Flexible flatfoot caused by an os tibiale externum (accessory navicular) deformity is readily visible upon radiographic analysis in the skeletally mature child and clinically diagnosable by observation and palpation of the skeletally immature navicular prominence. Neurological and syndrome disorders require thorough history-taking and clinical examination skills. Referral to an appropriate specialist may be necessary if undiagnosed neurological impairment or syndrome disorder is suspected.

Thorough history-taking and clinical examination will also identify iatrogenically induced pediatric flatfoot conditions. Similar measures may also be taken to identify mechanical causes such as Morton's syndrome, limb length discrepancy or forefoot varus. Equinus deficiencies are likewise assessed by clinical examination. The flexible pediatric flatfoot resulting from a congenital gastrocnemius–soleus equinus is distinguished from the developmental flatfoot by the inability to dorsiflex the foot beyond a right angle.

Pathomechanics

Significant faults in the static and dynamic functions of the developmental flatfoot may be seen on careful examination and demonstrate a foot that functions inefficiently. However, the developmental flatfoot is not necessarily a poorly functioning foot just because it is flat. The height of the arch is an unreliable indicator of foot function. Whether or not a child develops an arch upon weightbearing is not indicative of proper foot function later in life. Both the high-arched and the low-arched foot may function well, but it is only possible to determine this through a thorough painstaking musculoskeletal examination. The minimum components of this type of examination should include joint ranges and quality of motion studies of all the lower extremity articulations; strength and length determinations of the musculature; structural and postural analysis; stance and observational gait analysis as well as weightbearing radiographic evaluation.

One question this examination should answer is whether or not this developmental flatfoot is excessively pronated and if so, to what degree? Whether or not the foot is excessively pronated is linked to medial displacement of the line of weightbearing in the extremity and the associated postural malalignment. A plumb line dropped from the tibial tubercle should bisect the tibia and the talus. Should this line be carried forward, it would pass through the first or second toe. In a pronated foot, this line deviates medially thus allowing the talus to receive body weight at a medially deviated angle instead of at a right angle to the leg. In addition, in a normal individual a plumb line dropped from the center of the popliteal space would bisect the calf. It will also bisect and be parallel to both the talus and the Achilles tendon. In a pronated foot, the talus is tilted medially, the calcaneus is laterally displaced in relation to the line of gravity and there is a lateral bowing of the Achilles tendon (Fig. 12.9). This lateral bowing or Helbing's sign shortens the distance between the origin and

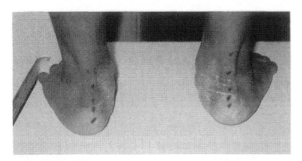

Figure 12.9 Marked displacement of body weight in a developmental flatfoot producing lateral bowing of the Achilles tendon.

insertion of the Achilles tendon and hence adaptive contraction occurs. It is a physiological law that when a normal tendon is overstretched, it becomes weaker, whereas when it is allowed to shorten, it usually contracts and becomes stronger. The peroneal tendons undergo this process of adaptive shortening and concomitant strengthening. Conversely, the anterior and posterior tibial tendons are overstretched and lose their effective power. Consequently, the lateral capsular and ligamentous structures around the ankle are shortened and contracted and the medial ankle ligaments and capsular structures are stretched and weakened. Gaps appear between the bones on the medial segment of the foot, with compression of the osseous structures on the lateral aspect. Transmission of body weight along the functional axis of joints and along the trabecular arrangement of bones becomes deleteriously deviated. All of these pathological forces occur in a foot whose osseous structures are immature and plastic and thus very susceptible to deformation. In addition, alteration of the functional axis of lower and, to some degree, upper extremity articulations causes these joints to function at a structural disadvantage during critical developmental years. The more marked the pronation, the more severe the postural derangement.

Medial displacement of body weight is one important factor in the production and retention of calcaneal eversion significantly beyond the vertical. Once body weight has been medially displaced, it is difficult for the developing foot, or for that matter any foot, to recover. The adage 'pronation begets pronation' is readily observable in most pronated feet. As a general rule, and particularly in the case of the developmental flatfoot, calcaneal eversion 5° beyond the vertical results in additional subtalar joint pronation to its maximum degree.[34] Body weight is one, if not the most powerful, of the pronating forces. Therefore, medial displacement of the line of weightbearing will make it increasingly difficult for the extremely malleable developing foot to function and to develop in an efficient fashion. In certain cases of developmental flatfoot, there is a compensatory toeing-in that may occur in an attempt by the child to recover the line of gravity over the supporting foot.[5] It is for this reason that children with intoe problems should be thoroughly investigated in order to rule out developmental flatfoot as the etiology.

MANAGEMENT OF DEVELOPMENTAL FLATFOOT

Objectives

The principal functions of the foot are:

1. to support the superstructure in static stance
2. to act as a mobile adaptor
3. to act as a rigid lever at appropriate phases of the gait cycle.

The static function is most efficiently achieved by alignment of the foot in a neutral to supinatory position while its dynamic functions are achieved through pronation and supination, respectively. The major functional deficit of the developmental flatfoot is that of excessive mobility. This deficit carries with it a concomitant inability for this foot to efficiently support the superstructure and to provide a reliable rigid lever for propulsion. Therefore, the management objectives for developmental flatfoot should be:

- to stabilize and align the osseous and soft tissue structures
- to neutralize excessive pronation
- to encourage the rigid lever function
- to promote ideal development.

Rationale

The literature reveals conflicting opinions as to which children with flexible flatfeet should be treated and which should be left to 'self-correct'.[5,8,9,33,35–37] Almost all authors agree that children with painful flexible flatfeet should be treated conservatively in the first instance with surgical intervention reserved for those cases that fail to respond.[3,5,9,33,35–37] However, if the child is to suffer any symptoms associated with flexible flatfoot, the child will not do so until the age of at least 3 to 5 years.[24] Those who say that only children with symptomatic flatfeet should be treated fail to recognize the important relationship between developmental deficiencies and foot dysfunction and deformity later in life. Lack of symptoms is an unreliable indicator of foot function in any age group but especially in the pediatric patient, therefore this philosophy is flawed. Once the deformity becomes established, the period of prevention is past. Corrective measures are, at this point, less effective attempts to reshape that which is already deformed. It should be remembered that, at best, correction is a poor substitute for prevention.[38]

'The earlier treatment is instituted, the more favorable is the prognosis', is a basic tenet in the treatment of pediatric foot disorders, i.e. the clinician should be conscious of not losing this so-called 'golden opportunity' to put into effect any treatment plans. Treatment of the developmental flatfoot should begin in infancy while the musculoskeletal system is immature and therefore plastic. Early in this period, the infant's extremities are not functional, i.e. children at this age are motile but not mobile. In the non-weightbearing infant, there is the added benefit, or detriment in the case of non-treatment, of little or no resistance being offered to destructive or corrective extrinsic forces. The human foot grows to one-half its adult length by the end of the first year of life.[39] The rapid growth that occurs during this first year may be influenced in a positive manner through treatment. Since the foot and leg complex of the infant follows the laws governing all growing things, the foot and leg will therefore adapt to the position assumed during growth. A wait-and-see attitude in the treatment of the developmental flatfoot is a serious mistake since it allows strength and maturity to accompany the rapid growth phase. This combination allows the deformity to become firmly set, making treatment increasingly difficult.

Benefits of early correction include bony remodeling to more favorable alignment.[21,35] According to Valmassy, 'if it is possible to maintain the bones of the foot in a normal relationship to one another during the growing years, regardless of whether the eventual outcome is a good arch or a flatfoot, the end result should minimize arthritic changes in later life.'[24] Rose[40] also agrees that if the foot is placed in a corrected position during the early growth years, 'cure will result' while at the same time preventing secondary arthritic changes later in life. Huurmann[41] is also in agreement with these authors as noted by his comment on treatment of the flexible flatfoot in the weightbearing child stating, 'growth and development can be effectively used to gain permanent correction as long as the orthotic device is worn faithfully and for a prolonged period of time.' Finally, it is better to err on the side of overtreatment in the management of the developmental flatfoot since the ultimate condition may be disabling.

The non-weightbearing flatfoot

The question of whether developmental flatfoot treatment is indicated is more readily discernible in the weightbearing pediatric population than it is in the non-weightbearing infant. Treatment of the non-weightbearing flatfoot is based on (i) structural assessment of the foot segments, (ii) the ranges of motion available in the joints of the foot, (iii) simulated 'weightbearing' pedal posture and (iv) family history of excessive pronation or joint laxity. In this population, examination of the developmental flatfoot will exhibit a subtalar and forefoot varus deformity. With the limbs in the hopscotch position, the feet and knees should point straight ahead and a longitudinal arch should be visible to the astute clinician.[38] This position readily reveals the presence of foot malposition, contracture or deformity.

Hyperflexibility of all the joints of the foot may be present. Once recognized, treatment of developmental flatfoot may begin at birth. Treatment at this point in development may include serial plaster immobilization and splinting along with appropriate footwear. Severe deformities may be serially immobilized in plaster with the rearfoot held in neutral subtalar joint alignment and the forefoot positioned perpendicular to a bisection of the calcaneus.[21,40] The cast extends from below the knee to the toes and is changed at bi-weekly intervals until the appearance of the foot is considered normal.[21,40,42] Rose[40] advocates this method of treatment in the newborn for those flexible flatfeet with an accompanying positive family history of ligamentous laxity or hyperpronated feet. Once correction has been achieved, it should be maintained for at least one-half the time needed to obtain it. Ganley[42] advises that correction be maintained for the same period of time necessary to achieve correction. This maintenance period may be augmented by the use of splints such as the Denis Browne bar[21,29] (Fig. 12.10). The Denis Browne bar should be bent in the center to allow the foot to be held in a supinatory position. The correction is maintained 22 hours a day and is reinforced by the further inversion created by the infant trying to kick the device off. In addition, the use of an orthotic device or a triplane, felt, rearfoot, varus wedge of approximately 4° inside the shoe will ensure

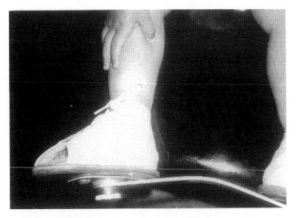

Figure 12.10 Denis Browne splint, bent in the center to maintain the foot in a supinatory position.

proper positioning of the non-weightbearing foot.[20]

The weightbearing developmental flatfoot

The latest time frame in which care for the developmental flatfoot should begin is from 7 to 9 months of age when the child first begins to bear weight. It is at this point that the developmental flatfoot exhibits its hallmark features. These features are those of an excessively pronated and significantly malaligned foot and include:

* marked calcaneal eversion
* medial protrusion of the talar head
* significant forefoot abduction.

Connolly[29] judges the need for treatment based on the medial stability of the talus. When a prominent, medially directed talar head is observed, then there is suggestive evidence of talonavicular joint instability. Other authors determine the need for treatment based on the observation of marked calcaneal valgus upon weightbearing.[8,9]

Radiographic evaluation

Weightbearing radiographs are important in the objective assessment of developmental flatfoot.[6,7,21,26] Radiographs allow an objective grading of flatfoot severity thereby determining the need for treatment while at the same time forming a baseline against which those cases requiring treatment may be measured and development monitored. Weightbearing radiographs in the anteroposterior and lateral projections are the standard views and can be obtained even in very young infants. Bordelon[6,21] employs a talar–first metatarsal bisection angle on a standing lateral radiograph in children between 3 and 8 years of age in order to determine whether or not treatment should be instituted in children with flatfeet (Fig. 12.11). The bisection forms a 0° angle in the 'neutral' foot and is increased as the talar head becomes plantarflexed. A mild flatfoot is depicted by 1–15° plantar angulation of

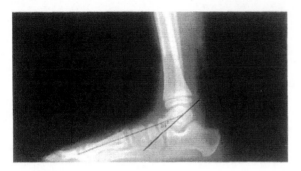

Figure 12.11 A talometatarsal angle of 24° in a 3¹/₂-year-old child with developmental flatfoot.

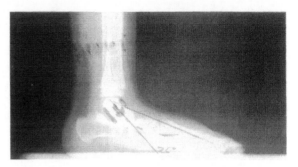

Figure 12.12 A 26° talometatarsal angle in an 18-month-old child with developmental flatfoot.

the talus in relation to the first metatarsal. A severe flatfoot is one that exhibits over 15° of plantarflexion angle of the talus in relation to the first metatarsal. In addition, Bordelon recommends no treatment or special footwear for 0° talometatarsal angle. Foot orthoses are considered in the 1–15° talometatarsal group if there is symptomatology or if the parents desire correction, and in the group with a talometatarsal angle over 15°, foot orthoses are prescribed[6,21] (Figs 12.12, 12.13). In the standing anteroposterior projection radiograph, the developmental flatfoot exhibits those features common to all hyperpronated feet and includes an increased talocalcaneal angle and a lowering of the calcaneal inclination angle, as well as an abducted position of the forefoot.

All of the above methods are employed to help identify an excessively pronated foot. Normal pronation allows the foot to adapt to the terrain and to absorb shock, as well as to place the plantar aspect of the foot in contact with the walking surface. The amount of this normal pronation is approximately 4–6° and not easily visible to the naked eye. The pronation we see in the developmental flatfoot is that of excessive pronation. Since excessive pronation is a poor postural position, which sets the stage for future disability, it should always be neutralized. When such a degree of pronation is easily visualized, it may be considered excessive.[10] Therapy in the weightbearing developmental flatfoot should be started in order to provide stability, align the osseous and soft tissue structures, neutralize

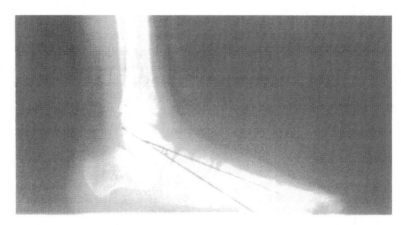

Figure 12.13 The same child as in Figure 12.12 after 2 years of treatment with functional foot orthotics. Note the reduction of the talometatarsal angle to 16°.

excessive pronation, and most importantly encourage ideal development. These objectives may be approached through the use of prescription foot orthoses in recommended footwear. Exercises are of no value in the treatment of a developmental flatfoot unless there is a demonstrated weakness of the foot musculature.[5,8,9,23,43]

PEDIATRIC FOOTWEAR

The effectiveness of any type of orthotic device is contingent upon an ideal foot-to-ground interface. Some of the more important considerations in prescribing footwear for the pediatric patient include a rigid counter to discourage calcaneal eversion, a rigid shank to limit subtalar and midtarsal joint pronation, and a flexible forefoot to encourage the development of the propulsive phase of gait.

For the most part, the problem in prescribing shoes designed for the early walker is that the sole of the shoe is either completely inflexible or, conversely, it is too flexible. It may take as much as 70 lb (31.7 kg) of pressure to flex the shoe of the beginning walker while the child may weigh only 25–40 lb (11–18 kg). Hence, parents often state that their child seems to walk better without shoes than with them. On the other hand, shoes with more flexible soles are not only flexible at the ball of the foot but at the midtarsal joint region as well. This midfoot flexibility offers nothing to restrict excessive pronation.

PEDIATRIC FOOT ORTHOSES

Various types of orthotic devices and shoe inserts have been utilized in the management of flexible pediatric flatfoot disorders ranging from the Whitman steel plate to the functional foot orthosis. Ideally, one would like to proceed with the prescription of an orthotic device to be used in a shoe with a rigid counter, rigid shank and flexible forefoot. Since it is not always possible to obtain a shoe with these characteristics, a flexible-soled shoe with a rigid counter, such as a well-made sneaker, may be used providing the material from which the orthotic device is made is essentially inflexible in the child's weight

range. Such inflexible orthotic devices, made of polypropylene or of graphite composite materials, will remedy the deficiency created by the lack of a rigid shank in the shoe. The prescription of similarly non-compressible but flexible orthoses such as those made of leather laminates, rubber butter or 'zote'-type materials would be inappropriate in these situations. Flexible orthoses in flexible footwear such as sneakers enable the entire system to bend in the midfoot region. This undesirable midfoot flexibility allows unimpeded oblique axis midtarsal joint pronation to take place.

Inflexible orthoses of the polypropylene or graphite composite-type possess low tensile strength and a moderate degree of elasticity, which provide the resiliency characteristic of this relatively inflexible group. Conversely, materials such as Rohadur (Rohadur, Rohm, Germany) or fiberglass possess a high-tensile strength and high degree of elasticity making them more prone to fracture in stressful situations when their elastic limit is exceeded, e.g. in running, jumping, hopping, skipping and bouncing. It is for these reasons that the essentially inflexible, low-tensile strength materials with a moderate degree of elasticity are more suitable for use in the management of the developmental flatfoot. Although a certain degree of elasticity in the device material is beneficial for use in the pediatric patient, too much elasticity will allow the module to compress which will have a negative effect on foot alignment and function. Thus, in the management of the developmental flatfoot, the recommended orthotic material should be one that is relatively inflexible and non-compressible.

Each child requires an individual amount of correction to be applied to the affected foot in order to achieve the optimum outcome. Therefore, the use of a mass-produced device is inappropriate. The prescription of custom-fabricated foot orthoses is a requirement in the treatment of most foot disorders and this is especially true in the pediatric patient. Whenever possible, the device should be fabricated from a subtalar joint neutral position plaster model of the child's feet. Although not as accurate, it may be necessary to utilize foam-impression casting in the younger or uncooperative child.

Shoes and shoe corrections by themselves have not been shown to be efficacious in the treatment of pediatric flatfoot.[35,37,44-46] The functional foot orthosis, the University of California Biomechanics Laboratory (UCBL) insert, the Blake inverted orthosis, and the dynamic stabilizing innersole system (DSIS) are among the most suitable prescription foot orthoses for use in the developmental flatfoot. Owing to the increased flexibility, increased subtalar joint range of motion and increased plantar fatty tissue noted in the young child, it is imperative to prescribe a device that will achieve the greatest control.

The functional foot orthosis was first developed by Merton Root in 1958 and is the model from which all other functional foot orthoses have been derived. The mechanism of action was in direct contrast to that provided by previously prescribed arch supports. The function of arch supports was to buttress the longitudinal arch with various materials in order to allow it to support the entire weight of the body. Unfortunately, these devices produced random supination of the entire foot, thereby unlocking the oblique axis of the midtarsal joint resulting in additional dysfunction. The Root functional device repositioned the foot in such a manner that optimum foot function could be achieved. The arch region of this device is usually lower than the observed arch region of the foot off-weightbearing. This is due to the fact that the Root functional orthosis achieves its effect by realignment of the rearfoot and forefoot, allowing those osseous segments that comprise the longitudinal arch to interlock and thereby support itself. In essence, the functional orthosis is a guide from which the foot may function, not a crutch for the superstructure to lean on. In order to enhance the effectiveness of this type of device, the incorporation of a medial and lateral flange as well as a deepened heel-seat may be prescribed. The resulting orthosis will then resemble a modified Roberts–Whitman device (Fig. 12.14).

Rearfoot and forefoot posting in the functional foot orthosis for the developmental flatfoot

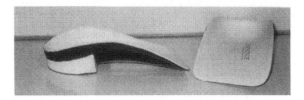

Figure 12.14 A typical functional foot orthotic device recommended for managing the developmental flatfoot. This device incorporates a high medial and lateral flange as well as the appropriate rearfoot and, if necessary, forefoot posting. The module is fabricated from a polypropylene-type thermoplastic.

should be individually determined and to some extent is age-dependent. In the adult foot, orthotic posting is prescribed in order to accommodate the full degree of deformity captured in the neutral position cast, which should be a direct reflection of the clinical examination findings. In the developing foot, complete neutralization of structural deficiencies noted in the neutral position cast may encourage the retention of prenatal imbalances by 'setting' the deformity in its abnormal position while at the same time discouraging ideal development. It must be remembered that since the major portion of the developmental process is not achieved until the child is 6 to 8 years of age (with a gradual tapering off so that complete developmental maturity may not occur in some individuals until they are 14 to 16 years old), complete neutralization of structural deficiencies in children under 8 years of age is ill-advised. Since most adults retain a minimum of 2–4° of subtalar varus, the addition of at least a 2 or 3° rearfoot varus post to the orthotic device is not contraindicated and may in fact enhance the effect of the orthotic. With regard to forefoot posting in the developmental flatfoot of the early walker, the approximately 10° of forefoot varus should not be completely neutralized. The degree of forefoot varus deformity that should be corrected is the minimum posting necessary to neutralize all visible pronation as well as to achieve neutral subtalar joint positioning. Another method of managing forefoot varus in the new walker is to plantarflex the medial column of the foot during impression casting, thereby lessening the forefoot varus deformity and increasing the medial arch of the negative and positive casts.

Management of the developmental flatfoot in the established walker from 2 to 4 years of age differs from that of the child who is just beginning to learn to walk in that structural deficiencies should be more closely observed. Inspection of individual developmental trends are important in ascertaining whether or not additional neutralization of these imbalances is indicated. No visible pronation should be permitted and the subtalar joint should be maintained in its neutral position. Since an adult-like mature gait with a heel-to-toe gait pattern is achieved by 3 years of age, the ability of this foot to provide a rigid lever for propulsion is of paramount importance in the management objectives for this age group.

In children aged between 4 and 8 years, the same caution must be exercised in the complete neutralization of structural deficiencies. Since we are closer to the point at which the majority of lower extremity developmental parameters should be achieved, additional neutralization of these deficiencies may be appropriate. The question then remains, should be structural deficiencies of the child over 8 years of age be neutralized? Since the developmental process does not abruptly end for some individuals but gradually tapers off throughout adolescence, complete neutralization of structural deficiencies may again be contraindicated. A clinical guide to the degree of neutralization necessary to achieve normal foot function in the over-8 years of age group would be the amount of posting required to re-establish ground contact with the rearfoot and forefoot while the subtalar joint is maintained in its neutral position. This structural repositioning will promote a normal sequencing of events during the gait cycle, thereby improving foot and leg function.

Another device that has been documented to be effective in the management of pediatric flexible flatfoot disorders is the UCBL insert.[44,47] Developed by the University of California Biomechanics Laboratory, it is fabricated from thin, lightweight, semi-rigid polypropylene and possesses high medial and lateral flanges which join

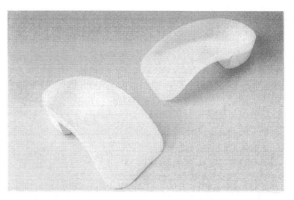

Figure 12.15 UCBL insert employed in the management of developmental flatfoot. Fabricated of thin polypropylene, it has a deepened heel-seat extending forward into high medial and lateral flanges.

in the heel region to form a deepened heel-seat (Fig. 12.15). This device differs from the Root-type device in that it depends on its contouring to resist abnormal motion rather than by encouraging normal foot mechanics.[20]

The Blake inverted orthosis is an aggressive varus correction of the standard off-weightbearing neutral position cast. This is achieved by plaster correction of the positive in the rear and forefoot regions. Corrections up to 75° may be achieved by this method with minimal tendency to lateral instability since the device contours well to the longitudinal arch. Additional modifications include a plantar fascial groove, a deepened heel-seat, as well as flat rearfoot posts. The typical foot orthosis for the pediatric patient usually requires a new prescription every 1 to 2 years or every two shoe sizes. Owing to its inverted heel-cup rather than forefoot or rearfoot corrections, together with its deepened, inverted heel contouring, the Blake inverted orthosis will accommodate the child's foot for over 3 years before a new prescription is necessary.[20]

The DSIS is indicated in the severely pronated weightbearing developmental flatfoot. The DSIS is an orthotic device that possesses a deep, offset heel-seat to cup the calcaneus[48] (Fig. 12.16). It maintains the calcaneus in approximately 5° of varus with high medial and lateral flanges which prevent lateral transverse plane drift of the first and fifth metatarsals, thereby increasing control.

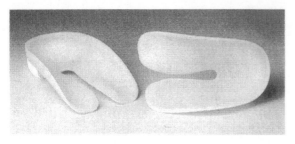

Figure 12.16 Dynamic stabilizing innersole system (DSIS) is effective in neutralization of excessive pronation which is typically seen in developmental flatfoot. Note the high, extended and separated medial and lateral arms, which provide unique, efficient and independent column control.

It is a semi-rigid device commonly fabricated of polyethylene–ortholene.

The goal of developmental flatfoot treatment is to achieve normal foot structure and function during stance and ambulation with all visible signs of pronation neutralized. Remission of symptomatology when present is not a criteria for cessation of therapy. Progress can be monitored objectively by means of periodic clinical examination, radiographic evaluation and, in the case of children over 3 years of age, by the use of computer-assisted gait analysis.[49] Since basic bone form and position are essentially complete by 7 to 8 years of age, this is the earliest time that cessation of therapy should be considered regardless of when treatment was started. As mentioned earlier, complete skeletal maturity does not occur until 13 years of age in girls and 15 years of age in boys. Therefore, it is prudent to maintain the correction obtained at least until this point in development. Existing observable structural deficiencies retained beyond this point require continuing care. Progress should be monitored throughout life.

REFERENCES

1. Day NR. Foot owners manual. Daly City: PAS; 1983.
2. Edmonson A, Greenshaw A. Campbell's operative orthopedics. St Louis: Mosby; 1980.
3. Mann RA. Surgery of the foot. 5th ed. St Louis: Mosby; 1986.
4. Salter R. Textbook of disorders of the musculoskeletal system. 2nd ed. Baltimore: Williams and Wilkins; 1983.
5. Tachdjian MO. Pediatric orthopedics, vol 4. Philadelphia: WB Saunders; 1990.
6. Bordelon RL. Correction of hypermobile flatfoot in children by molded insert. Foot Ankle 1980;1(3):143–150.
7. Paul RG. Common foot deformities in infancy and childhood. J Fam Pract 1976;3(5):537–543.
8. Powell HD. Pes planovalgus in children. Clin Orthop 1983;177:133–139.
9. Wernick J, Volpe RG. Lower extremity function and normal mechanics. In: Valmassy RL, ed. Clinical biomechanics of the lower extremity. St Louis: Mosby; 1996;13–15.
10. Tax HR. The evolutionary and phylogenetic development of the lower extremity in man. J Am Podiatr Assoc 1976; 66:363–371.
11. Trott AW. Children's foot problems. Orthop Clin North Am 1982;13(3):641–654.
12. Beck R, Andriacci T. Changes in the growth pattern of normal children. J Bone Joint Surg 1981;63:1452.
13. Katoh Y, Chao EYS, Laughman RK, et al. Biomechanical analysis of foot function during gait and clinical applications. Clin Orthop 1983;177:23.
14. McGraw M. Neuromuscular development of the human infant. J Pediatr 1940;17:741.
15. Shirley MM. Development of walking in the first two years: a study of 25 babies. Mineapolis: University of Minnesota; 1931.
16. Stantham M, Murray M. Early walking patterns of normal children. Clin Orthop 1971;79:8.
17. Sutherland DH, Olshen R, Cooper L, et al. The development of mature gait. J Bone Joint Surg 1980;62:336.
18. Pope A. Familiar quotations. 13th ed. Boston: Little Brown; 1955.
19. Hoerr N, Pyle I, Francis C. Radiographic atlas of skeletal development of the foot and ankle. Springfield: Charles C Thomas; 1962.
20. Wenger DR, Leach J. Foot deformities in infants and children. Pediatr Clin North Am 1986;33(6):1411–1427.
21. Bordelon RL. Hypermobile flatfoot in children. Comprehension, evaluation, and treatment. Clin Orthop 1983; 181:7–14.
22. Mantagine J, Clievrot A, Galmiche JM. Atlas of foot radiology. New York: Mason; 1981.
23. Barry RJ, Scranton PE. Flatfeet in children. Clin Orthop 1983;181:68–75.
24. Valmassy RL. Lower extremity treatment modalities for the pediatric patient. In: Valmassy RL, ed. Clinical biomechanics of the lower extremity. St Louis: Mosby;1996;442–443, 448.
25. Schuster RO, Port M. Abnormal pronation in children: an hormonal etiology. J Am Podiatr Assoc 1977; 67:613–615.
26. Preston ET. Flat foot deformity. Am Fam Physician 1974; 9(2):143–147.

27. Sharrard WJ. Intoeing and flatfeet. BMJ 1976;(6014):88–89.

28. Schuster RO. The effects of modern footgear. J Am Podiatr Assoc 1978;68(4):235–241.

29. Connolly J, Regen E, Hillman JW. Pigeon-toes and flat feet. Pediatr Clin North Am 1970;17(2):291–307.

30. Mehan PL. The flexible flatfoot. In: American Academy of Orthopedic Surgeons: Instructional course lectures 1982;31:261–262.

31. Morton DH. The human foot. New York: Hafner; 1935.

32. Tax HR. Podopediatrics. Balitimore: Williams and Wilkins; 1980.

33. Roper BA. Flat foot. Br J Hosp Med 1979; 22(4):35–37.

34. Sgarlato TE. A compendium of poditric biomechanics. San Francisco: California College of Podiatric Medicine; 1971.

35. Bleck EE. The shoeing of children: sham or science? Dev Med Child Neurol 1971;13:188–195.

36. Giannestras NJ. Foot disorders, medical and surgical management. 2nd ed. Philadelphia: Lea & Febiger; 1973.

37. Jhass MH. Atlas of orthotics: biomechanical principles and applications. St Louis: Mosby;1975;267–279.

38. Ganley JV. The hopscotch position. J Am Podiatr Med Assoc 1991;81(3):136–139.

39. Blais MM, Green WT, Anderson M. Lengths of the growing foot. J Bone Joint Surg 1956;38A:998–1000.

40. Rose GK. Pes planus. In: Jhass MH, ed. Disorders of the foot. Philadelphia: WB Saunders; 1982;486–520.

41. Huurmann WH. Congenital foot deformities. In: Mann RA ed. Surgery of the foot. 5th ed. St Louis: Mosby; 1986;542–543.

42. Ganley JV. Corrective casting in infants. In: Ganley JV, ed. Clinics in podiatry – podopediatrics. Philadelphia: WB Saunders; 1984;1(3):501–517.

43. Scougall J. Knock knees, in-toeing, and other common problems. Med J Aust 1977;1:21–23.

44. Bleck EE, Berzins VJ. Conservative management of pes valgus with plantarflexed talus flexible. Clin Orthop 1977;122:85–94.

45. Cowell H. Shoes and shoe corrections. Pediatr Clin North Am 1977;24:791.

46. Knittel G. The effect of shoe modifications for in-toeing. Orthop Clin North Am 1976;7:1019.

47. Mereday C, Dolan CM, Lusskin R. Evaluation of the University of California Biomechanics Laboratory shoe insert in 'flexible' pes planus. Clin Orthop 1972;82:45–48.

48. Jay RM, Schoenhaus HD. Hyperpronation control with a dynamic stabilizing innersole system. J Am Podiatr Med Assoc 1992;82(3):149–153.

49. D'Amico JC. The F-scan system with EDG module for gait analysis in the pediatric patient. J Am Podiatr Med Assoc 1998;88(4):166–175.

SECTION 4

13

Physical therapy

Jill Pickard

The objectives of physical therapy for any pediatric foot condition may be broadly stated as:

- to relieve pain and muscle spasm
- to increase range of movement at affected joints
- to increase the extensibility of shortened soft tissues
- to strengthen weakened muscles
- to normalize tonal abnormalities
- to re-educate balance and coordination
- to facilitate a normal gait pattern
- to restore normal movement and to allow the individual to be as functionally independent as possible.

This chapter will describe the main therapeutic measures employed in the management of pediatric foot conditions and the underlying principles governing them. Certain conditions most commonly treated by the physical therapist will then be discussed.

PSYCHOMOTOR DEVELOPMENT

The term psychomotor development is used to describe changes that occur in motor skills and intellectual complexity as a response to maturation of the central nervous system and it implies that there is a parallel development in both neuromuscular and psychological spheres.

For any treatment plan to be effective, a thorough knowledge of the sequence of psychomotor development of the child is essential as a basic foundation. This is especially important when dealing with children below the age of 5 years.

277

For instance, it would be inappropriate to use hopping activities in the treatment of a child who is not capable of such a task. Hopping requires a high degree of balance, coordination and postural control coupled with such understanding as is required to achieve the activity. Conversely, a child will soon tire of an activity which is neither physically demanding nor intellectually stimulating.

Within the first few months and years, an infant develops a wide range of motor and intellectual skills. An infant learns to sit, to crawl, to express needs and to show pleasure. The traditional view is that the movement of a newborn child is governed by a series of primitive responses. There is a progression from reflex to voluntary, from symmetrical to asymmetrical and from gross to precision movements as the increasingly mature cerebral cortex begins to exert its inhibition on the lower centers and spinal cord. The mechanisms underpinning the transition from reflex gross motor patterns to higher order control are still far from certain. More sophisticated and often asymmetrical responses develop as the infant matures.

Psychomotor development should not be viewed as being a linear function, and it is apparent that stages of physical, emotional and cognitive development are subject to spurts and periods of quiescence. Such development is now viewed as a dynamic process and is dependent upon external factors such as nutrition, sensory input, language acquisition and other environmental influences. It has been noted that there is a reciprocal relationship between nerve fiber myelination and function; myelination dictates the order in which specific activities develop. However, function may also facilitate and stimulate further myelination.[1]

The developmental sequence has commonly been considered to be fixed, i.e. all children pass through the same stages to achieve specific skills. However, if one considers an activity such as walking, it is apparent that not all children will crawl as an intermediate stage and those that do may crawl for variable amounts of time. There are certain stages of development that are essential for progression through the sequence, e.g. the child must be able to raise the head in prone before starting to crawl. Children who have a neurological impairment and who are unable to achieve head control will subsequently have difficulty continuing through the developmental sequence.

The human infant is born with an immature central nervous system and attainment of milestones reflects the maturation of the brain and spinal cord. At birth, myelination is not complete and is thought to have reached only the subcortical structures and not the cerebral cortex where motor activity is initiated.[2] Therefore, inhibition from the cortex occurs after birth.

The myelination process begins at the head and trunk and moves distally along the limbs, hence head and trunk control is gained before limb control. At birth, the brain volume is about 25% of the adult and this rises to 75% by the age of 1 year because of the increase in myelin present. As maturation is dependent upon physiological events, practice alone will not hasten the child's ability to perform a task until the sensorimotor system is sufficiently developed to produce controlled actions of the relevant muscles. Children who are born prematurely or with neurological impairment, e.g. cerebral palsy, will be delayed in their passage through this developmental progression. Those children who are severely impaired may not progress at all. The most important developmental milestones in locomotion are listed in Appendix VI.

MOVEMENT AND EXERCISE THERAPIES

Movement and exercise therapies are undoubtedly the most commonly used therapies when managing pediatric foot disorders. All congenital foot abnormalities that may be helped by physical therapy should be treated as soon after birth as possible. When they are not treated, secondary bony or joint changes may occur and these may lead to further deformity and loss of function. In the neonate, treatment must be entirely passive. However, as the child becomes older, more emphasis should be placed on play in order to reinforce favorable muscle action and appropriate joint positioning. Therefore, the objectives of treatment will depend upon the child's chronological age and level of psychomotor development.

Exercises cannot be prescriptive and great skill and ingenuity are required on the part of the therapist to make a movement regimen stimulating and fun. The attainment of small measurable goals will help to motivate the child and to maintain the child's interest.

TECHNIQUES TO INCREASE RANGE OF MOVEMENT AND SOFT TISSUE EXTENSIBILITY

Movement at joints in the foot may be limited for several reasons, e.g.:

1. *Damage to the articular surfaces and periarticular structures*, which may occur in children with conditions such as juvenile chronic polyarthritis. Such damage may manifest itself in the loss of movements such as inversion and eversion.
2. *Adaptive shortening* of soft tissues as might occur in the tendocalcaneus in certain congenital foot deformities; after prolonged immobilization; or as the result of neurological and rheumatological conditions. When a joint is immobilized for a short period of time, the muscles overlying that joint will adopt a shortened position and may lose extensibility. This is termed a contracture. When the contracted muscle is not treated, there will be a long-term faulty positioning of the joints over which that muscle passes. This may produce pain and loss of function. Similarly, when ligaments are immobilized, especially in a shortened position, they too may shorten and become fibrosed.
3. *Increased muscle tone* (hypertonia or spasticity) may lead to loss of range of movement because affected muscles resist lengthening. Such hypertonia may prevent normal joint positioning. When such tonal abnormalities are not treated, permanent joint changes may occur. This may be seen in the plantarflexed inverted foot of a child with spasticity. The fol-

lowing physiotherapeutic techniques are most commonly employed in order to increase joint range of movement and soft tissue extensibility:

a. passive muscle stretching
b. active muscle stretching
c. mobilizing exercises
d. proprioceptive neuromuscular facilitation (PNF)
e. mobilization techniques
f. soft tissue massage.

Passive muscle stretching

A muscle may be stretched when the range of movement at the joint is limited because muscles passing over the joint are shortened. In the child, stretching may be done in one of two ways: passively or actively. A passive stretch may be defined as a manual or mechanical stretch applied to the shortened tissues while the patient is relaxed or, in the case of small infants, well supported. This type of stretch is termed passive because the patient makes no contribution to the stretch. Such a technique is commonly used when the child is very young and is therefore unable to participate in the stretching process.

An active stretch occurs when patients provide the force for the stretch through their own muscular effort. This method may be employed with older children who are able to cooperate with the procedure. In order to ensure safe and effective treatment, two physiological mechanisms involved in muscle activity should be considered: the stretch reflex and the tendon reflex.

The stretch reflex – structure

Specialized stretch receptors are found within skeletal muscle, and are modifications of muscle fibers. These receptors are known as muscle spindles and are more numerous in small delicate muscles, e.g. of the hand and foot, than in the larger muscles, e.g. of the thigh. These specialized fibers are situated within a connective tissue capsule and are called intrafusal fibers in order to distinguish them from the usual type of muscle

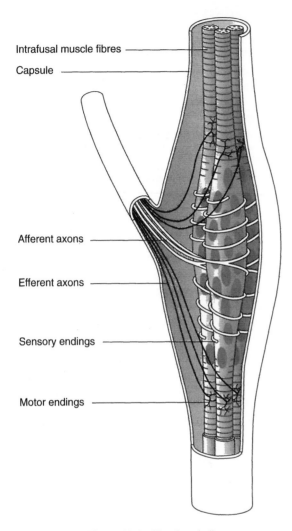

Intrafusal muscle fibres

Capsule

Afferent axons

Efferent axons

Sensory endings

Motor endings

Figure 13.1 Muscle spindle.

fibers called extrafusal. The intrafusal fibers lie parallel to the extrafusal muscle fibers and have contractile ends and a non-contractile center (Fig. 13.1). The contractile ends are innervated by small diameter gamma motor neurons. The non-contractile central portion is innervated by large diameter afferent fibers, which detect the stretch on the central portion. These fibers synapse in the spinal cord with the large diameter alpha motor neurons which in turn synapse with the extrafusal fibers of the muscle. They are also connected to the antagonist muscles via inhibitory interneurons.

Sensory and motor fibers synapse in the muscle spindle. The motor (efferent) fibers have a small diameter and synapse onto the contractile ends of the spindle.

The stretch reflex – function

When a muscle is stretched, the intrafusal and extrafusal fibers are lengthened and a stretch reflex is initiated. When a muscle is stretched quickly, the intrafusal fibers are deformed and the sensory fibers send impulses to the spinal cord where they synapse with the motor nerves supplying the muscle. Activation of the motor nerve causes the muscle to contract, thus relieving the tension on the muscle fibers. This series of events occurs very rapidly and is known as a stretch reflex and acts to prevent a muscle from being overstretched and possibly torn.

The degree of sensitivity of receptors can be modified by the action of the gamma motor fibers. These motor fibers cause the contractile ends of the intrafusal fibers to contract, thus increasing the tension on the central portion. When the central portion of the intrafusal fibers is taut, it is very much more sensitive to any changes in fiber length than would be the case if it were slack.

When a muscle is passively stretched, it is important that the stretch is applied slowly and smoothly. This action ensures that a stretch reflex mechanism is not initiated. It is suggested that when a muscle is stretched for 30 to 60 seconds, there is minimal activity of the stretch reflex.[3] When a stretch is applied too quickly, the muscle fibers may be torn as they contract against the lengthening force.

The tendon reflex – structure

The Golgi tendon organ is another receptor sensitive to muscle tension (Fig. 13.2) Golgi tendon organs are encapsulated nerve endings which may be found at the junction between the tendon and muscle.

Each tendon organs consists of the terminal fibers of a Ib sensory axon, being slightly smaller in diameter and slower than the sensory fibers that are found in the muscle spindle.

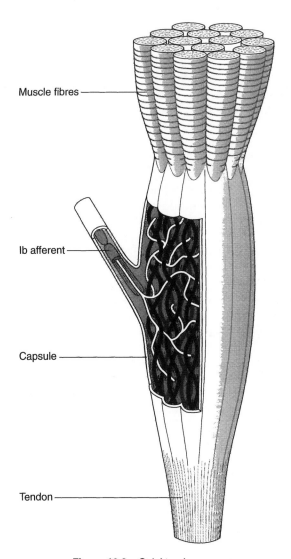

Muscle fibres

Ib afferent

Capsule

Tendon

Figure 13.2   Golgi tendon organ.

The nerve fibers of the Golgi tendon organ are intertwined around the collagen fibers of the tendon. Therefore, when there is increased tension on the tendon, there is compression of the tendon organ nerve fibers, which are then stimulated.

The tendon reflex – function

A tendon may be stretched by either a contraction of the muscle involved or by a passive stretch on the muscle and tendon. The Golgi tendon organ is more sensitive to stretch by muscle contraction because, during a passive stretch, the stretch will occur preferentially in the muscle, as these fibers are more elastic and extensible than those in the tendon.

When a tendon is stretched very strongly either by a muscle contraction or a passive stretch, the Golgi tendon organs are stimulated and impulses pass along the Ib afferent fibers to the spinal cord. In the cord, the fibers synapse with inhibitory interneurons that in turn synapse with the motor neurons that innervate the same muscles. Therefore, activation of the Golgi tendon organ inhibits the muscle activity and thus the tension is removed. In other words, the Golgi organ acts as a negative feedback mechanism to prevent overcontraction of the muscle. It is the mechanism of the muscle spindle and the Golgi tendon organ that underlie the techniques of muscle stretching.

Technique for passive muscle stretching

In this method of stretching, a force is applied in order to increase the range of movement at a joint that is limited by inextensible soft tissue. Passive stretching may only be used in children when there is a contracture because there is no necessity to stretch soft tissue that is of normal length. Indeed joints with immature ligamentous and muscular support may be traumatized if pushed beyond their normal anatomical limits. The child, often a newborn, should have all lower garments except a diaper removed, and should be positioned so that the maximum stretch possible may be obtained. The child's position will depend upon the stretch to be performed.

The muscle stretch will need to be undertaken regularly in order for the technique to be successful. Therefore, it is essential that the therapist explains to the parents or guardians the technique involved. The most common mistakes made are:

- not taking the muscle to the limit of its stretch
- not holding the stretch for long enough
- not localizing the movement to the appropriate joint or joints.

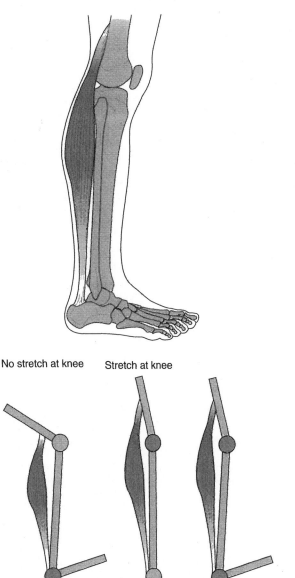

No stretch at knee   Stretch at knee

Stretch at ankle   No stretch at ankle   Stretch at knee and ankle

Figure 13.3   Sequence of muscle stretch – gastrocnemius.

When a muscle passes over more than one joint, e.g. gastrocnemius or flexor digitorum longus, each component of the movement that it performs must be stretched individually before

the whole muscle can be stretched over its entire length (Fig. 13.3).

The involved joint should be moved to the point of restriction. The therapist should then grasp either side of the joint in order to ensure that movement can only occur at that point. Constant pressure is applied slowly and firmly to the segment distal to the joint. The stretch should be maintained for at least 30 seconds, in which time the soft tissue tension will be felt to decrease. At this point, the soft tissues may be stretched a little further. The procedure must be repeated regularly as full range of joint movement frequently takes several weeks to achieve. Passive stretching is most commonly used for congenital foot deformities.

Small children will invariably cry when passive stretching is performed and great sensitivity is needed on the part of the clinician to what is a very distressing procedure for parents to watch and to undertake. In older children, a PNF technique is often used and will be discussed later in this chapter. The passive stretching that is undertaken for conditions such as talipes equinovarus are dealt with elsewhere in this book.

Active muscle stretching

Active stretching may be used with older children who are able to participate in treatment. When soft tissue is actively stretched, the patient participates in the procedure. Therefore, this method may only be used when a muscle is under the patient's conscious control; it cannot be used for neurological conditions such as hypertonia.

Mobilizing exercises

Exercises to increase range of movement at one or more joints can only be used with older children. Mobilizing exercises will only be successful when achievable goals have been set and the exercises are entertaining. The patient must be positioned so that the limb can move through its full available range. The limb must also be free from clothing in order to ensure that the therapist can:

- note how much movement is being achieved
- ascertain how much movement is occurring at the stiff joint
- determine if other joints are compensating for the loss of mobility
- observe which muscles are working.

The joint proximal to the joint that is to be mobilized must be fixed in order to prevent the occurrence of unwanted movement. For example, when the aim is to increase movement at the subtalar joint, the ankle joint will be fixed to prevent unwanted dorsiflexion and plantarflexion. Such fixation may be achieved manually by holding the relevant joint in a midrange position. Alternatively, a suitable starting position may be used in order to allow body weight or gravity to perform the task.

The joint should then be moved smoothly through the total available range of movement, taking care that the extremities of joint range are reached. This action is the basis of mobilizing exercises and is repeated regularly, the aim being to gain full range of movement at the joint.

Proprioceptive neuromuscular facilitation

Proprioceptive neuromuscular facilitation (PNF) is the term used for a group of treatment methods that aim to 'promote or hasten the neuromuscular mechanism through stimulation of the proprioceptors'.[4]

PNF employs the following physiological principles to influence neuromuscular activity:

Facilitation. PNF aims: (i) to decrease the threshold of excitability of the motor neurons in the spinal cord or (ii) to recruit the firing of extra motor neurons.

Inhibition. Inhibition may be regarded as the opposite effect to facilitation, where there is an increase in the threshold of the motor neurons in the spinal cord to the extent that firing may be prevented.

Facilitation and inhibition occur reciprocally in order to produce smooth and purposeful movement. In order for a movement at a joint to occur, the muscle producing the movement must be facilitated to contract and the antagonist muscle must be inhibited from contracting, thereby producing reciprocal relaxation. In PNF, the phenomena of reciprocal facilitation and inhibition are brought about by the use of maximal manual resistance to contraction, i.e. the most resistance to movement that can be applied by the therapist to the muscle while simultaneously maintaining a smooth muscle contraction and without preventing the full range of movement of that muscle.

Maximal contraction of the muscle produces two effects:

1. It facilitates recruitment of other motor units leading to overflow of activation into weaker muscles.
2. It facilitates the maximal relaxation of the antagonist at the same time and of the agonist directly after the contraction.

PNF hold-relax is an isometric technique that is used to obtain a lengthening reaction in shortened muscle and thus produces an increased range of movement where muscle tightness is the limiting feature. The principle of the technique is that by producing a maximal contraction of the tightened agonist muscles at the limit of the movement, there will be a subsequent relaxation and thus lengthening of the tightened agonists. For example, if there is muscle tightness in the plantarflexors, dorsiflexion will be limited. Therefore, the ankle joint is taken to the limit of available dorsiflexion and maximal resistance is applied by the therapist to the plantarflexors; the patient is instructed to 'hold' the joint in this position while the therapist maintains this position thus ensuring the maximal contraction of the muscle. This maneuver produces an isometric contraction of the plantarflexors. Having achieved maximum contraction, the therapist then instructs the patient to 'let go' and waits 10 to 15 seconds in order to allow relaxation of the agonists. The ankle joint may then be moved further into dorsiflexion brought about by the lengthened plantarflexors. The maneuver is repeated in order to gain a further increase in range. As the commands given need to be fairly specific, hold–relax techniques may only be used with older children who generally enjoy the procedure, especially when the hold phase is used as a show of strength as in arm-wrestling. The increased range achieved ought to be - regularly measured in order to provide small achievable goals.

Mobilization techniques

Loss of joint mobility may be treated by the manual application of graded oscillatory force in order to mobilize the peri-articular soft tissues and to increase the specific range of movement at that joint, usually termed as passive oscillatory movements. These techniques are not commonly used in pediatric foot conditions for several reasons:

- with small children, any limitation of movement is often caused by soft tissue tightness and may be most effectively treated with stretching and strapping
- small children find it impossible to keep sufficiently still for oscillatory movements to be applied to a specific joint and they are not able to report any alteration in the condition that this form of therapy has caused. However, it has been known for children of 8 years and over to be treated with passive oscillatory mobilizations when there is a musculoskeletal problem localized to an individual joint and when there are no other contraindications to the technique such as inflammatory joint disease or malignancy. These criteria are evaluated during initial assessment of the child's condition. Manual application of oscillatory movements at a joint are thought to:
  - stimulate mechanoreceptors which in turn inhibit the passage of painful stimulus to the brain by blocking the 'pain gate'[5]
  - increase the movement of synovial fluid within the joint thus enhancing its nutrition
  - elongate shortened soft tissues.
  - maintain or improve joint range of movement.

Passive oscillatory movements may be classified as either physiological or accessory. Physiological movements are those that normally occur at a joint and which can be performed by the patient, e.g. plantarflexion of the ankle. When such movements are limited, the therapist may achieve the same movements manually, e.g. in the case of plantarflexion by moving the talus on the tibia and fibula.

An accessory movement is one which must occur in order for normal joint movement to take place but which is not under the patient's control. A movement, such as dorsiflexion, may be limited by decreased gliding of the talus in the mortise. An anteroposterior movement of the talus performed manually by the therapist may resolve this problem.

There are very many different mobilizing techniques for the joints of the foot and ankle and similarly so for the other joints of the lower limb. The success of their outcome is dependent upon the careful assessment of the patient and the skill of the physical therapist performing the maneuver. It is impossible to cover this area in the necessary depth within this chapter, and it is suggested the reader refers to one of the specialized textbooks listed in the further reading section.

Soft tissue massage

Massage has been defined as 'hand motions practiced on the surface of the living body with a therapeutic goal'[6] and was first described over 4000 years ago. There are few contraindications to the use of massage. Massage should not be used over inflamed or delicate skin or where there is malignancy or deep vein thromboses. The possible therapeutic effects of massage are extensive.

Cardiovascular system

Massage to the body causes compression and distraction of the soft tissues as they are kneaded, squeezed and wrung. This leads to dilatation of superficial blood vessels and increased blood flow. Such vascular changes are mainly under the control of axon reflexes, and from the release of a histamine-like cell mediator from the tissues. The subsequent increase in circulation brings more oxygen and nutrients to the area thus aiding the healing process. Pressure on the thin walls of the veins and lymph vessels increases venous and lymphatic return, as fluid is pushed past the valves within the vessels. A decrease in tissue congestion also leads to an improvement in tissue perfusion. Therefore, massage is a valuable method of decreasing edema.

Immune system

Massage therapy has also been shown to have a positive effect on the immune system, increasing the numbers of natural killer cells and decreasing blood cortisol levels.[7]

Musculoskeletal system

Soft tissues are manually lengthened by certain techniques and are mobilized relative to the underlying tissues or the skin. These actions tend to stretch any adhesions that may be present thus increasing soft tissue mobility.

Nervous system

Massage is often used to relieve pain as it is thought to activate the 'pain gate'.[8] Relief of pain consequently decreases protective muscle spasm. The usual methods are effleurage and transverse frictions.

Relaxation

Massage is a recognized aid to relaxation,[9] the benefit of which may then be used by the therapist in order to gain the child's confidence and to increase the tolerance of the child to further less comfortable therapy. Massage may also be taught to carers as a means of helping them to participate in the management of the child. The most usual techniques used with children are:

Effleurage. The leg is elevated, and firm, slow, rhythmical strokes are applied to the leg from the toes to the groin, each stroke ending with a small increase in pressure into the popliteal or femoral lymph nodes. This technique increases venous and lymphatic drainage and decreases edema.

Kneading. Slow circular strokes are applied over the skin to mobilize the underlying tissues. Pressure is applied through a small part of the circle with the hands moving to cover the entire area. The whole hand may be used over larger areas such as the thigh or the posterior tibial muscles, while finger or thumb kneading may be more appropriate for localized areas such as the dorsum of the foot or around the malleoli.

Deep transverse frictions. A deep massage technique is applied at right angles or to tendon or ligamentous fibers that have become fibrotic, adherent or shortened. This technique aims to separate individual fibers both from each other and from neighboring structures, and therefore must be accurately delivered to the site of injury. Muscle fibers are treated with the muscle in a relaxed position, whereas tendons and ligaments are treated in a taut position. Although very effective in preventing and treating contractures and adhesions, deep transverse frictions are uncomfortable and the technique is only recommended with older children. More details of specific techniques can be obtained from more specialized sources (see Further reading).

FACILITATION OF NORMAL MOVEMENT

The normal functional ability of a child develops through normal movement. If a child walks on a plantarflexed foot that is not corrected, the child may never acquire a fully functional gait. Furthermore, the child may be unable to participate in a wide range of activities such as running, skipping and hopping. In addition, walking with a plantarflexed foot in effect lengthens the limb. Thus, there may be secondary compensatory postures at the hip, knee and trunk, which may cause the gait to become more abnormal. Such compensatory mechanisms may lead to a further decrease in function. Early detection and management of minor pediatric foot disorders are likely to facilitate the development of optimal function and thus prevent further deformity and disablement.[10]

The aim of physiotherapy is to gain maximal function by encouraging as normal a movement pattern as possible. However, there will be situations when quality of movement must be forsaken in preference for improved functional independence.

Musculoskeletal disorders

The main causes of musculoskeletal disorders in children are congenital in nature.[11] Any limited range of movement across joints or muscles that are weakened must be facilitated as early as possible by using recreational activities, movements and postures. For example, a child who is unable to dorsiflex fully at the ankle should be encouraged to kick, to pull on the toes in order to try to reach the mouth with the foot, and to stand on the heels. With rheumatological conditions, painful swollen joints must be protected by splints and treated appropriately while allowing the child to be as independent as possible.

Neurological disorders

Disorders of the nervous system may lead to abnormalities of muscle tone, of sensation and of coordination. Such dysfunctions may in turn lead to secondary difficulties such as poor balance, poor posture, gait abnormalities and diminished function. When the nervous system is damaged, reflexes that are usually superseded by more sophisticated and complex movement patterns may remain. In other words, an older child may exhibit reflexes and movement patterns normally found in small infants. Therefore, function will also be affected. The resting level of tension in a muscle, i.e. muscle tone, changes in response to body posture. For example, an individual will have greater general muscle tone when standing than when lying, fully supported on a bed. The physical therapist may utilize this phenomenon by positioning an affected child in such a way that either an increase or a decrease of tone is obtained. When the child is then encouraged to move within the bounds of such a therapeutic position, tonal abnormalities, posture, and movement may be improved and thus function can be enhanced.[12] This concept will be discussed in greater detail when considering individual conditions.

TECHNIQUES TO MAINTAIN OR INCREASE THE STRENGTH OF WEAKENED MUSCLE

The strength of a muscle or a muscle group may be defined as an increase in the amount of tension and thus in the resultant force that the muscle can produce whether statically or dynamically. Under normal circumstances, the child will develop muscle strength appropriate for normal functional activity. However, when there is a dysfunction in dynamic or static muscle activity, e.g. in the presence of congenital foot deformities or juvenile chronic polyarthritis (JCP), certain muscle groups may produce inadequate muscular force or weakness. When there is an imbalance between two opposing muscle groups (e.g. the dorsiflexors and plantarflexors), a secondary joint deformity is likely to occur, which may lead to inappropriate weight distribution and thus further problems. The following factors may lead to muscle weakness:

1. *Pain*. Pain on movement may lead to muscle inhibition, e.g. an acutely inflamed subtalar joint in a child with JCP will lead to inhibition of the invertors and evertors. It is essential that the physical therapist assesses the child thoroughly and is aware of the underlying pathology. The pain from an inflamed joint in a child with JCP will be treated very differently from the postimmobilization pain of an adherent ligament.
2. *Denervation of the muscle*. A muscle contracts when it is stimulated to do so by impulses passing along a motor nerve to the appropriate muscle fibers. If these impulses do not reach the muscle, it will not contract. The contraction will be weakened when only a few motor units (a motor nerve and the muscle fibers it innervates) are active. Therefore, total denervation of a muscle will lead to a complete loss of contraction, whereas partial denervation will lead to varying degrees of muscle weakness depending on the extent of the lesion.

3. *Alteration in normal skeletal leverage.* Shortening of the tissue of the tendocalcaneus may lead to weakness of both of the plantar and dorsi-flexors, because both muscle groups will be working at a mechanical disadvantage.
4. *Disuse.* A period of immobility may lead to muscle atrophy. Typically, such atrophy may be observed in the posterior tibial muscles after the lower leg has been immobilized in a below-knee plaster.
5. *Muscle damage.* Fibrotic changes that occur within a muscle or its tendon as a result of injury may prevent normal muscle contraction.

A muscle may work:

- *isotonically* where there is alteration in muscle length but not in muscle tone or
- *isometrically* where there is an increase in tone but not in length.

Both principles are employed when strengthening muscle.

Muscle strength may be measured in many ways. The following methods are those most commonly used by the physical therapist:

Oxford scale

Grade 0 is no contraction.
Grade 1 is a flicker of a contraction.
Grade 2 is an active movement with gravity eliminated.
Grade 3 is full range movement against gravity through available joint range.
Grade 4 is full range movement against gravity and with some resistance through available joint range.
Grade 5 is normal strength.

Isometric strength tests

Resistance is applied to an isometric contraction by means of a weight or a spring. The resistance that is applied in order to make the muscle work maximally is noted (usually in kilograms). This may be measured at any part of the range of muscle contraction, but not through the whole range of movement. This method is not commonly used with children.

Dynamic strength tests

The affected muscle moves through its full range with a known weight resistance applied. The amount of weight that can be moved in this way smoothly 10 times is known as the 10 RM (repetition maximum) and may then be used therapeutically.

Circumferential measurements

Circumferential measurements indirectly measure strength and are based on the premise that muscle strength is proportional to muscle bulk. In theory, when a muscle is weak, it will be atrophied and therefore smaller, and as a muscle becomes stronger, the fibers hypertrophy and the muscle bulk gets larger. The circumference of the thigh is often used as an indicator of quadriceps muscle strength. It is rarely used for muscle of the lower leg. However, the results must be treated with caution for several reasons:

— oedema may increase the measurement and disguise muscle atrophy
— reduction of swelling may disguise an increase in muscle bulk
— changes in size of other muscles of the thigh will influence the measurement.

Strength-testing machines

Other methods of strength testing, e.g. myometers and isokinetic machines, are not commonly used with children, owing to the need for maximal effort in undertaking the procedure and to difficulties in explaining the procedure to children.

Principles of muscle strengthening

The principle of muscle strengthening involves the application of specific resistance to a muscle contraction in order to either increase the size of muscle fiber or increase the number of motor units recruited. Thus the force of contraction (strength) is increased.

Care must be taken to ensure that strengthening techniques are not used when there is joint or muscle pain as these may be exacerbated and also that the muscle is allowed to relax completely between each contraction. The number of repetitions and the speed of a strengthening technique will vary according to the individual needs of the patient. However, the technique is generally performed in a slow controlled manner until there is evidence that the muscle is tiring. After the muscle has rested, the process will be repeated.

Muscle-strengthening techniques

The following are the most commonly used methods of strengthening muscles in the lower limb.

Manual resistance

The therapist applies resistance manually to the distal part of the segment to be moved while fixing the area proximal to the joint over which the muscle works. The resistance may be lessened by resisting nearer the moving joint and made more difficult by moving the hands further away. The resistance is applied at 90° to the moving bone throughout its arc of movement so that the resistance alters throughout the range of movement. Sufficient force is applied in order to oppose the required movement, e.g. to strengthen the dorsiflexors of the ankle, enough resistance is applied to the dorsum of the foot to resist the child's attempts at dorsiflexion. The therapist determines how much resistance is required to strengthen a muscle but generally maximal resistance for that muscle is applied and the technique repeated until the muscle begins to tire.

This technique is valuable for use with fairly young children and with very weak muscles. When the child is instructed to 'push away' from the therapist, the treatment may be used as an enjoyable game to play. Since the child does not need to remain in a fixed position throughout the treatment, the therapist can alter the application of the force as the child moves.

Mechanical resistance

The force used against the muscle contraction is produced by the application of weights, springs or pulleys. Although the resistance is measurable and easily progressed, the resistance is only maximal through part of the range of muscle contraction. Therefore, the force needs to be applied in such a way as to resist the weakest part of that range. This may need to be achieved by careful positioning of the child. However, this is often not possible with small children. Mechanical resistance is not suitable for either very weak muscles or for smaller muscles that may best be resisted manually.

As the amount of resistance is known, it is motivating for older children to note the increase in weight that they are lifting and this can make the treatment into a personal competition.

Gravity-resisted exercises

Muscles may be strengthened purely by contracting against the force that gravity may have on the body. An example of this might be a child standing on tiptoe for a set number of times in order to strengthen the plantarflexors. Such an activity requires the muscle to move the weight of the body with gravity resisting the movement.

PNF slow reversals

The techniques of slow reversals are part of a group which are known as PNF techniques. The principle of slow reversals is that maximal manual resistance is applied to stronger muscle groups which in turn leads to facilitation of contraction of weaker groups of muscles. Therefore, after maximal contraction of stronger muscles producing a movement pattern, there follows the opposite motor pattern using the weaker muscle groups. No relaxation is allowed between patterns in order to obtain maximal overflow. Mass motor movements are employed which are characteristic of normal movement rather than individual muscle movements. These motor patterns involve two angular movements and a rotatory component, e.g. one of the usual patterns of movement in the lower limb involves flexion, adduction and lateral rotation of the hip, with dorsiflexion, adduction and inversion of the foot and with the knee being either flexed or extended. For more detail on specific PNF patterns, refer to the textbooks listed in the further reading section.

Functional activity

It is important that strengthening exercises are fun and achievable and success is measurable. Exercises that have a functional purpose such as stair climbing, bouncing on a trampoline or cycling on an exercise bike are most suitable. Strengthening exercises may be made more entertaining by the use of equipment such as balls, hoops and bean bags. Children thrive on achieving small goals set for them in the treatment programme. The strengthening exercises that are included in the following section are a few examples for the lower limb muscles that could be given to children. However, the exercises prescribed must take into account other factors such as pain, joint range limitation or underlying pathology. Because of the constraints of space only one example of each exercise will be described.

TREATMENT OF SPECIFIC MUSCLE DYSFUNCTIONS

Hamstrings

When the hamstrings are weak, the child will not be able to lift the leg above the horizontal when leaning prone on to the end of a plinth with the opposite knee bent (Fig. 13.4) and may abduct or medially rotate the hip at the end of the range of motion. The weakness may manifest itself in the form of hyperextended knees or in a less efficient gait. If the medial hamstring is weak, there is a loss of stability on the medial side of the knee and this can give the appearance of a 'knock-kneed' gait. Muscle-strengthening exercises should be undertaken.

Tightness of the hamstring muscles is a more common occurrence than weakness and may cause restricted extension of the knee when the hip is flexed or in a flattened lumbar lordosis.

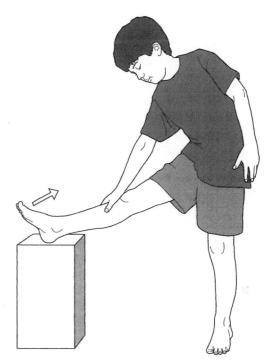

Figure 13.4 Active hamstring stretch. Child pulls foot up whilst leaning forward over leg,

When walking, the child may not gain full knee-extension in heel-strike and midstance phases, and as knee-flexion in effect shortens the leg, the foot may be plantarflexed or overpronated, with increased medial rotation of the hip. However, in many cases, these features may not be apparent, and specific muscle testing may be necessary.

Passive hamstring stretch

The child lies supine on the plinth with both legs extended. In order to stretch the hamstrings of the right leg, the therapist holds the left thigh down and gradually lifts the right leg to the limit of extensibility, making sure that the knee does not bend.

Active hamstring stretch

The child stands with the foot of the side to be stretched on the bottom stair or a small step. The child pulls the foot up and, with the other knee slightly bent, leans towards the foot (Fig. 13.4).

Strengthening exercise for the hamstrings

Holding on to a chair for balance, the child very slowly bends one knee towards the buttocks, and then very slowly straightens it down to the ground again. (This can be performed with a weight attached.)

Quadriceps

Quadriceps weakness, which is a common occurrence as a result of many lower limb disorders, presents with a decreased ability to straighten the knee against gravity. This will lead to difficulty rising from a chair, or in sitting down in a controlled manner, or in climbing up and down stairs. There may be an increased trunk- and hip-flexion at heel-strike to move the line of gravity forward anterior to the knee to improve stability. This may lead to hyperextension of the knee joint.

When the quadriceps are shortened, there will be a loss of hip-extension when the knee is flexed or in decreased flexion of the knee when the child lies prone with the hip extended. This is most commonly due to tightness of rectus femoris, a muscle that spans both the hip and the knee. Quadriceps tightness will cause some degree of leg shortening, most commonly apparent at the hip.

Passive quadriceps stretching

The child lies on one side or on the therapist's lap with the leg to be stretched uppermost. One hand of the therapist is placed over the anterior hip joint and, while the forearm supports the weight of the uppermost leg, the other arm fixes the pelvis. The child's leg is then moved backwards into extension (Fig. 13.5). This movement stretches the rectus femoris. The knee may be passively flexed if necessary by movement of the therapist's hands so the 'pelvic' arm fixes the thigh and the other arm moves the lower leg.

Active quadriceps stretching

The child is instructed to hold onto a chair or suitable piece of furniture. The child then grasps the ankle in such a manner as to bring the foot as

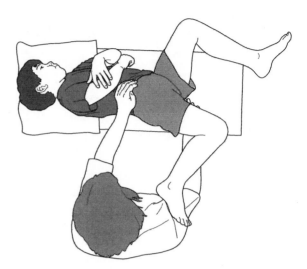

Figure 13.5 Passive quadriceps stretch.

close to the buttocks as possible. The child's thighs should be in alignment. A greater stretch may be achieved by moving the thigh backwards in order to extend the hip (Fig. 13.6).

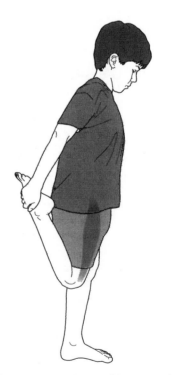

Figure 13.6 Active quadriceps stretch.

Strengthening exercise for the quadriceps

The child sits upright on a high plinth or table and slowly straightens and lowers each leg alternately, dorsiflexing the foot at the same time. The leg is held for a count of 10 and then slowly lowered.

Iliotibial tract

The iliotibial tract can be shortened and this may lead to pain along the lateral aspect of the thigh.

Passive iliotibial stretch

The patient lies on the back with the knee to be stretched bent up. The therapist stands on the affected side, stabilizing the uppermost iliac crest and slowly pushes the bent knee downward toward the plinth.

Active iliotibial stretch

The child sits on the floor with the legs outstretched and the arms on the floor behind the back. The child is then instructed to bend the leg to be stretched across the other leg so the foot is placed on the floor next to the outer surface of the

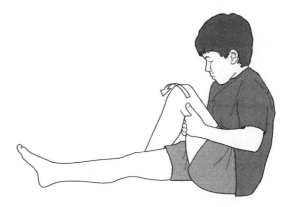

Figure 13.7 Active iliotibial stretch.

opposite knee. The child pushes this bent knee towards the straightened leg using the opposite elbow (Fig. 13.7).

Hip adductors

Tightness of the adductor muscle group of the hip leads to limited hip abduction and lateral deviation of the pelvis in walking. Children with adductor spasticity may carry the leg across the midline, narrowing the base of support, and have

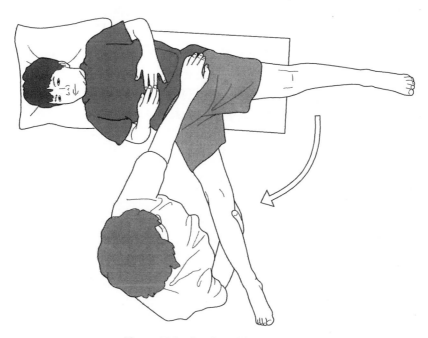

Figure 13.8 Passive adductor stretch.

a decreased stride length, or, if the condition is bilateral, they may demonstrate 'scissoring'.

Adductor weakness may also manifest itself with lateral pelvic tilting during walking.

Passive adductor stretch

The child lies supine and one arm of the therapist is used to fix the child's pelvis and the other arm to support the child's leg, which is carried out to the side and held at the limit of movement (Fig. 13.8).

Active adductor stretch

The child sits on the floor with the knees bent and the soles of the feet touching. Gentle pressure is exerted on the knees (Fig. 13.9).

Strengthening exercise for hip abductors and adductors

The child lies on one side and lifts and then lowers the uppermost leg very slowly. This is then repeated with the other leg.

Ankle plantarflexors

Plantarflexors that are either contracted or tight are a common finding presenting as a loss of range of ankle dorsiflexion when the knee is extended or in a loss of knee-extension when the foot is dorsiflexed. In walking, there is limited

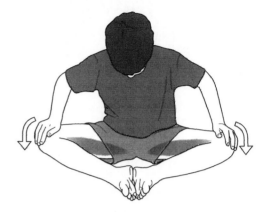

Figure 13.9 Active adductor stretch.

dorsiflexion in the stance phase and heel-strike may also be affected.

Passive plantarflexor stretch

The child lies or sits with the legs outstretched on the treatment couch. The therapist controls hip and knee movement with one hand and the heel and the tendocalcaneus with the thumb and fingers of the other hand. The plantarflexors are stretched by the therapist pulling distally on the tendon while pushing the foot into dorsiflexion with the forearm. The knee can be gradually moved into extension to stretch both gastrocnemius and soleus (Fig. 13.10). The pull on the tendocalcaneus may be directed laterally in order

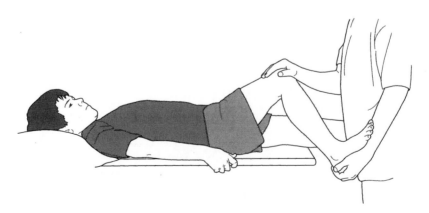

Figure 13.10 Passive plantarflexor stretch.

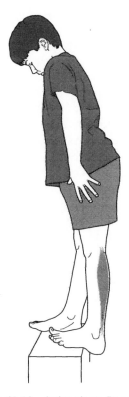

Figure 13.11   Active plantarflexor stretch.

to increase the stretch on the medial tissues of the foot which may be tightened.

Active plantarflexor stretch

The child stands on the bottom step with both heels over the edge. The child is then instructed to lower the heels slowly toward the ground (Fig. 13.11).

Strengthening exercises for the plantarflexors

The child stands holding on to a chair. The child is then instructed to go up onto tiptoe, hold, and then come down again very slowly.

Anterior tibials

The most common affectation of this muscle group is weakness. Such weakness decreases the child's ability to dorsiflex the ankle joint, which can affect heel-strike and the swing phases of gait.

Strengthening exercises

The child sits on a chair with one foot placed over the other. The child is then asked to lift the underneath foot while the uppermost foot prevents any movement.

THE ORTHOPEDIC SURGICAL PATIENT

Surgery on the foot and on the lower leg may be undertaken for various conditions in the child, e.g.:

- correction of a persistent talipes equinovarus
- joint fusion
- metatarsal osteotomy
- tendon lengthening
- tendon transfer.

For these forms of surgery, it is likely the child will spend a period of time in fixation, e.g. plaster of Paris or some lighter material such as Baycast. This period of immobilization will depend upon the surgical procedure undertaken and upon the wishes of the surgeon. Physiotherapy management may be divided into:

a. preoperative management
b. postoperative management in fixation
c. postoperative management out of fixation.

Preoperative management. If the child is to be non-weightbearing after surgery, a frame or elbow crutches should be correctly measured in advance. A wheelchair with leg support may be provided in order to allow the child to be mobile before the child is able to walk with a suitable aid. All such aids should be explained to the family and the child should be given the opportunity to practice using them in advance.

Postoperative management in fixation. Following surgery, it is likely that the surgical site will be immobilized in order to allow healing of cut bones and soft tissue. The duration of fixation will be variable as will its form.

Usually, it is not necessary to undertake exercises to maintain range of movement at unaffected joints as the child will soon be active and use all unaffected joints normally. However, when there is an underlying rheumatological condition, exercises to maintain range of movement may be necessary. Fixation may cause other joints to become overstressed and painful, therefore pain-relieving modalities such as ice or heat may be of value.

In order to maintain the strength of muscles that pass over immobilized joints, static muscle activity is employed. For example, when the knee is immobilized, static quadriceps and hamstring contractions will be undertaken and similar activities for the muscle groups around the ankle joint will be performed when the ankle is temporarily fixed.

The parents should be advised on how to care for the method of fixation used and to encourage the child to be as functionally independent as possible. Small children will be given frames and those over the age of about 6 years will be able to use crutches. Trolleys may also be supplied so that the child may lie prone and be able to move around the floor. It is usually necessary to teach methods for climbing stairs using the mobility aid, but small children must obviously be carried.

Postoperative management out of fixation. Initially, the child will require to use the walking aid in order to bear some body weight. However, as the joints become more mobile and the muscles become stronger, the support that the aid gives may be reduced and may finally be removed. The child will usually decide when it is right for this to happen. Overall objectives of treatment will be to:

- restore as much movement as is possible to the joints that have been immobile
- strengthen any muscles that are weakened – frequently those that pass over the site of surgery
- rehabilitate the child to as full functional ability as possible within the limits of ability and development
- educate the parents or guardians in maintenance of the child's condition and establish follow-up appointments as necessary.

JUVENILE CHRONIC POLYARTHRITIS

This term is used to describe a group of poly-arthropathies that occur before the age of 16 years. In order for a differential diagnosis to be made, the child must be under 16 years old and have a 6-week history of joint pain, tenderness and swelling with an associated rise in temperature and limitation of movement at the joint, which cannot be attributed to any other cause such as trauma, infection or neoplasm.[14]

Severe inflammatory changes may occur in the foot in JCP, and most commonly arise in the forefoot, eventually moving more proximally to involve the joints of the hindfoot. Such changes in the architecture of the foot lead to abnormality of the biomechanical forces acting on the lower limb which may then produce effects on the ankle, knee, hip and lumbar spine. These more proximal joints are also susceptible to the development of deformities, e.g. flexion contractures of the knees, and adduction and flexion deformities of the hip.

It is important that the therapist is involved from the earliest stage possible in the management of such a child. Physical therapy plays a vital part in the management of these conditions in association with drug therapy.

The aims of intervention in the child with lower limb involvement will be:

- to relieve pain and muscle spasm
- to maintain or improve range of movement at affected joints
- to maintain or improve muscle strength over affected joints
- to prevent deformity
- to improve function.

In the acute phase, irrespective of whether the child is in hospital or at home, full bed rest should be avoided unless the child is febrile and systemically ill. It is often sufficient for the child to have regular rests throughout the day in order to conserve energy. At this stage, good posture should be emphasized. Parents should be advised that although placing a pillow under the child's knees may be more comfortable, such a course of action may lead to flexion contractures.

Similarly, a bed cradle should be used to avoid the weight of the covers pulling the foot into plantarflexion.

Throughout this stage, the therapist must aim to prevent contractures and to maintain soft tissue extensibility. Contractures may be avoided by ensuring that each joint is moved through its full available range each day. Pain relief may be afforded by the application of ice packs to inflamed joints, and exercises should be timed with analgesia when necessary. This daily routine of active or assisted movement should be carefully taught to the child and the carers in order that the exercises can be continued at home. Great sensitivity and encouragement may be required to instigate a daily maintenance routine, which should be as brief and as simple as possible in order to ensure that everyone involved is motivated to implement it. When one considers the number of joints that may be potentially affected in JCP, a regimen that includes movement of every joint several times daily may take so much time that it may not be appropriate to the daily life of the child.[14] In this situation, some well-performed stretches to maintain movement and functional activities such as hair brushing, stair climbing or toe tapping may be preferable. The carers at this stage will be very involved in the physical management of the child's condition and must be able to discuss with the therapist any difficulties that arise.

Hydrotherapy may be used in the early stages in order to relieve pain, maintain joint range and to facilitate normal movement before this is possible on dry land. Once the child is ambulant, some form of walking aid with gutter handles to prevent extra strain on the hand joints should be provided. As the joints become less acute, more active movement may be undertaken and movement therapy should be progressed when appropriate.

In the chronic phase when pain has subsided, the child may be left with stiffened joints, weakened muscles and some degree of deformity. Hydrotherapy is again valuable in improving range of movement with buoyancy-assisted activities. Serial splintage may be used to stretch contracted soft tissue; this form of splintage is more commonly required for the knee than for the foot and ankle. Orthoses or ultimately surgical intervention may be required to overcome deformity and to provide a functional foot position. The child should attend for regular maintenance check-ups and treatment 'top-ups' if indicated.

SPINA BIFIDA

In spina bifida, there is incomplete closure at midline of the neural tube or its covering. The defect varies in degree of severity. There may be no more than a puckering of the skin or a bifid spinous process, or, in the most severe form, there may be disruption of the spinal cord, vertebral bone structure and overlying tissues.

In cases where there is neurological impairment, there is normal innervation down to the affected level, flaccid paresis of the muscles innervated by the affected nerve roots and spastic paresis of the muscles below the level of the lesion. The muscle paresis usually affects the lower limbs, the severity depending on the extent of the lesion. It may vary from mild weakness of one motor group to paraparesis. Accompanying the motor paresis, sensory disturbances tend to be similarly distributed and, in addition, urinary and/or fecal incontinence frequently occurs. Spina bifida is often accompanied by spinal deformities that may lead to decreased respiratory function and to difficulties using the upper limbs. Uneven paralysis and the resultant muscle imbalance that occurs may predispose the child to the development of contractures and deformities of the lower limbs and should be treated as soon after birth as possible. There is a danger that deformities will worsen and that other bony changes may ensue if poor postures caused by abnormal muscle tone are perpetuated as the child develops. Such bony changes may include femoral antetorsion when there is prolonged increased tone in the hip flexors and adductors, or leg shortening when an asymmetrical posture is maintained. Therefore, it is very important that the therapist maintains soft tissue extensibility by the use of full range passive movements and techniques in order to normalize tone and educate posture. Parents should also be taught how these activities should be performed and they should also be advised of their importance.

The type of deformity that may occur in the lower limbs will depend upon which muscle actions are unopposed and upon other external factors that may influence joint position. The following are examples of common deformities that may occur:

1. calcaneovalgus or varus deformity may be caused by weakness in the plantarflexors relative to the dorsiflexors
2. equinovarus deformity may be the result of weak evertors and dorsiflexors
3. flexion of the metatarsophalangeal joints may be caused by weak lumbricals
4. a flexion deformity of the forefoot may be caused by an uncorrected calcaneal deformity with associated effects of gravity and pressure of bedclothes
5. a flexion deformity of the knees may be caused by weakness of the knee extensors
6. hyperextension of the knee may occur by unopposed action of the quadriceps. It may not be possible for physical therapy to assist in the correction where deformities are brought about by abnormal muscle pull. In such cases, orthotic management or orthopedic surgery is indicated.

The physical therapist will encourage the child to move through the development sequence beginning at a level appropriate for the child's abilities. Movement may be used to encourage head control at a very early age and this may lead on to assisted rolling or other activities. It must be remembered that there is likely to be altered tone below the level of the cord lesion and this makes the use of the lower limbs difficult. Therefore, all body movements are affected.

Some form of mobility aid will probably be required by the child with spina bifida. Such aids may be in the form of calipers (with or without pelvic and thoracic bands), crutches or wheelchairs, the level of support being dependent upon the level of the lesion. Most children should be ambulant with some form of aid. Irrespective of the walking aid used, children will require to develop the musculature in the upper limb, shoulder girdle and trunk in order to enable them to bear their body weight and to propel themselves. The physical therapist will therefore devise a suitable exercise regimen to strengthen these affected muscles.

As with all pediatric conditions, it is very important that the parents are informed and are involved in the management of their child and that they are always aware that they can contact the physical therapist for help and advice when problems arise. As there is likely to be some degree of sensory loss, parents must be aware of the damage that may be caused by the pressure exerted by wrinkled socks or ill-fitting shoes. Similarly, parents ought to be advised about the dangers of using excessively hot water when bathing, which can lead to skin damage and the development of pressure sores and ulcers.

CEREBRAL PALSY

Cerebral palsy (CP) is the term used to describe a disorder which is caused by a variety of factors including trauma, infection and developmental disorders of the brain occurring around the time of birth. Such neurological damage leads to abnormalities in muscle tone, in sensation, in balance and in coordination and there may be associated epilepsy and problems involving speech, sight and perception. There are many manifestations of this condition. The clinical features will depend upon the area of the brain involved and the severity of the brain damage. Although it is almost impossible to outline the role of the physical therapist in the management of CP, the therapist's responsibilities may be broadly categorized as:

1. *Prevention of deformities.* Deformities commonly occur in the child suffering from CP as the result of increased muscle tone since the muscles are rarely fully stretched. Treatment of deformities has already been discussed under spina bifida.
2. *Facilitation of normal movement.* Normal movement may be only performed with normal tone and sensation. Therefore, the therapist

will aim to assist the child to move through the developmental sequence by trying to alter tone to a more normal level and to use techniques to improve sensory awareness.

3. *Re-education of gait*. This may be undertaken only in conjunction with normal movement activities. Although there is always an emphasis on maximizing function, walking on a hypertonic, inverted and plantarflexed foot will ultimately lead to an increase in tone, resulting in greater deformity and to an even more abnormal gait pattern in an affected child.

REFERENCES

1. Zelazo PR. The development of walking: new findings and old assumptions. J Motor Behav 1983;15(2):99–137.
2. Gassier J. A guide to the psychomotor development of the child. Edinburgh: Churchill Livingstone; 1984.
3. Kisner C, Colby LA. Therapeutic exercise: foundations and techniques. Philadelphia: FA Davis; 1985.
4. Knott M, Voss DE. Proprioceptive neuromuscular facilitation. New York: Harper & Row; 1973.
5. Melzack R, Wall P. The challenge of pain. Harmondsworth: Penguin; 1982.
6. Gifford J, Gifford L. Connective tissue massage. In: Wells PE, Frampton V, Bowsher D, eds. Pain: management and control in physiotherapy. London: Heinemann; 1988.
7. Ironson G, Field T, Scafidi F, et al. Massage therapy is associated with enhancement of the immune system's cytotoxic capacity. Int J Neurosci 1996; 84:205–217.
8. Bowsher D. Modulation of nociceptive input. In: Wells PE, Frampton V, Bowsher D, eds. Pain: management and control in physiotherapy. London: Heinemann; 1988.
9. Valentine KE. Massage in psychological medicine – modern use of an ancient art. N Z J Physiotherapy 1984;12:15–16.
10. Levy LA. Podopediatrics: beginning of the natural history of adult foot disorders. J Am Pod Med Assoc 1991;81:155–156.
11. Silman AJ. Musculoskeletal disorders in childhood. Br Med Bull 1985;42: 196–199.
12. Carr JH, Shepherd RB, Ada L. Spasticity: research findings and implications for intervention. Physiotherapy 1995;81(8):421–429.
13. Melvin JL, ed. Rheumatic disease in the adult and child. 3rd ed. Philadelphia: FA Davis; 1989.
14. Swezey RL. Rheumatoid arthritis: the role of the kinder and gentler therapies. J Rheumatol 1990;17(suppl 25):8–13.

FURTHER READING

Alter MJ. The science of stretching. Illinois: Human Kinetics Books; 1988.
Cyriax J. Textbook of orthopedic medicine, vol 2. 11th ed. London: Baillière Tindall; 1984.
Inman VT, Ralston HJ, Todd F. Human walking. Baltimore: Williams and Wilkins; 1981.
Janda V. Muscle function testing. London: Butterworths; 1983.
Kendall FP, McCreary EK, Provance PG. Muscle testing and function. 4th ed. Baltimore: Williams and Wilkins; 1993.
Melvin JL. Rheumatic disease in the adult and child. Philadelphia: FA Davis; 1989.
Shepherd R. Physiotherapy in paediatrics. London: Heinemann;1974.
Shumway-Cook A, Woolacott M. Motor control: theory and practical applications. Baltimore: Williams and Wilkins; 1995.
Smidt GL, ed. Gait in rehabilitation. Clinics in physical therapy. New York: Churchill Livingstone; 1990.
Whittle M. Gait analysis: an introduction. 2nd ed. Oxford: Butterworth Heinemann; 1997.

14

Serial casting

Laurence J. Lowy

This chapter will give explicit step-by-step instructions on the application of casts to the four most common lower extremity deformities for which serial casting is an appropriate form of therapy. The ability to correct a deformity by this method is great. However, the possibility of damaging the lower extremity by means of the clinician's carelessness or inexperience is equally great. Therefore, the clinician must have a thorough understanding of the deformity, of the structures involved and of the proper techniques employed before attempting to cast the child's foot. Serial casting is open to modification and personal preference. However, as long as the clinician adheres to the overall principles and is mindful of possible iatrogenic complications, no harm will be done.

Serial immobilization casting refers to the application and re-application of a holding material, usually plaster of Paris or fiberglass, to a body part in order that it may heal or remain in a corrected position, e.g. in the treatment of fractures or tendon lengthenings. In the context of this chapter, the technique may be defined as the sequential, gradual correction of congenital foot pathologies through manipulation, with maintenance of the new position by means of a cast applied to the part.

HISTORY

The concept of serial immobilization casting has been present as a medical modality since the beginning of modern medicine. Hippocrates is credited with being one of the first clinicians to use manipulation, bandaging materials and immobilization in order to treat talipes equinovarus.[1] J. Hiram Kite is generally considered one of the first clinicians to advocate gentle, rather than forceful, manipulation for foot deformities. Prior to Kite, Elmslie,[2] Guerin[3] and Browne,[4] among others, practiced forceful correction under general anesthesia, followed by splinting or casting. Kite found that such techniques resulted in joint stiffness, joint incongruity and decreased joint space so he proposed a more subtle correction.[5,6] He recommended gradual, repeated correction to be maintained by retention casts. Kite appears to be the first to recognize the need to elongate soft tissue structures slowly. While many have questioned some of his techniques and philosophy, most still adhere to the general principles he proposed and practiced for more than 30 years.

GENERAL CONSIDERATIONS

The podopediatrician must understand and be able to implement the basics of serial casting prior to applying it for a particular pathology.

Rationale for serial casting

Much of the orthopaedic literature over the years has advocated little or no treatment of foot and leg pathologies unless they are particularly severe. Controversies abound as to the treatment of asymptomatic flatfoot, internal tibial torsion, metatarsus adductus and calcaneovalgus.[7,8] While there is evidence that active treatment alleviates or prevents more serious complications, many authors maintain these conditions are 'outgrown.' Serial casting is often reserved for the more severe deformities.

However, most podopediatricians and many orthopaedists recognize the need to be proactive in treatment. Not only have they found that the deformities are frequently *compensated for*, not outgrown, but also that the early phase of a child's life is the ideal time to correct any problems.[9] In infancy, bones, cartilage and epiphyseal plates are soft and malleable – more so than tendon and ligaments.[10] Manipulation and maintenance will cause stresses to the bone, the cartilage, the epiphyseal plates and the soft tissues, which in turn

will effect change in these structures. Growing epiphyses will yield to stress by changing the direction of the growth. Bone will remodel according to Wolff's law.[11] Such changes can be long lasting when maintained over a period of time. To allow deformities to remain untreated will result in the bone and soft tissue becoming stronger, essentially maintaining the deformity throughout the child's life. By the time the pathology begins to limit the type of shoegear patients may wear, the activities they may participate in, or cause pain with simple ambulation, correction will only be achieved through surgery. Therefore, it appears to make better sense to address the problem when correction is relatively painless. It should also be kept in mind that most authors and clinicians who maintain that deformities are outgrown admit that a certain percentage will persist into later life.[12] Therefore, the inability to predict which child's deformity will 'resolve' and which will not almost demands treating all such cases in order that each child may have an equal opportunity to develop a normal lower extremity.

Age, severity, flexibility

Most clinicians involved in serial casting agree that casting should begin before the first year of life, and preferably within the first 6 months when the structures involved are most malleable.[9] It is also maintained that casting should begin before the child takes the first step. Weightbearing hastens the bone-strengthening process as well as muscle and tendon contraction. Casting after the age of ambulation may lead to failure, although on occasion the severity of the pathology may warrant this course of action. The clinician's judgment and experience will dictate the approach and course in those circumstances. Both the length of treatment and the prognosis of the problem are related to the severity of the deformity; more severe pathologies will usually require longer duration of casting and of maintenance. In addition, such deformities may not respond to treatment as well as one that is less severe and the final correction may not be as complete or ideal. This principle is important for clinicians to understand in order that they do not demand an outcome that they cannot achieve.

More importantly, the parents must be made aware of the guarded prognosis in order that their expectations do not exceed what the podiatrist and patient are able to achieve.

Similarly, a more flexible pathology will generally respond well to casting and correction may be effected early. However, such a foot may just as easily lose the correction if casting is not carried out for long enough or it is not maintained by other modalities. Flexibility is an asset but not a guarantee of complete success.

Preparation

Preparation for serial casting refers not only to having all the appropriate materials ready but also being in the right environment, preparing all the parties involved and, ideally, obtaining pre-casting radiographs.

The appropriate environment should be a warm treatment room that is free from distractions. There should be sufficient room for all the people involved to perform their respective tasks comfortably.

People involved

Essentially there are four parties involved in a serial casting: the parent or parents, the patient, the clinician and an assistant.

The parents must be prepared on many levels. At the first encounter, prior to casting, the clinician must thoroughly explain the reasons for casting, the method of casting, the expectation of outcome, and the parent's involvement in the process. If the clinician believes surgery may be necessary at a later date, e.g. in cases of talipes equinovarus, the parents should be made aware of this possibility early on. The parents should also be advised that the foot might not be corrected to normal, but that it will be improved and made more functional.

Length of treatment

Invariably, the parents will ask how many casts will be needed, or how long the process will take. Unfortunately, any timeframe can only be an esti-mate and is relative to the severity of the problem. However, it must be made clear to the parents that abandoning therapy prematurely will most likely result in failure. Parents may also be worried that their child will be delayed in achieving certain milestones such as walking. This may happen, but the delay is usually minimal and most children catch up quickly. The parents should be advised that their child will eventually walk (assuming no neuromuscular impairments) and that the casting will not permanently affect the child. Indeed, most children try to walk while in the casts, even when the cast is above the knee.

Psychologically, the parents should be prepared for the reaction of their child to serial casting. Most children cry at some point during the process as a result of the stretch on soft structures and from an overall fear of the procedure. The parents should be assured that the manipulation involved is gentle and slow and that the foot is not being unduly stressed.

Finally, the parents must be prepared to remove the casts themselves at home. It is in the child's best interest that the casts are gently soaked off in warm water or a warm water/white vinegar solution. The latter should be mixed in a 4:1 ratio, as the vinegar may be too caustic at higher dilution. The vinegar helps accelerate the process of softening the plaster. However, the parents should be advised that the soaking and removal may take an hour or more, especially on the first occasion. As the parents become more proficient, soaking time may decrease to half-an-hour or less. Certain clinicians prefer to remove the casts themselves with a cast saw but such practice introduces two possible problems: (i) although it is unlikely that the saw will cut the child, an agitated child may be at risk from a burn or from an abrasion; (ii) the noise and vibration may also be sufficient to frighten the child to such an extent that subsequent castings may be impossible.

It may be useful to schedule the child's appointment just prior to a feed as this may act as a useful distraction for the child and may help to pacify the child. For the same reason, the child should have access to a favorite toy or comforter.

While the parents will be responsible for preparing the child, the clinician will also be responsible for preparing in advance, by having all the necessary materials and the room ready. Ideally, the casting should be performed without interruption. An assistant is indispensable at the time of actual casting. A good assistant can distract the child when necessary, as well as help to maintain the foot and leg in alignment as the clinician applies the casting material. A variation on this is to have the assistant apply the material while the clinician holds the foot and leg.

MATERIALS

Prior to the application of cast materials, a skin preparation is generally used. The most common of these are Betadine (Purdue Frederick, Norwalk, CT), skin lotion or tincture of benzoin. The rationale behind utilizing Betadine is to increase traction when applying cast padding and to provide antisepsis should the skin be compromised under the cast. Tincture of benzoin has also been used to provide traction, as well as adhesiveness, which allows tighter application of cast padding. Skin lotion may be employed to maintain skin suppleness and thereby possibly prevent skin breakdown owing to dryness under the cast. It should be kept in mind that *not* using a skin preparation is also an option as any topical preparation applied to a baby's skin under occlusion may result in dryness, maceration, dermatitis or allergic reaction.

Tubular gauze material such as Surgitube (Glenwood Inc., Tenafly, NJ) or Tubegauze (Scholl Co., Chicago, IL) should then be placed over the limb. This material is folded over the edges of the cast, and provides a soft interface between the skin and the cast and hence minimizes irritation. The gauze will also prevent the child from picking at and possibly eating the plaster. Finally, the gauze helps prevent the cast from fraying at the edges. For most children, #2 Surgitube is adequate for the lower leg and #3 Surgitube is good for the thigh.

Cast padding is essential prior to the application of plaster in order to prevent the skin from irritation or from being compromised. Many brands and types of cast padding exist and use of any particular one becomes a matter of personal choice based upon experience. Johnson & Johnson Specialist Cast Padding (J & J Professional, Inc., Rayham, MA) provides softness and good contouring of the foot and leg, while providing important breathability under cast materials. Webril (The Kendall Company Hospital Products, Boston, MA) is also suited to serial casting because of its soft texture and relatively high tensile strength. It allows a good amount of tension to be applied, helping to maintain the body part in the corrected position after manipulation.

Cast paddings come in various sizes. The widths used most frequently in serial casting are 1, 2 and 3 inch (2.5, 5 and 7.5 cm). As a rule of thumb, 1 inch is suited to the neonate up to the first or second month of life. For infants under 8 months old, 2 inch is appropriate for the foot, ankle and lower third of the leg and 3 inch is good for the upper leg and thigh. For children older than 8 months, 3 inch cast padding may be used throughout, although better maneuverability will be achieved when 2 inch is used on the foot. Again, experience and preference will dictate which should be used and in what situation. For the novice, it is probably better to use 2 inch as maneuvering around the heel, ankle joint and knee become difficult with larger sizes.

For years, plaster of Paris has been the material of choice for casting but there have been improvements that have produced new and possibly better synthetic casting materials. Of particular interest for serial casting is 3 M Scotchcast (3 M Health Care, St Paul, MN) which is a semi-rigid fiberglass material. When compared with plaster, this material has the advantages of fiberglass, including lighter weight, faster setting time, radiolucency, durability and cleaner application. In addition, it has better moldability and flexibility than regular fiberglass and is easily removable with soaking.[13] However, its disadvantages may preclude its use for extensive serial casting. As it has a shelf life of only 2 years, it cannot be stored long term. In addition, its ability to shape and contour does not match plaster. Finally, the cost of Scotchcast is far greater than plaster of Paris. Given that serial casting usually entails many applications, cost is an important factor. Thus, plaster of Paris remains first choice because it is relatively easy to work with, easily moldable, easily available, has a very long shelf life and is inexpensive.[14]

Speed is of the essence when manipulating and applying a cast to a squirming baby, therefore materials which set faster are better. For serial casting, it is advantageous to utilize the 'extra-fast' setting plaster which sets in approximately 2 to 4 minutes as opposed to the 'fast' setting type which takes approximately 5 to 8 minutes to harden. As with cast padding, plaster is available in various sized rolls. Personal preference and size of the child determine choice of size. While 3-inch (7.5-cm) plaster rolls are easier to handle and will cover the leg faster, 2-inch (5-cm) rolls are better for the early clinician because of the ability to shape them around the smaller features of a baby.

RADIOGRAPHY

Prior to beginning treatment, radiographs should be obtained, not only to aid in the diagnosis of the pathology but also to monitor the progress of the casting. While some authors believe clinical improvement is the determinant of success, most support radiographic change as the hallmark of correction.[15,16] Kite strongly favored clinical assessment and usually did not X-ray his patients. However, Heywood notes that the 'corrected' clubfeet of Kite were not radiographically corrected.[17] It appears prudent to take pre- and post-casting X-rays, as well as one or two intermediate X-rays, in order to determine overall progress and to monitor for iatrogenic complications.

Taking X-rays of an infant presents a particular challenge to the clinician. The standing X-ray units most podiatrists use are usually inappropriate in the case of an uncooperative, non-standing baby. It must be remembered that because of radiation exposure to the child, poor quality X-rays are worse than no X-rays. Therefore, it is better to have the images taken at a facility that has X-ray tables. Such an arrangement may make it more difficult for the podiatrist to view the results immediately but the overall quality will be improved and the purpose served. If at any time improper correction is viewed, casting should be stopped immediately, the technique should be re-evaluated and the problem should be addressed.

MANIPULATION

The importance of manipulation cannot be over-emphasized. It is manipulation that brings about change in the body parts, not the casting. The cast merely holds or maintains the corrected position achieved by manipulation. If the child's foot has not been manipulated adequately, optimal change will most likely not occur. A displaced fracture will not heal properly, no matter how well a cast is applied, if it has not been reset. Similarly, a congenital deformity must be distracted and re-aligned with appropriate pressure in order to effect better anatomical relationships.

While some clinicians prefer placing the child on an examining table for application of manipulation and casting, it is probably better to have a parent holding the child on a lap. This not only gives the baby a sense of comfort, but the parent can act as an additional set of hands in stabilizing the child's body. Manipulation is effected when clinicians place their hands at appropriate points on the child's foot and exert gentle, gradual force to the bones and soft tissues. For each deformity, the placement and movement of the clinician's hands is different. Specifics will be covered later with respect to each pathology. Commonly, manipulation should be performed for 5 to 10 minutes per foot and leg. The effectiveness may be appreciated by shaking the limb to its relaxed state and noting if the foot and leg rest in better anatomical position. This is also good practice to assess overall change when the child presents for the next casting.

It is extremely important to bear in mind the moderation that must be employed when manipulating the child. Structures, especially cartilage and bone, are very fragile and subject to deformation with too much exertion. Serial casting must be viewed as a slow process with incremental, not monumental, changes at each session. Patience is paramount.

Certain authors have advocated involving the parents in the manipulation procedures when the deformities are mild to moderate in severity in order to avoid serial casting. However, owing to the possibility of doing harm when carrying out manipulation, it is recommended here that parents do not manipulate at home.

CASTING

Once correction has been obtained through manipulation, the attitude is sustained with casting. This entails use of the tubular gauze, cast padding and plaster. Most clinicians involved in casting pull tubular gauze over the full length of the foot and leg. This serves no purpose in the center portion of the cast and only adds extra material to the overall process. Therefore, it is suggested that two pieces of the gauze be cut of sufficient length in order that they may be placed over the distal and proximal portions of the cast only (Fig. 14.1).

Webril or other suitable cast padding is then applied from the distal aspect of the toes to the proximal end point, pulling with sufficient tension to make it snug. The padding should be pulled off the limb and against the deformity. Neurovascular compromise will not occur with padding, as it will tear if too much tension is placed upon it. Three to four layers are appropriate at the distal and proximal portions of the cast to help protect the skin from the edges of the plaster. Elsewhere, only two layers are applied, overlapping half the width of the previous turn.

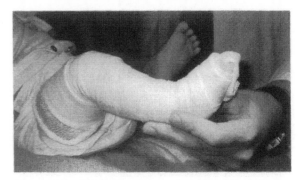

Figure 14.2 Webril is applied in a distal to proximal direction with even tension.

The padding is laid on with even tension and no wrinkling (Fig. 14.2).

Particular attention should be paid to the plantar and posterior aspects of the calcaneus as these areas are frequently underpadded. When necessary, a strip of padding may be placed at these sites, and extended to the malleoli. Care should be taken not to carry these strips to the anterior ankle, which would produce more bulk. It is very important to apply minimal amounts of the padding as too much may allow movement, thereby decreasing the effectiveness of the treatment and possibly allowing the child to wriggle free of the cast. Too much bulk or improperly placed padding may also result in pressure necrosis, irritation, blistering or ulceration of the skin. It is important to apply the padding while both the foot and leg are held

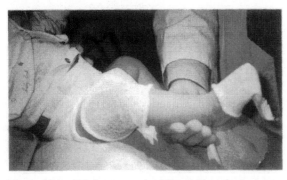

Figure 14.1 Tubular gauze should be cut in order to cover the most distal and proximal portions of the cast only.

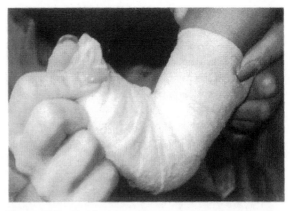

Figure 14.3 Padding should be applied with the foot and leg held in the corrected position in order to prevent wrinkling which may subsequently result in a pressure necrosis.

in correction. Otherwise, the padding will wrinkle and it may pinch the underlying skin when the foot and leg are subsequently placed in the desired position (Fig. 14.3). Such pinching frequently produces a pressure necrosis usually of the anterior ankle that leaves the child with hyperpigmentation for a considerable length of time at the site. While this does not have any serious effect, parents are often dismayed at the perceived 'scarring' on their child's foot.

A container of lukewarm-to-warm water should be made ready for applying the plaster. Cooler water will result in a longer drying time, which may make it difficult to sustain a good leg and foot position in a moving baby. Owing to the considerable exothermic reaction of plaster, hotter water may result in the child becoming agitated or, worse, it may result in a burn. Holding the end of the plaster so that it does not get melded with the roll, the bandage is held in the water long enough to saturate the inner layers, usually until bubbles have stopped forming. The roll is then removed from the basin and lightly squeezed to get rid of excess water, maintaining a creamy, wet consistency. The bandage is then immediately rolled onto the limb, starting from distal and working proximal. It is important to leave $^1/_4$–$^1/_2$ inch (0.63–1.27 cm) of cast padding free distally and proximally so that a soft interface may be achieved. It should be remembered that unlike cast padding, plaster of Paris can compromise neurovascular structures if applied too tightly. Therefore, it should be rolled directly on to the foot and leg and not pulled off the limb. Essentially, the roll is passed from one hand to the other. Three to four layers of bandage are initially applied at the distal and proximal portions for strength. As with the padding material, each turn of the plaster overlaps the previous one by a half.

The bandage should be applied evenly, with no wrinkles, and the foot and leg should be maintained in the corrected positions. The plaster should be rubbed smooth so that all layers form one unit. How far proximally one goes with the first roll depends upon the size of roll used, the type of deformity and the size of the child. Once the first roll is applied, the foot and leg are held in position as the plaster sets (Fig. 14.4). It is

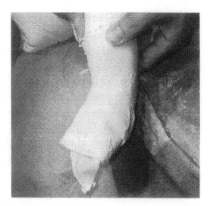

Figure 14.4 The foot and leg are held in a position as the first roll of plaster sets.

very important not to exert too much finger pressure at this stage as this may cause high points within the cast leading to irritation. Once dry, the cast material is brought proximally and the tubular gauze is pulled over the edges of the padding and plaster. Care should be taken to visualize the posterior aspect of the thigh in long leg casts, as it is a common error to apply the plaster more proximal than the padding. The final roll or rolls are then applied, and a tag or lump of plaster is created at the end so that the parents can find the end and unravel the softened cast more easily (Fig. 14.5).

The toes are checked for any impingement and the capillary filling time is evaluated. The parents are given instructions to check the toe color and remove the cast if there is a chance of

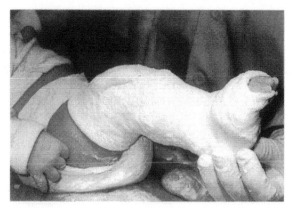

Figure 14.5 It is important to finish with a tag of plaster, which will facilitate ease of removal of the cast by the parents.

vascular compromise. The parents are also given instructions on soaking the cast off.

In the newborn or infant under 3 months of age, the casts should be changed at least weekly and possibly every 4 to 5 days because of the rapid growth these babies undergo. During this period, a cast could become too tight because of the growth, putting the child at risk. Beyond 3 months, casts should initially be changed every week to effect the most rapid change. Once correction is being acceptably attained, casts may be changed every 2 weeks.

CONTRAINDICATIONS TO CASTING

There are few contraindications to serial casting, but one must be mindful of them when they present.

1. If severe irritation, rash, blistering or ulceration is evident, the condition should be allowed to heal before applying a cast.
2. If the child is ill.
3. When a child is due for immunizations. A long leg cast may interfere with the inoculation site. Furthermore, a child may exhibit irritable behavior following immunization. With a cast, parents are unable to distinguish whether the child's irritability is due to the cast or to the immunization.
4. Hip dysplasia.

PROBLEMS AND ERRORS

Serial casting is not without its dangers or problems. As mentioned, there is the possibility of harming the skin, especially with prolonged casting. Iatrogenic complications may occur including over-correction, dislocation, rocker-bottom foot, fracture and flattop talus.[18] In addition, the casts interfere with bathing; diaper changing; clothing the baby; and childhood movements and activities are curtailed.[19]

Errors in casting may include using too much cast padding; applying the padding or plaster too loosely; wrinkling of materials; stopping the casting too soon; and failure to retain correction postcasting.[9]

MAINTENANCE

Once correction has been accomplished, it should be maintained for a period of time. Correction should be assessed using clinical and radiographic criteria. It is suggested that maintenance should be for at least as long as the child can tolerate the maintaining device. However, the period should be no less than the length of time it took to bring about the correction.[9] By what means the limb is best maintained in its new position is not well documented. It is usual for clinicians to continue casting for half the amount of time it took to correct, then utilize other methods of bracing. Certain clinicians will abandon casting after correction and use other methods exclusively. It is best to use one's judgment based upon the severity of the deformity and the likelihood of recurrence. Common devices used to preserve the limb are the Denis Browne splint, the counter rotational system (CRS), (Langer Biomechanical Group, Deer Park, NY), straight last shoes, reverse last shoes, and orthoses.

The clinician must be vigilant for relapse or recurrence of the deformity. In such circumstances, the clinician must initiate manipulation and casting again as soon as possible, especially if the child is still not ambulating. Two of the biggest mistakes made in serial casting are abandoning the treatment too early and failure to aggressively treat relapse.[20]

SPECIFIC DEFORMITIES

What follows are step-by-step instructions on performing serial casting for the four most common congenital foot pathologies:

- metatarsus adductus
- talipes calcaneovalgus
- talipes equinovarus
- tibial torsion.

One must bear in mind the general principles presented earlier when implementing these techniques. In each, hand positions and the force used are outlined for manipulation but these should be maintained for casting as well. It is important to have the cast reflect most, if not all, of the manipulations. This will ensure the cast is continuing appropriate retentive force at critical areas of the foot and leg. Where multiple pathologies are involved, e.g. talipes equinovarus with an associated internal tibial torsion, one may choose to treat each one separately or combine casting techniques at the same session.

Metatarsus adductus

Despite its relatively high presence in the patient population, metatarsus adductus is frequently not aggressively addressed, especially with respect to serial casting. However, justification for correction of the 'hooked or C-shaped' foot does exist. Left untreated, metatarsus adductus has been implicated in hallux valgus formation, pain on the lateral border of the foot, and intoe.[21] Since non-treatment has an unpredictable outcome, it is sensible to treat this condition earlier in life.[22] Bleck[23] found that the earlier a patient was treated the better the outcome. Other clinicians also believe metatarsus adductus should be treated as soon as possible.[20,24–26]

Method

1. The clinician's opposite hand holds the calcaneus of the involved foot, i.e. the clinician's left hand would hold the child's right calcaneus. The thumb is placed at the calcaneocuboid joint, proximal to the styloid process and parallel to the fibula (Fig. 14.6A). The index finger is placed flat against the talar head plantarly and medially (Fig. 14.6B).
2. The rearfoot is held in slight varus. This will counteract any valgus force the clinician's other hand may place on the rearfoot.[25] On occasion, metatarsus adductus is associated with a rearfoot valgus. In these circumstances, it is sufficient to hold the rearfoot in neutral position, but in the midst of other manipulations and with a small calcaneus, it may be difficult to determine whether the hindfoot is in neutral. Therefore it is better to err on the side of varus.

3. The clinician's other hand is placed in such a manner that the index finger is on the dorsal aspect of the metatarsal heads, the thumb is on the plantar aspect of the metatarsal heads and the first web space is against the first metatarsal head medially (Fig. 14.6C). The fingers maintain the metatarsals on the same plane to prevent a 'log jam' effect when a transverse force is applied.
4. A transverse force is directed laterally against the first metatarsal head by the web space, maintaining alignment of the metatarsal heads. The thumb of the opposite hand provides counterforce laterally and the index finger prevents subluxation of the talonavicular joint. When there is a metatarsus/forefoot varus associated with the adductus, the same hand as the foot can exert a valgus effect so that the forefoot is perpendicular to the rearfoot.
5. Padding is rolled dorsally from lateral to medial. As the roll passes around the longitudinal arch an abductory force is placed on the metatarsals (Fig. 14.6D). The ankle joint should be held at 90°. Padding is carried to the proximal tibia as a short leg cast (SLC) will be applied to the child in this case.
6. The cast is applied in a similar manner to the padding and hand positions and influences are repeated. When finished, the foot should be straight or in slight abductus with the ankle at 90° (Fig. 14.6E).
7. Correction can be maintained utilizing straight last shoes padded with $1/4$ inch (0.63 cm) felt padding placed at the calcaneocuboid joint and the first metatarsal head. It may be necessary to place a third pad at the medial heel in order to prevent a retrograde valgus force on the calcaneus. The shoes should be worn at all times.

Talipes calcaneovalgus

It should be remembered that calcaneovalgus, the so-called 'up and out' deformity, is a form of clubfoot. Although the medical literature tends to favor non-intervention, serial casting for calcaneovalgus is justifiable for many reasons. Turco[27] advises early intervention as it is innocuous. He

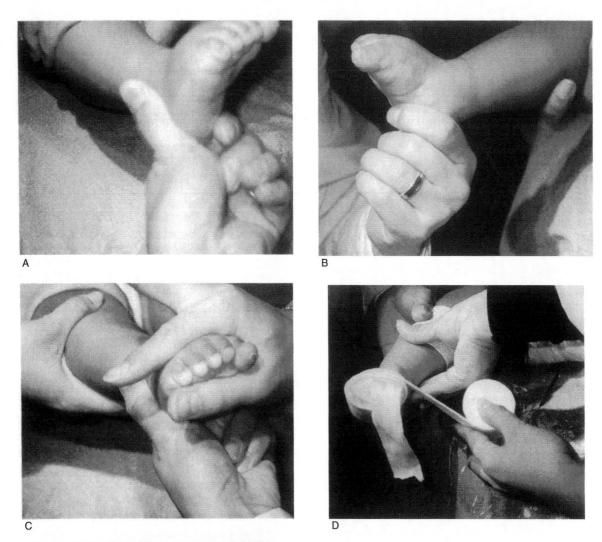

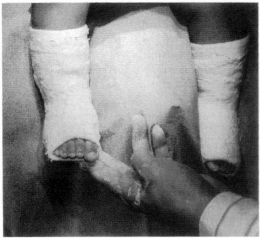

Figure 14.6 (A) Casting for metatarsus adductus. Clinician's thumb is placed on the calcaneocuboid joint proximal to the styloid process and parallel with the fibula. (B) The rearfoot is held in slight varus. (C) With the foot held in the correct position a transverse force is applied at the level of the 1st metatarsal head. (D) Padding is applied in a lateral to medial direction. (E) The foot should be straight or in slight adductus with the ankle at 90 degrees.

reports cases where untreated calcaneovalgus result in a plantarflexed talus because of soft tissue contractures. Wetzenstein[28] observes that, in a significant number of cases, flatfoot is a consequence of a congenital valgus heel. Likewise Tachdjian[29] and Giannestras[16] noted that there was a high degree of correlation between calcaneovalgus and flexible flatfoot in the older child. Untreated calcaneovalgus leads to unstable talonavicular and subtalar joints, which in turn may produce muscle imbalances.[30] In addition, a rearfoot that begins in valgus will remain in valgus when a child takes its first steps. Body weight and ground reactive force will serve to retain the valgus attitude.

Method

1. The same side hand (i.e. left foot–left hand) holds the calcaneus of the affected foot. The thumb is placed plantar to the talar head (Fig. 14.7A) and the index finger is curled around the lateral aspect of the calcaneus (Fig. 14.7B).
2. The calcaneus is inverted while the thumb slightly dorsiflexes the talus. It is important to

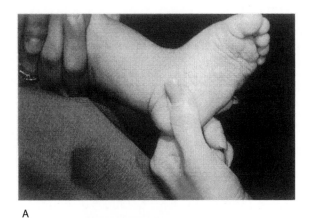

A

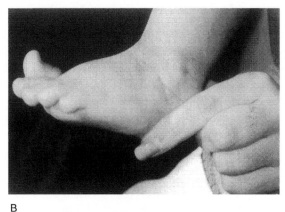

B

C

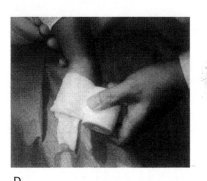

D

Figure 14.7 (A) Casting for Talipes calcaneovalgus. The clinician's thumb is placed plantar to the talar head. (B) The index finger is curled around the lateral aspect of the calcaneus. (C) The forefoot is plantarflexed and slightly everted. (D) Padding is applied dorsally in a medial to lateral direction. (E) On completion the foot should be inverted and plantarflexed.

E

be able to invert the calcaneus with this hand alone. It is a common error to believe that this inversion can be accomplished with the other hand during the plantarflexion of the forefoot.

3. The clinician's opposite hand is placed with the thumb on the plantar aspect of the metatarsals and the remaining fingers on the dorsal aspect of the child's forefoot. The forefoot is plantar-flexed and slightly everted so that the forefoot is relatively perpendicular to the rearfoot (Fig. 14.7C). In the newborn with extreme con-tracture, daily stretches are recommended prior to casting. However, this maneuver must be carried out very slowly and carefully in order to avoid the possibility of skin necrosis.

4. Padding is rolled dorsally from medial to lateral, maintaining the ankle in a plantar-flexed position (Fig. 14.7D). Since an SLC will be applied in this case, padding is carried to the proximal tibia.

5. The cast is applied in a similar fashion to the padding and the hand positions and forces exerted on the foot are repeated. When casting is completed, the foot should be inverted and plantarflexed on the leg (Fig. 14.7E).

6. Owing to relative straight alignment of the cast and the child's baby fat, an SLC may slip off. If this should be the case, then on sub-sequent visits a long leg cast (LLC) would be applied, flexing the knee to 30–90°. Cast padding is carried to the proximal thigh in these circumstances.

7. Maintenance may be achieved with varus heel-wedges in rigid soled shoes, a Denis Browne bar with a varus bend, CRS, and/or prefabricated or custom UCBLs.

Talipes equinovarus

Few question the efficacy of serial casting with respect to talipes equinovarus as early interven-tion with serial casting may obviate the need for surgical management.[31,32] In a child with club-foot, many clinicians subscribe to Kite's original protocol of first correcting the forefoot, then the rearfoot and then the equinus.[5,33] The rationale behind this approach is to avoid a midtarsal joint breach resulting in a rocker-bottom foot. Certain authors advocate correcting the forefoot and rearfoot together, and then the equinus;[21,34] while others recommend addressing all three at once.[35–37] As a result of the strength of the posterior tendons and the relative weakness of the cartilage, some believe it prudent to perform an Achilles tendon lengthening early on in order that future casting may then maintain the new length.[9] If acceptable results are not being achieved by serial casting, one must consider surgery in conjunction,[18,32] e.g. posteromedial release.

What follows is an approach designed for optimal correction with minimal casting, while avoiding iatrogenic complications. However, both the parents and clinician should be pre-pared for prolonged casting and possibly a less than perfect result. The parents must understand that surgery may be necessary at some point in the treatment. The clinician must understand that clubfoot casting is the most difficult form and requires much skill and patience. It should also be borne in mind that forceful manipulation may be more radical than surgery.[37] The rearfoot and forefoot components of talipes equinovarus can be addressed at the same time if one is careful in manipulation. The equinus should be continuously assessed and surgery performed if no change is noted after 4 to 5 casts.

Method

1. The child's heel is held by the clinician's oppo-site hand, with the thumb placed at the cal-caneocuboid joint (Fig. 14.8A) and the index finger placed flat against the plantar talar head on the medial aspect (Fig. 14.8B). A valgus motion is applied to the heel, main-taining the index finger underneath the talar head. In both calcaneovalgus and talipes equinovarus, it is essential that rearfoot cor-rection is done with the hand that holds the rearfoot and not to depend on the forefoot manipulation to bring this about. Failure to do this will result in subluxation at the midtarsal joint. When the maneuver has been carried out successfully, wrinkling of the skin will be noted on the lateral aspect of the ankle.

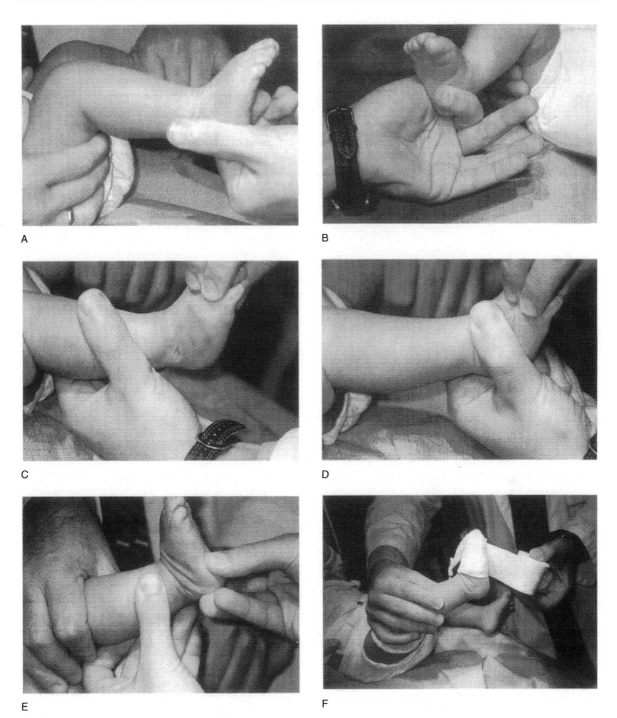

Figure 14.8   (A) Casting for Talipes equinovarus. The clinician's thumb is placed on the calcaneocuboid joint. (B) The index finger is placed against the plantar talar head on the medial aspect. (C) The forefoot is gently pulled distally and an abductory force is applied. (D) The thumb of the rearfoot hand exerts medial pressure to the lateral aspect of the talar head. (E) The anterior calcaneus is dorsiflexed whilst the posterior aspect is pulled down. (F) Padding is applied dorsally in a lateral to medial direction.

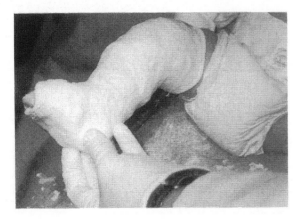

G

Figure 14.8 (G) The cast is extended to the proximal thigh, flexing the knee to 30–90 degrees.

2. After adequate reduction of the rearfoot varus, the forefoot is then held by the metatarsal heads with the other hand; the thumb on the plantar aspect and the other fingers on the dorsum. The forefoot is gently pulled distally and an abductory force is applied (Fig. 14.8C) while the thumb of the rearfoot hand exerts medial pressure to the lateral aspect of the talar head (Fig. 14.8D). The thumb is placed just anterior and distal to the lateral malleolus, in the area of the sinus tarsi. This maneuver relocates the talar head with the cartilaginous navicular. A slight eversion of the forefoot may be attempted to reduce the forefoot varus, but the early emphasis should be on the adductus deformity.

3. The equinus may be addressed initially if it is performed carefully and aggressive casting for it is postponed. Utilizing the forefoot hand, the thumb is placed on the plantar aspect of the calcaneocuboid joint and the remaining fingers are positioned on either side of the calcaneus posteromedial and posterolateral. The thumb is then pushed into the anterior calcaneus, thereby dorsiflexing it, while the posterior aspect of the calcaneus is pulled down by the other fingers (Fig. 14.8E). In effect, the clinician is attempting to increase the calcaneal inclination angle. As the adductus and varus components are corrected, the dorsiflexion

alone may be performed in the above maneuver, combining it with dorsiflexion of the entire foot on the ankle with the other hand. Merely dorsiflexing the foot on the ankle allows the Achilles tendon to plantarflex the calcaneus, not only perpetuating the equinus but also risking a rocker-bottom foot.

4. Cast padding is applied dorsally from lateral to medial (Fig. 14.8F). At the ankle joint, it is advantageous to reverse directions to counteract the internal tibial torsion that frequently accompanies talipes.

5. Most clinicians propose an LLC for clubfoot, decreasing a child's ability to pull out of the cast, reducing movement in the cast, controlling talus rotation and relaxing the gastrocnemius component of the Achilles.[20,38] There are some who believe a 'well-molded' SLC is sufficient.[35] Given the small 'bean heel' found in clubfoot and the considerable plantarflexed attitude of the foot, the likelihood of cast slippage appears greater with an SLC. With the added benefit of eradicating gastrocnemius pull, it seems prudent to initially apply LLCs and reserve the SLC for when correction has progressed to an acceptable level.

   When applying the cast, a short leg segment is affixed first. The forefoot and rearfoot are manipulated as above, initially sparing the equinus component. However, in order to prevent further contraction of the Achilles tendon, the foot should be lightly dorsiflexed to the point of resistance. Dorsiflexing the foot in this manner will take up the slack on the Achilles tendon.[20,34] Later, the calcaneus may be manipulated in the cast as previously described. Finally, the cast is then extended to the proximal thigh, flexing the knee to 30–90° (Fig. 14.8G).

6. More than any other pathology, correction for talipes equinovarus must be adequately maintained owing to a high incidence of recurrence. Casting beyond correction seems sagacious. After casting, other forms of maintenance that have been used have been straight last shoes, reverse last shoes, Denis Browne bars, CRS, custom supramalleolar orthoses and custom ankle–foot orthoses

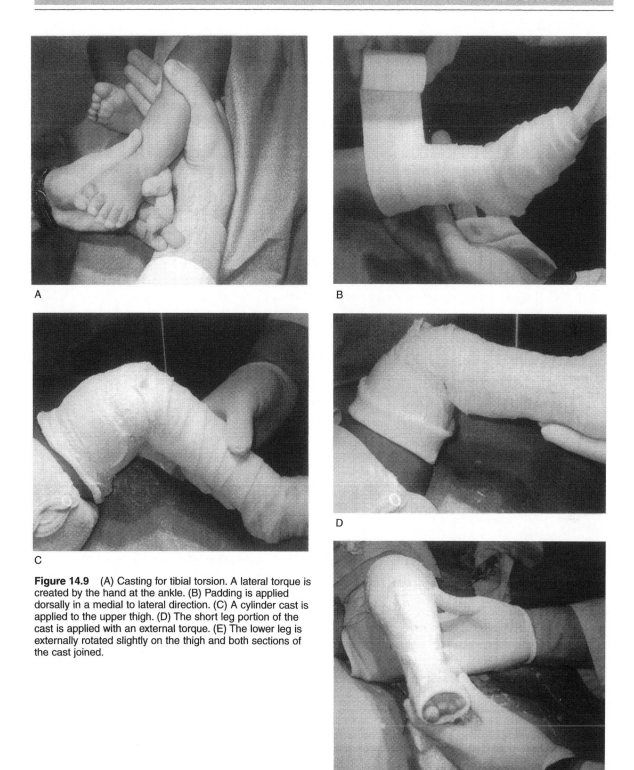

Figure 14.9   (A) Casting for tibial torsion. A lateral torque is created by the hand at the ankle. (B) Padding is applied dorsally in a medial to lateral direction. (C) A cylinder cast is applied to the upper thigh. (D) The short leg portion of the cast is applied with an external torque. (E) The lower leg is externally rotated slightly on the thigh and both sections of the cast joined.

(AFO). Only the last two devices address the equinus and only the AFO does this adequately. A solid AFO with an ankle dorsal strap to hold the heel in place is an appropriate modality but with a rapidly growing child, it becomes very expensive. A compromise is a pre-fabricated AFO modified by an orthotist to include the ankle strap.

7. The clinician must be willing to re-cast as appropriate at the first sign of a recurrence of the deformity.

Internal tibial torsion

Internal tibial torsion is perhaps the most controversial deformity with respect to serial casting. Most of the literature cites this problem as being outgrown or benign. Those who recognize it as a problem resort more to bars and splints, in the belief that no change can be effected through casting. However, serial casting for internal tibial torsion is successful when performed properly.[39] Most clinicians who cast for tibial torsion do so by manipulating the lower leg on the thigh at the knee. When executed gently, this is an effective correction for soft tissue at this level; however, this form of manipulation does not address the more distal pathologies. Therefore a modified version of this technique will be described.

Method

1. With the proximal portion of the tibia and fibula held from behind by the opposite hand, the same side hand grasps the malleoli from behind with the thumb medial and the other fingers lateral. With the leg stabilized proximally, a gentle lateral torque is created by the hand at the ankle (Fig. 14.9A). This movement will effectively stretch the distal soft tissues that become contracted in tibial torsion – specifically tibialis posterior and the long flexors. In addition, especially in the younger child, there is possibility of effecting change at the physis due to Wolff's law.

2. Padding is applied dorsally from medial to lateral so that at the leg, tension externally rotates the limb (Fig. 14.9B). This is continued to the proximal thigh.

3. Casting may be done from distal to proximal but it is better to start with a cylinder cast on the upper thigh (Fig. 14.9C). The short leg portion is applied distally with an external torque applied as above (Fig. 14.9D). Then, using the cylinder cast as a stabilizer, the lower leg is externally rotated slightly on the thigh and both sections are attached (Fig. 14.9E).

4. Correction may be maintained with a Denis Browne bar or CRS.

CONCLUSION

Manipulating and correcting pediatric foot deformities help avoid the sequelae of untreated feet. When casting is applied successfully, the child's overall quality of life may be improved to the extent that the child may be able to participate in activities that would have otherwise been precluded by the foot deformity.

REFERENCES

1. Hippocrates. The genuine works of Hippocrates. Baltimore: Williams and Wilkins; 1939.
2. Elmslie RC. The principles of treatment of congenital talipes equinovarus. J Orthop Surg 1920; 2:669–686.
3. Guerin M. Division of the tendon Achilles in clubfoot. Lancet 1935;ii:648.
4. Browne D. Modern methods of treatment of clubfoot. BMJ 1937;5:570–572.
5. Kite JH. Non-operative treatment of congenital clubfeet: a review of one hundred cases. South Med J 1930;23:337–345.
6. Kite JH. The treatment of congenital clubfoot. JAMA 1932;99:1156–1162.
7. Sullivan JA. The child's foot. In: Raymond TM, Weinstein SL, eds. Pediatric orthopaedics. 4th ed. New York: Lippincott-Raven; 1996.

8. Tolo VI. The lower extremity. In: Raymond TM, Weinstein SL, eds. Pediatric orthopaedics. 4th ed. New York: Lippincott-Raven; 1996.

9. Ganley JV. Corrective casting in infants. Clin Podiatr 1984;1(3):501–516.

10. Denham RA. Congenital talipes equinovarus. J Bone Joint Surg Br 1967;49:583.

11. Arkin AM, Katz JF. Effects of pressure on epiphyseal growth. The mechanism of plasticity of growing bone. J Bone Joint Surg Am 1956;38:1056–1076.

12. Rushforth GF. The natural history of hook forefoot. J Bone Joint Surg Br 1978;60(4):530–532.

13. Coss HS, Hennrikus WL. Parent satisfaction comparing two bandage materials used during serial casting in infants. Foot Ankle 1996;17(8):483–486.

14. Adkins LM. Cast changes: synthetic versus plaster. Pediatr Nurs 1997;23(4):422,425–427.

15. French S, Niespodziany J, Wysong D, et al. A radiographic study of infant metatarsus adductus treatment by serial casting. J Foot Surg 1985;24(3):222–229.

16. Giannestras NJ. Recognition and treatment of flatfeet in infancy. Clin Orthop 1970;70:10–29.

17. Heywood AWB. The mechanics of the hindfoot in clubfoot as demonstrated radiographically. J Bone Joint Surg Br 1964;46:102–107.

18. Weseley MS, Barenfeld PA, Barrett N. Complications of the treatment of clubfoot. Clin Orthop 1972;84:93–96.

19. Tax HR. Podopediatrics. 2nd ed. Baltimore: Williams and Wilkins; 1980.

20. Kite JH. Errors and complications in treating foot conditions in children. Clin Orthop 1967;53:31–38.

21. Lovell WW, Price CT, Meehan PL. The foot. In: Lovell WW, Winter RB, eds. Pediatric orthopaedics. 2nd ed. Philadelphia Lippincott; 1986.

22. Fagan JP. Metatarsus adductus. In: DeValentine SJ, ed. Foot and ankle disorders in children. New York: Churchill Livingstone; 1992.

23. Bleck EE. Metatarsus adductus: classification and relationship to outcomes of treatment. J Pediatr Orthop 1983;3:2–9.

24. Farsetti P, Weinstein SL, Ponseti I. The long-term functional and radiographic outcomes of untreated and non-operatively treated metatarsus adductus. J Bone Joint Surg Am 1994;76(2):257–265.

25. Galluzzo AJ, Hugar DW. Congenital metatarsus adductus: clinical evaluation and treatment. J Foot Surg 1979;18(1):16–22.

26. Reiman I, Werner HH. Congenital metatarsus varus: a suggestion for a possible mechanism and relation to other foot deformities. Clin Orthop 1975;110:223–226.

27. Turco VJ. Nonidiopathic clubfoot and other foot deformities. In: Clubfoot. New York: Churchill Livingstone; 1981.

28. Wetzenstein H. The significance of congenital pes calcaneo-valgus in the origin of pes plano-valgus in childhood. Acta Orthop Scand 1960;30:64–72.

29. Tachdjian MO. Pediatric orthopedics. 2nd ed. Philadelphia: WB Saunders; 1990.

30. Ganley JV. Calcaneovalgus deformity in infants. J Am Podiatr Assoc 1975;65(5):405–420.

31. Ikeda K. Conservative treatment of idiopathic clubfoot. J Pediatr Orthop 1992;12(2):217–223.

32. Nather A, Bose K. Conservative and surgical treatment of clubfoot. J Pediatr Orthop 1987; 7(1):42–48.

33. Preston ET, Fell TW. Congenital idiopathic clubfoot. Clin Orthop 1997;122:102–109.

34. Rodgveller B. Talipes equinovarus. Clin Podiatr 1984;1(3):477–499.

35. Coleman SS. Complex foot deformities in children. Philadelphia: Lea & Febiger; 1983.

36. DeValentine SJ, Blakeslee TS. Congenital talipes equinovarus. In: DeValentine SJ, ed. Foot and ankle disorders in children. New York: Churchill Livingstone; 1992.

37. Tachdjian MO. The child's foot. Philadelphia: WB Saunders; 1985.

38. Ponseti IV, Smoley EM. Congenital clubfoot: the results of treatment. J Bone Joint Surg Am 1963;45:261–275,344.

39. Schoenhaus HD, Poss KD. The clinical and practical aspects in treating torsional problems in children. J Am Podiatr Assoc 1977;67:620–627.

15

Orthotic management

Barbara Resseque

INTRODUCTION

Many factors must be considered in the orthotic management of the pediatric patient. The podiatric physician must be thoroughly familiar with the normal developmental trends of the growing child before attempting to assess abnormality. A complete history and physical examination, including gait analysis, are essential. The 'simple flatfoot' or 'intoe' is not always so simple. Neurological assessment and the application of one's knowledge of those systemic disorders that affect foot and leg function are integral parts of the pediatric workup.

In cases of severe flexible flatfoot, one must rule out such conditions as benign congenital hypotonia, muscular dystrophy, Down syndrome, Marfan syndrome, osteogenesis imperfecta and Ehlers–Danlos syndrome. Not only must podiatric physicians be familiar with biomechanics, they must be thoroughly cognizant of the neurological and medical conditions that present as orthopedic problems.

PEDIATRIC FOOT ORTHOSES: PRESCRIPTION CONSIDERATIONS

Once the etiology of the problem has been determined and distinguished from the normal developmental 'unwinding' of the child's foot and leg, there are important factors that must be considered before prescribing orthoses:

- the age of the child
- the symptomatology
- the biomechanical examination findings

- orthotic materials
- the shoegear.

Age of the child

Whether prescribing a night-time splint or a foot orthosis, the age of the patient and an understanding of normal ontogeny are important. Altman[1] observed a trend towards a decreasing degree of pronation from the beginning ambulator to the child aged 6 years. Decreasing talar declination angles and increasing calcaneal inclination angles were noted in his 138 pediatric subjects.[1] Valmassy[2] describes a normal reduction in the degree of calcaneal eversion up until 7 years of age. Since the normal reduction of calcaneal eversion is approximately 1° per year, Valmassy uses the following formula to determine the degree of normal calcaneal eversion for a particular age: 7° minus the child's age equals normal calcaneal eversion.[2] For example, a 3-year-old child would normally have 4° of calcaneal eversion. Tax[3] states that the forefoot varus in the child tends to decrease until 6 years of age. Therefore, before considering orthotic intervention, it is especially important in a child under 7 years of age to differentiate between normal and abnormal degrees of pronation.

Symptomatology

Many pediatric patients will present with a lack of symptoms. Often the chief complaint is the parents' concern about their child's flatfoot or intoe gait. However, when the child does present with a specific painful complaint, the orthosis should be designed to relieve that complaint. For example, a painful calcaneal apophysitis is often relieved with the use of a foot orthosis that reduces abnormal pronation and includes a heel-lift and a deep heel-seat.[4]

Biomechanical lower extremity examination

Equinus

It is extremely important to examine for equinus influences because of their propensity for caus-

ing deformity. The presence of an equinus may be determined by evaluating muscle tightness at the ankle, at the knee and at the level of the hip joint. Stretching exercises in order to improve joint range of motion in conjunction with the use of heel-lifts to accommodate the equinus may be factors the clinician may wish to consider in the management of the patient. Equinus may also limit the degree of orthotic control that can be tolerated by the patient.

Torsional and rotational abnormalities

Torsional and rotational abnormalities of the lower extremity may result in compensatory pronation of the foot[5] (see Ch. **11**). Occasionally, the forefoot abduction that accompanies foot pronation will mask the true extent of the intoe gait. This pronatory compensation will often cause the gait of a child who has medial leg rotation or metatarsus adductus to appear straight or significantly less intoed. Such compensation 'perpetuates an illusion of successful observational management'.[6] In general terms, every degree of calcaneal eversion controlled by an orthosis results in 1° of adduction of the foot. Hence, orthotic control of the pronated foot in a child with a medial femoral torsion or internal tibial torsion will actually cause the gait to appear more intoed. Therefore, when an orthosis for such a patient is being designed, this effect on the gait angle must be taken into consideration. When the child demonstrates a heel-to-toe propulsive gait, a gait-plate orthosis may be an option. Such a device has an angulated distal border which can alter an abductory or adductory gait angle (see gait plates, p. **326**).

Varus and valgus abnormalities

Clinical measurements should be utilized in order to assess frontal plane deformities of the foot and leg. Dynamic compensation for these imbalances should be evaluated by examining the patient in stance and during gait. Posting of the orthosis may be used to control these compensations. Posting limits compensatory pronation or supination by altering the contact relationship of the foot to the ground. By raising the ground to meet the plantar surface of the foot, undesirable compensatory movement is reduced or eliminated.

Navicular differential measurement

Schuster[7] describes a navicular differential measurement as an indicator of excessive pronation, particularly midtarsal joint compensation. The patient's navicular is marked at its apex or most prominent spot. Care must be taken to mark the same spot on each side, and two measurements are taken from the navicular to the supporting surface. One measures the distance from the patient's navicular to the supporting surface with the patient's foot placed in the neutral calcaneal stance position. The second measurement measures the distance from the navicular to the ground with the patient in a relaxed calcaneal stance position. The navicular differential is the difference between these two measurements. Schuster found that differentials greater than $^3/_8$ inch (0.95 cm) suggested excessive pronation in all pediatric age groups. When the measurement exceeds $^3/_8$ inch (0.95 cm), it is considered to be an indication for orthotic intervention.

Joint ranges of motion

Joint ranges of motion of the foot are indicators of how the foot may function dynamically and of possible underlying pathology. For example, a limited subtalar joint range of motion in a child between the ages of 8 and 13 years is suggestive of tarsal coalition. Conservative management of tarsal coalitions includes the use of orthoses fabricated from pronated casts. A rigid device with a deep heel-seat, high medial and lateral flanges and 0° posting is often prescribed.[8] Over time, an orthosis with varus posting may be used based on the patient's tolerance. This type of conservative orthotic therapy is more successful in calcaneonavicular bars than in talocalcaneal coalitions.[9]

In the case of the child who presents with midtarsal joint hypermobility, the clinician should consider methods by which this joint may be stabilized by reducing excessive motion. For example, long medial and lateral orthotic flanges act to limit excessive forefoot abduction.[4] Midtarsal pronatory motion is triplanar. Restriction of pronatory motion on the transverse plane will also restrict pronatory motion on the sagittal and frontal planes.

Another effective orthotic modification in order to limit abnormal pronation is to increase the calcaneal pitch. This is achieved by means of an enhanced lateral arch contour incorporated into the orthotic shell in the area corresponding to the calcaneocuboid articulation. The calcaneal inclination angle modification serves to stabilize the lateral column of the foot.[10] The author has found this modification to be particularly effective in the management of pediatric patients with excessive subtalar and midtarsal joint pronation.

Neutral and relaxed calcaneal stance position measurements

The neutral calcaneal stance position is a measurement of the angle formed between a line representing the bisection of the posterior aspect of the calcaneus and the vertical plane when the subtalar joint is placed in the neutral position. The relaxed calcaneal stance position is a measurement of the angle formed between the heel bisection and the vertical plane when the patient is in a relaxed standing position. The relaxed calcaneal stance position is the weightbearing position of the calcaneus after compensation for foot and superstructural imbalances has occurred. One guide to the amount of correction necessary in order to achieve more normal foot function in a child over 6 to 8 years of age is to calculate the difference between these two measurements. The amount of posting required to re-establish ground contact with the rearfoot and forefoot while the subtalar joint is in its neutral position is one useful guideline.[11]

Gait analysis

Analysis of how the foot and leg function in gait is one of the most important parts of the biomechanical examination. Orthotic design must be geared towards dynamic function. Therefore, superstructural influences upon the foot must also be evaluated in the context of gait as well as in static examination.

Orthotic materials and posting

The choice of materials used in the fabrication of foot orthoses has undergone considerable change over time. Emphasis has shifted away from metal alloys and leather to plastics. Plastics may be categorized as either thermosetting or thermoplastic. Thermosetting materials are liquid in their original state, solidify when mixed with a catalytic agent and will not soften when reheated. Thermoplastics are available in sheets and become moldable with the application of heat.

Thermoplastic materials may be divided into high-temperature and low-temperature thermoplastics. The high-temperature thermoplastics include the polyolefins and acrylics. The polyolefin class includes polypropylene and polyethylene. Polypropylene pediatric foot orthoses are particularly popular. This material is easily modified and has a low breakage rate. Although over a period of time polypropylene will not retain its shape as well as other materials, this is less of a problem in lighter weight pediatric patients than in heavier weight adults. Acrylics such as Polydor are polymers of methyl methacrylate. Acrylics have greater stiffness and retention of shape than the polyolefins but have a greater rate of breakage.[12] Foams are thermoplastic materials, e.g. Plastizote, Pelite and Aliplast. High-density Plastizotes may be used in the fabrication of the orthosis shell. Lower density Plastizotes are often used as a soft tissue supplement material to accommodate plantar lesions. Poron, Ovaflex and Vylite are examples of open cell foams. Such foams exhibit durability, excellent shock absorption and good retention of shape. In addition to their use as soft tissue supplements, they may also be used for forefoot extensions and reinforcing longitudinal arch fillers.

The posting material of an orthosis may be rigid, semi-rigid or shock absorbing. Dental acrylic is a rigid posting material usually combined with a polydor shell. High-density ethyl vinyl acetate, or EVA, is a semi-rigid posting material. Medium density EVA has more shock-absorbing posting material. EVA forms a fairly effective bond with the polyolefins such as polypropylene and polyethylene.

The rearfoot post provides increased frontal plane stability of the orthosis as well as frontal plane control of the foot. Rearfoot posts are incorporated into the design of the vast majority of functional foot orthoses. Most rearfoot posts allow a certain degree of calcaneal eversion during the contact phase of gait. This is referred to as a post with motion. This type of post is constructed with a biplanar grind-off, i.e. it is shaped in such a way that the medial and lateral aspects of its plantar surface are at different frontal plane angles. This grind-off allows for normal pronation at heel-strike, yet resists abnormal pronation. As the foot moves into the midstance phase of gait, the rearfoot varus post applies a force beneath the sustentaculum tali which in turn limits excessive calcaneal eversion. Limiting calcaneal eversion helps to control abnormal compensatory subtalar joint pronation and it also stabilizes the midtarsal joint during midstance. The most common rearfoot post is a 4° varus post with 4° of motion, i.e. the post is fabricated to allow for 4° of calcaneal eversion during early contact phase while resisting excessive pronation later in the stance phase.[13]

The amount of control provided by the rearfoot post is dependent on many factors:

- the stiffness of the material
- the anterior–posterior length of the post
- the width of the post
- the number of degrees of posting.

A stiffer, wider, longer post has more control than a more flexible, narrower, shorter post. Many factors including the patient's chief complaint, the biomechanical examination findings and the gait analysis will all determine the number of degrees of rearfoot posting that is required. For an adult patient with an average sagittal plane inclination angle of the calcaneus, a 4° varus post is usually recommended.[5] For the more supinated foot with a higher sagittal plane inclination angle of the subtalar joint axis, a 0–2° rearfoot post is often incorporated into the orthotic design. For the adult hyperpronator with a low sagittal plane inclination of the subtalar joint axis, a 5–6° varus rearfoot post with motion is often prescribed.[14] As a general rule, pediatric patients require greater correction than adults for the same degree of calcaneal eversion. In cases of younger children under 7 years of age with excessive pronation, often several anti-pronatory methods must be used in addition to sufficient rearfoot posting to adequately control the foot.

A forefoot post is less frequently used than a rearfoot post and is generally not recommended for the child under 7 years of age. A child's normal ontogeny may reduce a congenital forefoot varus. A forefoot post used in a child under 7 years of age may perpetuate a forefoot deformity, and therefore should not be used.[11] Kirby[15] states that posting the forefoot in a varus position in a young child with a flexible flatfoot creates a large dorsiflexion moment on the medial metatarsal rays. This increased dorsiflexory force may cause longitudinal arch collapse and subsequent excessive subtalar joint pronation.

Decision-making factors in the choice of materials for the patient include the weight of the patient, the activity level of the patient, the joint range of motion, and the aim of treatment. Is the goal of treatment accommodation or biomechanical control? Is the child involved in a particular sport that requires shock-absorbing materials as well as functional control? Will a material that is semi-rigid for an adult-sized patient function as a rigid material in a lighter weight pediatric patient? Questions such as these must be addressed in choosing the orthotic design best suited for the patient.

Shoegear

The ubiquitous use of athletic shoegear in the pediatric population is particularly advantageous for the clinician prescribing foot orthoses. Most running shoes have adequate depth to easily accommodate orthoses. However, if a child does not wear 'orthotic friendly' shoegear, this must be considered when prescribing and designing foot orthoses. Orthotic modifications that increase the bulk of the devices such as full-length top covers and longitudinal arch fillers must be used judiciously relative to the shoe that will be worn by the patient. In addition it is important that orthoses are used in shoegear with firm counters and midsoles. Flexibility of the ball area of the shoe is also important for normal gait function.

EFFICACY OF PEDIATRIC FOOT ORTHOSES

The evaluation and treatment of the pediatric 'flexible flatfoot' deformity has been debated within the medical community for over 100 years. Certain clinicians believe that flatfeet in children tend to correct themselves spontaneously. However as Helfet[16] states 'a visit to any orthopedic department dealing with adults … will rapidly dispel such an illusion'[6] (see also Ch. 12).

The main function of the foot is to support the superstructure in stance and to act as a mobile adaptor and rigid lever during appropriate phases of gait.[11] The excessively pronated foot can neither sufficiently support the superstructure nor act as a rigid lever at propulsion. It has been documented that more than 80% of Americans will suffer from some type of foot problem at one point in their lives.[17] Many of these problems begin in childhood although symptomatology may not occur until much later in life. Therefore, it would appear logical to consider orthotic intervention even in the asymptomatic, young child with the excessively pronated foot. In a prospective study of 71 cases of patients with flexible pes valgus with plantarflexed talus, Bleck & Berzins[18] found a clinical and roentgenographic improvement in 79% of the patients treated with orthoses. Basta & Mital[19] studied 50 children with symptomatic, flexible flatfoot. They concluded that pain could be relieved with conservative management that included shoes, foot orthoses and padding. Mereday et al[20] reported the results of treatment of 12 children with a pes valgus deformity. In this study, a University of California Biomechanics

Laboratory (UCBL)-type of foot orthosis was used over a 2-year period. Results included the relief of diffuse foot pain as well as the relief of localized anterior tibial muscle pain, an improvement in gait and improved shoe wear.[20]

TYPES OF FOOT ORTHOSES

Historically, one of the earliest descriptions of conservative treatment for a pes valgus deformity was given by an English chiropodist named Durlacher. In 1845, he described the use of a built-up leather inlay in order to alter the position of the foot within the shoe. In 1874, Hugh Owen Thomas, an English surgeon, described the use of leather sole additions in the management of foot disorders. The Thomas heel, an elongation of the medial side of the shoe's heel, is still prescribed today.[21]

Whitman brace

In 1889, Royal Whitman, an American orthopedic surgeon, was one of the first physicians who attempted to describe foot pathomechanics and to correlate foot function to painful postural complaints. Dr Whitman referred to the flexible flatfoot as a 'weak foot' that could be corrected with muscle strengthening.[22] He designed a metal foot brace that was fabricated over a plaster cast taken of the foot in a supinated position. It had medial and lateral flanges, a narrow front and a short rounded heel (Fig. 15.1). The Whitman brace tended to rock into inversion upon weight-

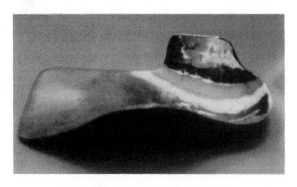

Figure 15.1 Whitman brace.

bearing. This resulted in a painful stimulus in the medial talonavicular area. Whitman believed that this painful stimulus would cause the patient to repeatedly supinate the foot, thereby strengthening weak muscles and correcting the flatfoot deformity. Later research would indicate that muscles were not the prime supporters of the arch and that in most patients the muscles of the pronated foot were not physiologically weak. The Whitman brace was seldom used in its original form because it caused excessive pain. However, it still represents one of the early attempts at orthotic foot control.

Roberts brace

In 1914, Percy Roberts designed another rigid device that was very similar in design and theory to the Whitman brace. The Roberts device had a higher medial flange than the Whitman brace. Roberts also placed a varus heel-wedge onto the device. He observed coronal sections of the calcaneus and noted that the weightbearing portion of the heel resembled the shape of a ball. Just as a ball will roll on a slope, Roberts theorized that a varus heel-wedge would increase the ground reactive forces on the medial aspect of the heel, thereby causing inversion.[23] This varus heel-wedge was a precursor to what is described today as rearfoot posting.

Shaffer brace

In 1897, Shaffer described a metal sole plate that functioned as a true arch support. This type of appliance covered the plantar surface of the foot from the heel to the metatarsal heads as well as the medial arch area. The convexity of the medial longitudinal arch corresponded to the navicular tuberosity.

Whitman–Roberts brace

In the early 1900s, Otto F. Schuster, a bracemaker and chiropodist, combined the Whitman brace with the Roberts brace to produce the Whitman–Roberts brace. This combination device was more effective and better tolerated by the patient than the original Whitman brace or Roberts brace. It caused less pressure over the medial talonavicular tuberosity than the Whitman brace and spread the corrective force over a larger surface area than the original Roberts brace.

Levy mold

In 1950, Dr Ben Levy, a podiatrist, described a technique for producing an arch support that was similar to the innersole of a molded shoe. The Levy mold consisted of a full-length leather shell that extended from the heel to the end of the digits. It also included a digital crest. The leather was wet-lasted to a plaster model of the patient's foot and the formed contours were supported by a latex and wood mixture known as 'rubber butter'. The mold functioned to increase the weightbearing surface area of the foot.[24]

Heel stabilizers

In 1956, Helfet, an orthopaedic surgeon, described a 'heel-seat' specifically designed to limit calcaneal eversion. Helfet[16] stated that 'with the heads of the first and fifth metatarsals bearing weight normally in the shoe, correction of the eversion of the heel corrects the flatfoot. A vertical heel gives the flat foot a normal arch.' Helfet believed that the growing foot would develop and function according to the shape in which it was held. He believed that children who used his orthoses would 'develop a strong arch and foot' over time.[16] Over the years, many orthoses have been designed to restrict subtalar joint pronation by reducing calcaneal eversion (Fig. 15.2). The heel stabilizers used today are based on Helfet's early design and are usually fabricated of polypropylene or fiberglass. In general, heel stabilizers are better tolerated by the beginning ambulator and young child than by adolescents or adults.

Functional foot orthosis

Dr Merton Root, a podiatrist, developed the functional foot orthosis over a 12-year period spanning 1954 to 1966. It was developed during

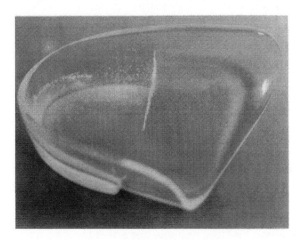

Figure 15.2 Heel stabilizer.

a time when criteria defining a normal foot were established and 'specific structural abnormalities were identified and their effects on foot function became evident.'[25] Structural deformities of the foot, such as rearfoot varus, forefoot varus and forefoot valgus were identified and measured. For example, a patient may have exhibited a structural rearfoot varus deformity off-weightbearing that caused excessive subtalar joint pronation on-weightbearing. A foot orthosis with a rearfoot varus post and high medial heel-cup could have been employed to resist this excessive subtalar joint on weightbearing pronation. In addition, abnormalities of the lower extremity proximal to the foot, i.e. internal tibial torsion, femoral anteversion, and hip flexor equinus, were also evaluated in the context of how they affected foot function. All of these factors began to play a role in the design of the functional foot orthosis.

The goal of the Root functional orthosis is to maintain the stability of the joints of the foot by resisting those ground reaction forces that cause abnormal skeletal motion to occur during the stance phase of gait. The orthosis is designed to ensure that the subtalar joint is neutral or as close to neutral as possible, at the end of the midstance phase. The foot is then better prepared to function efficiently when forces increase during propulsion. Also, the orthosis helps to ensure that the midtarsal joint is fully pronated during midstance, thereby stabilizing the forefoot and enabling first-ray plantarflexion at propulsion.[14]

During the period 1958 to 1959, Dr Root began to attempt to improve upon the then very popular Levy leather mold. Although this device could control pronation, it was not very durable and became unhygienic with time. Root searched for a thermoplastic material that was rigid enough to afford good foot control, yet flexible enough to resist fracture. The answer came with the discovery of a German import called Rohadur. This material could be heated and pressed over a plaster model of the foot to form a lightweight, durable and controlling foot orthosis.

In the early stages of the development of the functional foot orthosis, abnormal foot pronation was controlled with the use of a cork triplanar heel-wedge glued directly into the heel-seat of the shoe. A triplanar heel-wedge affects foot function on all three body planes. It promotes frontal plane inversion of the calcaneus, transverse plane abduction of the talus and sagittal plane dorsiflexion of the talus and calcaneus.

By 1961, Root was in the process of developing the rearfoot post with the use of dental acrylic material. A range of elevations for various heel heights was also developed so that the orthosis could be fitted more accurately with shoes of different heel heights. The heel-cup was placed into the acrylic and the orthosis was inverted to the required number of degrees. Once the acrylic was set, the post was ground on its medial plantar surface to allow for normal subtalar joint pronatory motion during the contact phase (Fig. 15.3).

During this same period of development of the functional foot orthosis, Root and others also developed the off-weightbearing neutral subtalar joint casting technique. In this method, the subtalar joint is maintained in a neutral position and the midtarsal joint is maintained in a maximally pronated position around both of its axes. The cast captures any forefoot varus or valgus deformity inherent in the patient's foot structure.

Numerous modifications of the Root orthosis have developed over the years. With regard to the use of this device for pediatric patients, special considerations must be addressed. Typically, this device is prescribed to children older than 3 to 4 years of age. Since this device functions at specific points of a heel-to-toe gait cycle, it is recommended for a child who has a propulsive gait.[2] The device is generally outgrown after two full shoe size changes.

In children younger than 6 to 7 years of age, a variation of the standard Root off-weightbearing neutral subtalar joint neutral position is recommended. Tax[3] states that orthotic devices for children should not be posted to hold the forefoot in a varus position as the forefoot varus in a young child normally reduces from birth to 6 to 7 years of age.

Posting the inverted forefoot position of a young child may perpetuate the deformity. Therefore, the casting technique should be modified to reduce this forefoot varus position. Tax[3] recommends that while maintaining a subtalar joint neutral position and loading the fourth and fifth metatarsal heads, a mild plantarflexory force

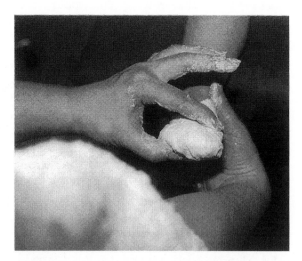

Figure 15.4 Casting technique – the subtalar joint is maintained in neutral and the first metatarsal is plantarflexed.

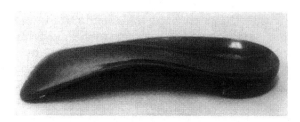

Figure 15.3 A functional Root orthosis.

should be applied to the dorsum of the first metatarsal head (Fig. 15.4). This maneuver reduces the forefoot varus imbalance in the negative cast. When casting for a foot orthosis for a pediatric patient, a plaster cast impression taken off-weightbearing is preferred to one that is taken semi-weightbearing. When a child is cast semi-weightbearing, there is often distortion of the forefoot to rearfoot relationship and the subtalar neutral position in the cast impression. The semi-weightbearing impression of the child's plump foot is also often wider than the off-weightbearing cast impression because of the soft tissue splay out that occurs when a child's foot is casted in this manner.

Orthotic modifications may be used to enhance the effectiveness of the orthosis in the control of excessive pronation in the pediatric patient under 7 years of age. Kirby[15] recommends pouring the negative cast 5–10° inverted rather than the standard Root vertical heel position. The more inverted the orthosis, the greater supination moment the orthosis can exert on the foot, thereby gaining greater control of foot pronation. However, this inverted cast technique also inverts the forefoot as well as the rearfoot. Supinating the longitudinal midtarsal joint axis destabilizes this joint and can cause increased medial arch collapse. To counteract the varus influence on the forefoot created by this inverted casting technique, Kirby[15] recommends plantarflexing the medial metatarsal heads during negative casting. This combined use of a modified negative cast impression and inverted positive cast offers greater control of excessive pronation without excessively supinating the longitudinal midtarsal joint.

In the pediatric patient under 7 years of age with excessive pronation, a polydor or polypropylene ($^3/_{16}$ inch (0.48 cm) or $^4/_{16}$ inch (0.6 cm)) shell is often recommended for greater pronatory control. The less rigid materials, such as a $^2/_{16}$ inch (0.32 cm) polypropylene or $^2/_{16}$ inch (0.32 cm) polyethylene, are generally well tolerated by the patient and are easy to adjust. However, these more flexible materials may not provide sufficient resistance to the deforming force exerted by the hypermobile, excessively pronated foot. A deep medial and lateral heel-cup and a long rear-foot post with a medial flareout are also examples of anti-pronatory measures. Long, high medial and lateral flanges limit forefoot abduction and assist in stabilizing the midtarsal joint. When fabricating an orthotic device using $^3/_{16}$ inch (0.48 cm) or $^4/_{16}$ inch (0.6 cm) polypropylene, the polypropylene plastic that will form the flange area may be pulled thinner than the plastic used to form the plantar aspect of the orthotic shell. Thinner, more flexible flanges are often better tolerated by the patient than thicker, stiffer flanges. An increased calcaneal pitch may also be incorporated into the shell of the orthosis at the calcaneocuboid articulation to stabilize the lateral segment of the midtarsal joint. It is important that modifications should be geared to the specific needs of the patient.

Today, there are many adaptations of the original Root functional foot orthosis. Such modified versions are the most commonly prescribed orthoses in podiatry.

University of California Biomechanics Laboratory

In 1967, W. H. Henderson and J. W. Campbell, while working at the University of California Biomechanics Laboratory, developed a polypropylene foot orthosis with high medial and lateral flanges and a high heel-cup. The flanges extended to an area just proximal to the first and

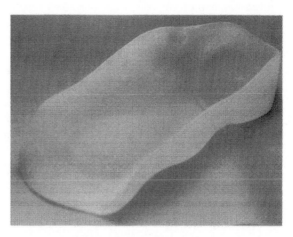

Figure 15.5   A UCBL orthosis.

fifth metatarsophalangeal joints (Fig. 15.5). This semi-rigid plastic laminate was originally fabricated from a negative mold made with plaster of Paris while the foot was compressed by a balloon and the tibia was medially or laterally rotated to give the desired subtalar joint position. The casting was performed with the foot bearing weight and a heel-elevator was applied that was equivalent to normal heel height.

Henderson and Campbell believed that this device was superior to other devices because it applied corrective forces to the midfoot and forefoot in addition to the rearfoot. Its long flanges blocked forefoot abduction and talar adduction associated with hyperpronation. Depending on the needs of the patient, the forefoot could be held supinated, pronated or neutral relative to the rearfoot. In their study of 93 subjects, Henderson & Campbell[26] found the UCBL orthosis to be the most successful device used in patients with flexible foot deformities. Success was achieved in those patients whose main requirements were the restriction of excessive motion in the subtalar joint and maintenance of the neutral position of the foot. In more severe foot deformities, the orthosis was used to maintain correction after other procedures such as surgical intervention, night splinting, and physical therapy were performed.

The UCBL device has become the orthotic of choice for the pediatric patient with a severely pronated foot. In a radiographic and clinical study of 71 children with a flexible pes valgus and plantarflexed talar position, Bleck & Berzins[18] recommended UCBL orthoses in cases which demonstrated a talar plantarflexion angle of 45° or greater. A deep heel-seat was recommended for those children who had a talar plantarflexion angle of 35–45°.[18] Down syndrome children with severely pronated feet and select cerebral palsied children with equinovalgus foot deformities are other examples of patients that may benefit from a modified UCBL orthosis.

Gait plates

The gait-plate orthosis is a rigid device employed to physically alter the cosmetic appearance of an intoe or out-toe gait. In 1967, Schuster[27] described

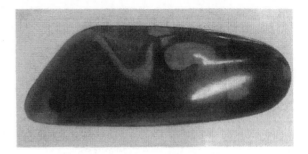

Figure 15.6 A left gait-plate orthosis.

the gait plate as a device consisting of rigid material, cut to the outline of the insole and contoured directly to the shoe. The anterior border was angulated to alter the break in the shoe. Normally, a shoe 'breaks' or flexes at a right angle to the walking direction. The gait plate is designed to alter this break in the shoe, thereby altering the gait angle.[27]

A gait plate to encourage out-toe extends distal to the fifth metatarsophalangeal joint and proximal to the first metatarsophalangeal joint (Fig. 15.6). In gait, weight passes along the lateral aspect of the foot, across the ball and through the hallux. When a child with an intoe gait wears a gait plate to induce an out-toe position, the rigid plantar lateral extension inhibits the child from pushing off the lateral aspect of the foot. The foot must perform an abductory 'twist' to allow propulsion over the medial side of the plate. Conversely, a device to encourage intoe extends distal to the first metatarsophalangeal joint and proximal to the fifth metatarsophalangeal joint. The rigid plantar medial extension induces a greater adductory gait angle in the out-toeing child.

The gait-plate orthosis is effective during the propulsive phase of the stance phase of gait. Therefore, gait plates are recommended for use in a child older than $3\frac{1}{2}$ to $4\frac{1}{2}$ years of age with an established propulsive gait pattern. For the gait plate to be effective, the child must also have a minimum of 25° lateral femoral rotation with the hip extended.[28] The device will not be effective in altering the gait angle of a young child who is apropulsive and has only 5° of lateral femoral rotation with the hip in extension. Because the gait-plate orthosis is effective during the propulsive phase of stance, some of its influence is lost during the swing phase. However, the device still exerts enough influence on the foot during the stance phase to improve the gait angle by 5–20°.[27] The gait-plate device is also most effective in a shoe or sneaker that bends easily at the ball of the foot area. Although the original gait plates were made directly into the shoe, a gait-plate extension can be incorporated into any orthotic device. If a child demonstrates both an intoe gait and excessive pronation, an orthosis with a gait-plate extension can be fabricated over a neutral position cast of the child's foot. It is important to note that the more the orthosis controls excessive pronation, particularly abduction, the less will be the cosmetic improvement achieved with the gait plate extension. For every degree of correction of calcaneal eversion, there is a corresponding 1° increase in forefoot adduction. Anxious parents of children with intoe gait should be instructed concerning the long-term importance of controlling foot pronation in addition to improving the child's angle of gait.

Blake inverted functional foot orthosis

In 1986, Dr Richard Blake first described his inverted functional foot orthosis as a device for those patients whose excessive subtalar joint pronation and associated symptomatology could not be controlled with a Root functional orthosis.[29] Although it was later used for the pediatric population, the inverted orthosis was originally designed to control abnormal pronation in runners and other athletes.

Blake stated that the main distinction between the inverted functional orthosis and the Root orthosis was the difference in cast modifications. In the case of the inverted functional orthosis, the positive cast is poured and balanced in an inverted heel position instead of the standard Root heel vertical position. A modification to the heel, arch and forefoot areas of the positive cast allows the cast to be inverted between 15° and 75°. 25° is the standard amount of inversion for a moderately pronated patient. Based on changes observed in the resting calcaneal stance position

and video gait analysis, Blake believed that a 5° positive cast correction could achieve a 1° heel position change. Therefore, based on this 5:1 ratio, a 25° inverted platform would be necessary to correct a calcaneus that was everted 5°. The second main cast modification difference between the Blake inverted orthosis and the Root orthosis is the medial arch platform. A significantly greater medial arch platform is added to the inverted orthosis than the Root orthosis. Blake states that this platform helps to avoid problems that might otherwise occur with this aggressive casting modification.

Dynamic stabilizing innersole system (DSIS)

In 1992, Jay et al[30] described a new orthosis, the DSIS, for the management of hyperpronation. This orthosis is characterized by a deep, offset varus heel-seat that maintains the calcaneus in approximately 5° of varus while still allowing normal pronation to occur during early stance phase. As in the UCBL design, long medial and lateral flanges extend proximal to the first and fifth metatarsal heads to limit the transverse spread and motion of the foot when weight is shifted from the rearfoot to the metatarsal heads. In particular, the flanges limit both talar head adduction and abduction of the forefoot relative to the rearfoot.[30]

A central, longitudinal split is incorporated in the plantar aspect of the shell. This split is designed to provide independent function of the medial and lateral columns of the device as well as greater flexibility in the forefoot area. Jay et al hypothesized that in a device with a rigid forefoot segment, the medial column of the foot may still be maintained in a varus position as the lateral column of the foot is contacting the ground, which may perpetuate a forefoot varus deformity in a young child. Theoretically, the independent motion of the flanges of the DSIS allows for independent plantarflexion of the medial column while the lateral column of the foot is contacting the ground.

Jay et al[30] studied the neutral calcaneal stance position and relaxed calcaneal stance position of 50 children with and without the DSIS. The ages ranged from 20 months to 14 years of age, with an average of 5.5 years of age. Their study showed a statistically significant correction of hyperpronation. They found this device to be well tolerated and effective in the treatment of pediatric patients between 2 and 16 years of age who had flexible pes planovalgus deformities.

SPLINTING AND BRACING: TREATMENT CONSIDERATIONS

Age of the child

In the management of rotational and torsional deformities of the lower extremities, the ideal age for treatment with splinting is when the patient is less than 1 year old. In young children, the bones of the lower extremities are preformed in cartilage and are rapidly growing. Therefore, they are more receptive than the bones of older children to a gently applied manipulative force.[31] Correction of such a deformity may still be achieved up until 2 or 3 years of age when the growth rate is still relatively rapid. However, tolerance becomes more of a problem as the child becomes older. In addition, by this age, the child is probably intelligent enough to know how to remove the shoes and splint during the night. After 2 or 3 years of age, it becomes increasingly more difficult for most children to tolerate night-time splinting.

Once the child begins to walk independently, the daytime use of splints is generally restricted to naptime. However, in order to assure correction of the deformity, the child should wear the splint for approximately 8 to 12 hours per day during night and nap times. The pre-ambulatory child may wear the splint for a longer period during the day depending upon the type of splint used. Correction may be expected in a shorter time in the pre-ambulatory child who wears the splint for a longer period during the day than in the ambulatory, older child who wears the splint only 8 to 12 hours per day.

Before the initiation of treatment, the clinician must be thoroughly familiar with the normal ontogenetic development of the lower extremities. For example, a mild internal tibial torsion in

a 3-month-old child may be expected to improve spontaneously by 6 years of age. However, a severe internal tibial torsion in an 18-month-old child may merit splinting intervention. In other words, a mild deformity in a younger child is more likely to correct spontaneously with age than a more severe deformity in an older child.

Type of deformity

Braces and splints may be used to correct rotational or positional deformities or to maintain correction of a deformity after serial plaster immobilization. Controversy still exists as to their need and to their effectiveness in the management of various deformities. Braces and splints are generally considered to be more effective in the treatment of soft tissue deformities, such as medial tibiofibular rotation, than in the treatment of bony deformities such as medial femoral torsion. McCrea[32] states:

These splints will primarily provide: help in avoiding a sleeping position that will promote a positional or soft tissue contracture; a varus or valgus position to the foot–ankle with the bending of the bar when necessary; a stretch to the soft tissue structures around the hip with full extension of the limbs; a stretch to the soft tissue structures around the knees when the knees are maintained in a flexed position.

Night-time splints such as the Denis Browne bar and Langer Counter Rotation System splint (Langer Corp., Deer Park, NY) are primarily indicated for medial tibiofibular rotation and internal tibial torsion. These deformities may be treated with splinting as a primary means of treatment or as a means of maintenance of correction following serial plaster casting. For example, a pre-ambulatory child with metatarsus adductus and medial tibiofibular rotation may first be treated with above-knee serial plaster casts and then followed with straight last shoes attached to a night-time splint. A child with a talipes equinovarus and internal tibial torsion will often be treated initially with casts and surgical intervention and then followed with ankle–foot orthoses and a night-time splint.

Ideally, any congenital foot deformity associated with a torsional or rotational abnormality should be initially treated with serial plaster casting where 'constant and unremitting corrective force'[31] may be applied to the deformed foot 24 hours per day. If the child is already walking, then serial plaster casting, especially above-knee casting, may not be feasible. Ambulatory children do not tolerate casts as well as pre-walkers do and will often break the cast. If a child with a congenital foot deformity is already walking, treatment will depend on the nature and severity of the foot deformity. For example, an ambulatory child with a calcaneovalgus deformity may benefit from a controlling foot orthosis. A child with a congenital talipes equinovarus who has been casted for several months and is now ambulating should be evaluated for surgical intervention. A 1-year-old ambulatory child with internal tibial torsion and metatarsus adductus might be a candidate for straight last shoe therapy during the day and a splint for night-time.

In general, medial and lateral femoral torsion problems do not respond well to splinting techniques. Tachjdian[33] states that Denis Browne splints are specifically contraindicated in cases of femoral torsional deformities 'as they will cause secondary deformities in the segments distal to the hip joint; namely, pes valgus, lateral torsion of the tibia, and genu valgum. The deforming influence and harmful effects of the Denis Browne splint in the treatment of femoral anteversion cannot be overemphasized.'

A splint attached to the feet will exert its influence on the midtarsal joint, subtalar joint, ankle joint and knee joint before it can exert an effect on the hip joint. Figure 15.7 shows a 13-year-old male with patellofemoral arthralgia. This patient was treated with twister cables for medial femoral torsion. Note that he still demonstrates a medial femoral position with a secondary genu valgum deformity and an excessive lateral tibiofibular rotation induced by the twister cable bracing.

With regard to soft tissue abnormalities at the level of the hip, debate exists regarding the benefit of splinting. It has been argued that night splints may exert an influence by altering the sleeping position and possibly causing a stretch on soft tissue contractures.[34] However, caution is

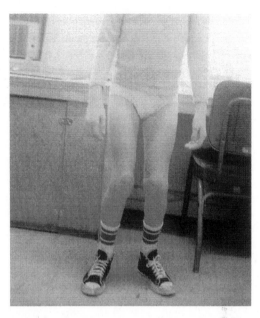

Figure 15.7   This boy was treated with twister cables. Note the lateral tibiofibular rotation, genu valgum and persistent medial femoral torsion.

advised because of the possible negative influence of these splints on the more distal joints. It is estimated that only 10% of the population will retain a medial femoral torsion into adult life.[35] Since femoral torsion generally will resolve by 8 years of age and because there is a potential risk of causing secondary deformities with splinting, the clinician may prefer to consider alternative treatments for the management of medial femoral torsion and rotation. Activities that are designed to encourage lateral femoral rotation such as roller-skating and ballet, when used as an adjunct to orthotic control for compensatory foot pronation, are viable alternative treatments. The use of orthoses with gait-plate extensions is another treatment alternative for select patients with a heel-to-toe propulsive gait and sufficient lateral femoral rotation.

Length of treatment

The length of treatment will depend on the severity of the deformity and the age of the patient. Generally, a child less than 18 months of age, who is in a very rapid growth period, will achieve faster correction than an older child whose growth rate is slower. In addition, a more severe deformity generally requires a longer period of treatment than a milder deformity. For example, when splinting is used as the initial form of treatment in cases of medial or lateral tibiofibular rotation, it may be expected that treatment may last for approximately 3 to 6 months.[2] Time is required to achieve correction as well as to maintain the correction once splinting is discontinued. Deformities may recur when insufficient maintenance time is prescribed for the patient.

When splinting is used as a secondary mode of treatment, e.g. after serial casting, a shorter period of splinting is usually required than on those occasions where splinting is used as the primary means of correction. Generally, a splint or brace is used for approximately twice as long as the period of time required for serial plaster casting. However, in cases of tibial torsion rather than position, a longer period of splinting is generally required. In this case, 12 to 18 months of night-time splinting may be required if splinting is chosen as the primary mode of treatment.[2] With regard to combined foot and leg deformities, the length of the splinting period should be based on the severity of the deformities and on whether or not serial plaster casting has been used as an initial treatment. If casting has been used initially, splinting should be used for at least twice as long as the casting period. In more severe deformities, especially those requiring surgery, the splinting period may be three times longer than the casting period or more. In more severe deformities such as clubfoot, an ankle–foot orthosis in conjunction with night-time splinting may be prescribed.

Degree of correction

Correction of rotational deformities should be applied gradually. In cases of medial tibiofibular rotation, it is usual to initially set the splint at a low degree of external rotation, e.g. 20–25°. The correction is increased 5° every 1 to 2 months to a maximum of 45°.[3] The clinician must be careful not to exceed the range of lateral femoral rotation since cases of avascular necrosis of the femoral head have been reported with excessive lateral

correction of the limbs.[36] When the deformity is unilateral, the night-time splint may be set asymmetrically. For example, when a 10-month-old child has a unilateral internal tibial torsion deformity of the left leg, the splint might be initially set at 25° external for the abnormal left leg and at 15° external for the normal right leg. Over the course of several months of treatment, the correction could be increased to 45° on the left side and maintained at 15° on the normal right side.

Treatment of excessive lateral femoral rotation and excessive lateral tibiofibular rotation is less common. Generally, clinicians are more aggressive in the treatment of excessive medial tibiofibular rotation and medial femoral rotation than in the treatment of excessive lateral femoral and tibial rotation. It must be remembered that in normal infants, lateral rotation averages 60° and medial rotation averages 0–20°. After 2 years of age, the amount of medial rotation begins to approximate the amount of lateral rotation.[3] If the position of a limb is truly excessively laterally rotated and splinting therapy is initiated, care must be taken to avoid aggressive limb adduction and possible hip subluxation. It is important to note that an infant's hip is most stable in abduction and lateral rotation. Medial rotation and adduction place the hip in a less stable position. Valmassy[2] recommends setting a night-time splint approximately 25–45° external to alter a lateral femoral or tibial segment. A negative or internal value has the greatest chance of causing a hip subluxation.[2]

SPLINTS AND BRACES

Denis Browne splint

The Denis Browne splint is essentially a bar with shoes attached to metal screw plates at both ends (Fig. 15.8). By rotating the shoes internally or externally, the clinician attempts to achieve rotation of the limbs. The bar exerts its greatest effect on rotational problems originating below the knee. Hutter & Scott[37] first described the use of the Denis Browne splint for the treatment of tibial torsion in 1949. Weseley et al[38] endorsed its use for select patients with internal tibial torsion in their study of 5000 patients over a 20-year

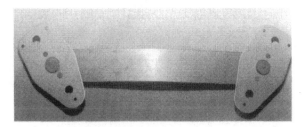

Figure 15.8 Denis Browne bar.

period. The splint is also used as a primary treatment for congenital foot problems but this remains controversial. Tachjdian, for example, does not recommend the Denis Browne bar or its variants in the treatment of metatarsus adductus because of its potential pronatory effect on the foot.[39] The creator of the splint, Sir Denis Browne, originally designed the splint in 1934 for the treatment of congenital talipes equinovarus. The original design consisted of two L-shaped pieces of aluminum attached to a horizontal connecting bar. Browne believed that the foot could be kept active while its shape was being corrected and that the position of one foot could control the other foot during treatment.

In the treatment of internal tibial torsion, rotational adjustment on the bar should be done gradually up to the limit of the patient's tolerance. Correction should not exceed 45°. The length of the bar should be equal to or slightly greater than the width of the pelvis. A standard measure is the distance from the anterior superior iliac spine to the anterior iliac spine plus 1 inch (2.54 cm). A splint that is too wide may result in a genu valgum deformity. A splint that is too narrow may result in hip instability.[3] The Denis Browne bar, as well as other nighttime splints, may cause possible subluxation of the joints of the foot. To reduce this potential problem, a bend of approximately 15° is placed in the middle of the bar. A varus wedge in the heel-seat of the shoe is also recommended.

Fillauer bar

The Fillauer bar (Markell Corp., Yonkers, N.Y.) is a variant of the Denis Browne bar. The main difference between these two splints is in the manner by which the shoes are attached to the splints. The Denis Browne bar uses a screw plate as the means of attachment; the Fillauer bar uses a clamp. This modification allows the patient to re-use the shoes after splinting is discontinued.

Ganley splint

The Ganley splint was developed by James Ganley in order to treat combination foot and leg disorders.[31] The splint consists of four footplates, two shank bars and one torque bar. The length of the torque bar is altered by sawing off segments of the bar (Fig. 15.9). When treating the foot deformities, the midsole sections of the shoes are removed to allow for proper placement on the four footplates; two plates for each shoe. Nails are then used to mount the shoes to the plates.

The Ganley splint represents the first splint design that attempts to alter the forefoot to rearfoot relationship. The split shoe and sectioned footplates allow for such an alteration in both the frontal and transverse planes. For example, in the case of a metatarsus adductus foot structure, the shoes are split at the Lisfranc's joint, and a 7–10° bend in the shoe shank bar is made. This results in an abductus position of the forefoot relative to the rearfoot. In addition, a varus wedge is placed in the heel-seat of the shoe in an attempt to counteract pronatory influences. In cases of calcaneovalgus, the shoes are split, the rearfoot is inverted, and the forefoot is plantarflexed and adducted relative to the rearfoot.

When patients present with medial or lateral tibiofibular rotation or torsion deformities, adjustments are made to the central torque bar.

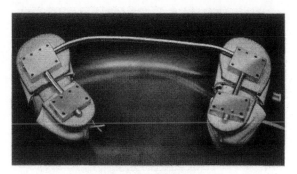

Figure 15.9 Ganley splint.

The torque bar is attached to the two rearfoot plates. When treating lateral tibiofibular rotations or torsion, the torque bar is attached to the two forefoot shoeplates. The angle of correction in the transverse plane is set with an Allen wrench and a varus bend is placed in the torque bar to minimize subluxatory influences on the foot. There is no need to split the shoes in patients who present with a tibial problem and no associated foot deformity.

Counter rotation system (CRS)

Because of its unique design, the CRS or counter rotation system is a very mobile and well-tolerated splint (Fig. 15.10). It comprises two moveable rectangular pattern crossbars and two adjustable footplates. The two crossbars are composed of a series of three hinged joints and eight circular rotation joints.[40] The footplates may be

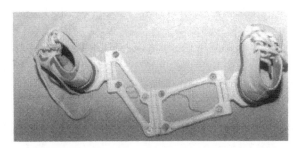

Figure 15.10   Counter rotation system splint.

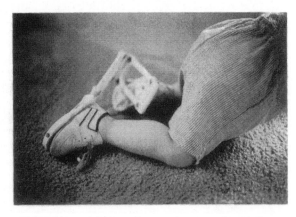

Figure 15.11   A child crawling wearing a counter rotation system splint.

adjusted to the desired medial or lateral position. Two straps are also placed in the rectangular crossbars system to limit medial and lateral rotation. While limiting rotation, the splint allows significant flexion and extension as well as adduction and abduction of the limbs. Therefore, the mobility of the CRS design affords a child a variety of movements. Whereas the Denis Browne bar allows only a 'bunny hop' type of crawling pattern, the CRS permits the alternate flexion and extension of the limbs required for normal reciprocal crawling (Fig. 15.11). Children who demonstrate poor tolerance to the Denis Browne bar at night may be switched to the CRS with the likelihood of increased tolerance.

Any type of shoe or sneaker may be applied to the CRS footplates. In place of screws, clamps or nails, the CRS system uses an adhesive for shoe attachment. The central two rectangular crossbars may be detached from the shoes while the shoes remain on the child's feet. This is accomplished by spring catches on the footplates that allow the parents to remove the central portion of the splint without having to remove the child's shoes. Parents appreciate this feature, especially when the splint must be removed for diaper changes or for other reasons. This feature allows for easier application of the splint, since the shoes may be applied to the child's feet first and then the central portion of the splint may be easily snapped onto the footplates.

The CRS is available in one size that automatically adapts to the width of the child's pelvis. No measurements are required. A bend in the middle portion of the splint to counteract pronatory influences is not necessary. The footplates move easily on the frontal plane, and can be inverted to adapt to the varus neutral rearfoot position of most younger pediatric patients. The footplate itself is also split to allow for altering the forefoot to rearfoot relationship on the frontal plane. However, it does not adjust for adductus or abductus deformities of the forefoot to the rearfoot. The CRS is sometimes referred to as the more humane treatment for rotational deformities, and generally the acceptance of this splint by the child and the child's parents is excellent.[36]

Wheaton brace

The Wheaton brace is a lightweight polypropylene device initially designed for the treatment of metatarsus adductus (Fig. 15.12). It may be used as a primary treatment modality or as a postcasting maintenance splint. It is also used for the treatment of talipes equinovarus. The age range for patients who might benefit from the Wheaton brace is from infancy to 4 years of age. Chong, a pediatric orthopedic surgeon, designed the splint following the well-established three-point fixation principle.[41] The first point of fixation is the rearfoot, which is securely retained to prevent subtalar joint pronation. The second point of fixation is the distal portion of the first metatarsal and the hallux. The third point of fixation provides the corrective force on the lateral border of the foot at the apex of the lateral convexity. A strap is used on the lateral side of the foot to provide the third point of fixation. The brace is available in a variety of sizes based on a child's foot length. The Wheaton brace is used for pre-ambulatory children with a metatarsus

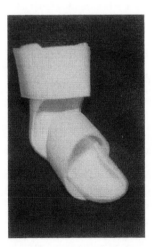

Figure 15.12 Wheaton brace.

adductus and is constructed so as to retain the foot in a plantarflexed position at the ankle. When the Wheaton brace is used for an ambulatory child or for a child with a talipes equinovarus deformity, the splint is constructed so as to retain the foot at a 90° ankle position.

Wheaton bracing system

The Wheaton bracing system consists of the Wheaton brace plus a polypropylene upper leg component. It is recommended in the treatment, or in the postcasting or postsurgical maintenance of metatarsus adductus, talipes equinovarus and internal or external tibial torsion. The upper leg segment maintains the knee in 90° of flexion and is designed to correct internal or external tibial torsion. This splint allows for the correction of unilateral deformities. It also isolates the tibial segment without twisting the femur or hip.[2]

SUMMARY

The management of foot and leg problems of the pediatric patient can be a challenging and rewarding experience. However, the clinician who works with this patient population must have a thorough knowledge of normal developmental trends and of the neurological and medical conditions that may manifest as orthopedic problems. Technology and an expanding knowledge of biomechanics have resulted in a variety of treatment modalities that must be customized to the individual needs of the patient. Parents with foot and postural problems will often ask their clinicians if there is anything that can be done so that their children will not suffer the same fate. The answer is that if we can provide children with early treatment, we have a better chance to reduce or eliminate foot and postural malalignment problems that are so common later in life.

REFERENCES

1. Altman MI. Sagittal angles of the talus and calcaneus in the developing foot. J Am Podiatr Assoc 1968;58(11):463–470.
2. Valmassy R. Lower extremity treatment modalities for the pediatric patient. In: Valmassy R, ed. Clinical biomechanics of the lower extremities. St Louis: Mosby; 1996;425–441.
3. Tax H. Podopediatrics. Baltimore: Williams and Wilkins; 1985.
4. Philps JW. The functional foot orthosis. Edinburgh: Churchill Livingstone; 1990.
5. Root M, Orien W, Weed J. Normal and abnormal function of the foot. Los Angeles: Clinical Biomechanics Corporation; 1977.
6. Bleck E. Metatarsus adductus: classification and relationship to outcomes of treatment. J Pediatr Orthop 1983;3:2–9.
7. Schuster RO. Children's foot survey (Harpursville). NY State J Podiatr 1956; July and October.
8. Valmassy R. Biomechanical evaluation of the child. In: Valmassy R, ed. Clinical biomechanics of the lower extremity. St Louis: Mosby; 1996;244–277.
9. Spencer A, Person V. Casting and orthotics for children. Clin Podiatr 1984;1(3):621–629.
10. Wernick J, Cusack J, Wernick E. Spontaneous rupture of the posterior tibial tendon: a conservative approach. Curr Podiatr Med 1989;June–July:11–15.
11. D'Amico J. Developmental flatfoot. Clin Podiatr 1984;1(3):535–546.
12. Berenter R, Kosai D. Various types of orthoses used in podiatry. Clin Podiatr Med Surg 1994;11(2):219–229.
13. Kirby K. Troubleshooting functional foot orthoses. In: Valmassy R, ed. Clinical biomechanics of the lower extremities. St Louis: Mosby; 1996;327–348.
14. Anthony R. The manufacture and use of the functional foot orthosis. Basel: Karger; 1991.
15. Kirby K. Foot and lower extremity biomechanics: a ten year collection of precision intricast newsletters. USA: Precision Intricast, Inc.; 1997.
16. Helfet A. A new way of treating flat feet in children. Lancet 1956;262–264.
17. Day NR. Foot owner's manual. Daly City California: PAS Publishing; 1983.
18. Bleck EE, Berzins BA. Conservative management of pes valgus with plantarflexed talus, flexible. Clin Orthop 1977;Jan–Feb(122):85–94.
19. Basta NW, Mital MA, Bonadio O, et al. A conservative study of the roles of shoes, arch supports, and navicular cookie in the management of symptomatic mobile flat feet in children. Int Orthop 1977;1:143–148.
20. Mereday C, Dolan C, Lusskin R. Evaluation of the University of California Biomechanics Laboratory shoe insert in 'flexible' pes planus. Clin Orthop 1972;Jan–Feb(82):45–58.
21. Kirby K, Green D. Evaluation and nonoperative management of pes valgus. In: Valentine S, ed. Foot and ankle disorders in children. New York: Churchill Livingstone; 1992;295–310.
22. Whitman R. The importance of positive support in the curative treatment of weak feet and a comparison of the means employed to assure it. Am J Orthop Surg 1913;11(215):598–601.
23. Starrett C. Historical review and current use of the Whitman/Robert's orthoses in biomechanical therapy. Clin Pod Med Surg 1994;11(2):231–239.
24. Schuster RO. A history of orthopedics in podiatry. J Am Podiatr Assoc 1974;64(5):332–334.
25. Root M. Development of the functional orthosis. Clin Podiatr Med Surg 1994;11(2):183–210.
26. Henderson WH, Campbell JW. UC-BL shoe insert casting and fabrication. Bull Prosthet Res 1969;Spring:215–235.
27. Schuster RO. A device to influence the angle of gait. J Am Podiatr Assoc 1967;57(6):269–270.
28. Jordan RP. Therapeutic considerations of the feet and lower extremities in the cerebral palsied child. Clin Podiatr 1984;1(3):547–561.
29. Blake R. Inverted functional orthosis. J Am Podiatr Med Assoc 1986;76(5):275–276.
30. Jay R, Schoenhaus H, Seymour C, et al. The dynamic stabilizing innersole system (DSIS): the management of hyperpronation in children. J Foot Ankle Surg 1995;34(2):124–131.
31. Lynch F. The Ganley splint: indications and usage. Clin Podiatr 1984;1(3):517–533.
32. McCrea J. Pediatric orthopedics of the lower extremity. An instructional handbook. Mount Kisco, NY: Futura; 1985;330.
33. Tachdjian M. Pediatric orthopedics, vol 2. Philadelphia: WB Saunders; 1972;1452.
34. Volpe R. Evaluation and management of intoe gait in the neurologically intact child. Clin Podiatr Med 1997;14(1):57–85.
35. Schuster RO. Intoe and outtoe and its implications. Arch Podiatr Med Foot Surg 1976;3 (4):25–31.
36. Valmassy R, Lipe L, Falconer R. Pediatric treatment modalities of the lower extremity. Am Podiatr Med Assoc 1988;78(2):69–80.
37. Hutter CG, Scott W. Tibial torsion. J Bone Joint Surg 1949;31A:511–518.
38. Wesele MS, Barenfeld PA, Eisenstein AL. Thoughts on in-toeing and out-toeing: twenty years experience with over five thousand cases and a review of the literature. Foot Ankle 1981;2:49–57.
39. Tachdjian M. The child's foot. Philadelphia: WB Saunders; 1985;297.
40. Milgrom C, Porat S. The pediatric counter rotation system (CRS) – an improvement on the Denis Browne splint for post club foot release splinting: a report of two cases. Orthop Rev 1987; XVI(10):762–763.
41. Chong A. A new device for the treatment of metatarsus adductus. Clin Invest Med 1986;9:3.

16

Sports injuries

Steven Subotnick

INTRODUCTION

With an ever-increasing number of children participating in organized activities, the number of adolescent podiatric sports medicine injuries will continue to rise. Both intrinsic and extrinsic factors play a role in a child's risk of musculoskeletal injury. Extrinsic factors include the environment, equipment and training program. Intrinsic factors include musculoskeletal strength, flexibility and bulk, associated disease states and the potential for growth.[1] This potential for growth, as well as the adolescent growth spurt, make adolescent anatomy and physiology uniquely different from that of adults.

Although the adolescent's musculoskeletal system has the ability to heal and remodel injury faster than adults, the open growth plates and rapid growth of musculotendinous units and the bones present a unique set of musculoskeletal injuries. While a young child and adolescent can completely remodel a poorly reduced long bone metaphyseal fracture in the plane of a joint, severe growth plate injuries in a young child or adolescent can result in complete cessation of growth and major deformity and disability.

When adolescents go through a growth spurt, it is normal for the bones to grow longer first which will result in a relative tightness of the muscles and tendons. Such tightness may produce functional limitations of motion across certain joints. In the case of a functional equinus, abnormal forces are produced that cause excessive and/or premature pronation of the foot leading to a myriad of overuse injuries. In addition, the rapid growth period can produce 'growing pains' in the thigh or leg. Furthermore, soft tissue musculotendinous tightness which accompanies these growth spurts may be responsible for excessive pressures on the anchoring of tendons into the apophyseal growth plates causing apophysitis which becomes more pronounced during sports.

Sports-related injuries can broadly be classified into two categories:

1. high-energy macrotrauma
2. repetitive microtrauma.

Macrotrauma includes acute fractures, dislocations, sprains and ligament tears. Repetitive microtrauma is responsible for such injuries as stress fractures and apophysitis. Both rapid growth and relative inflexibility may predispose the adolescent athlete to overuse injuries.[1]

An understanding of the unique anatomy and physiology of the adolescent athlete as well as the extrinsic factors contributing to the potential for musculoskeletal injury will assist in rapid diagnosis and appropriate treatment of sports injuries of the lower extremity in children. The aim is to use this knowledge to prevent injury. This chapter reviews the diagnosis and treatment of some of the common adolescent sport injuries of the lower extremity.

INJURIES TO THE PELVIS AND HIP

The podiatric sports medicine specialist must be aware of the various pathologies and injuries to the hip and pelvis which may present in the adolescent patient. These injuries may be secondary to malposition or to excessive abnormal biomechanical forces beginning at the feet, and therefore they respond well to a podiatric approach. On the other hand, there may be primary pathology within the hip or pelvis, which will necessitate referral to an orthopedic specialist.

Acute pelvis and hip fractures are rare in children. When these fractures occur, they usually result from high-energy trauma. The pediatric pelvis is more elastic and flexible than the adult pelvis, and therefore it can tolerate greater defor-

mation prior to acute fracture. Thus, pelvis fractures in children can be associated with significant injuries to the viscera, major blood vessels and nerves. Rapid evaluation and treatment may decrease the high rate of associated morbidity and mortality.[2]

As mentioned earlier, hip fractures are rare in children, and comprise less than 1% of all frac-

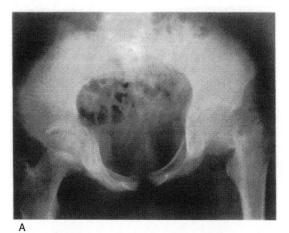

A

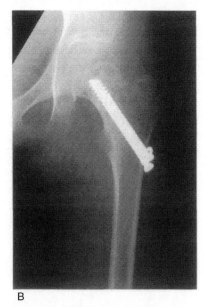

B

Figure 16.1 (A) Anteroposterior view of the pelvis demonstrating displaced femoral neck fracture in a 10-year-old girl, left side of pelvis (reproduced from Widmann & Micheli[6]). (B) Reduced fracture.

tures. Such fractures are also often associated with other injuries but may require urgent treatment. Rapid evaluation, diagnosis and treatment of acute physeal fractures as well as femoral neck fractures will decrease the incidence of late complications such as avascular necrosis, growth arrest, non-union and progressive deformity and degenerative changes (Fig. 16.1A, B).

Avulsion fractures of the pelvis and hip

Avulsion fractures of the pelvis and proximal femur result from vigorous muscle contractions or stretch across an open apophysis. Such injuries include avulsion of:

— the hamstring from the ischial tuberosity
— the iliopsoas from the lesser trochanter
— the erector femoris from the anterior inferior iliac spine
— the sartorius from the anterior superior iliac spine
— the abdominal muscles from the iliac crest.

Avulsion fractures typically occur in children between the ages of 13 and 17 years, after the appearance, but prior to the fusion, of the secondary center of ossification.[3] This developmental stage corresponds to a period of rapid growth inflexibility.[1] Although historically boys

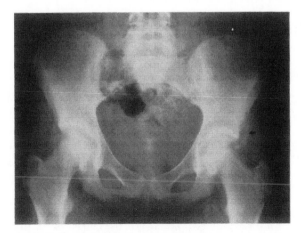

Figure 16.2 Displaced anterior inferior iliac spine fracture (reproduced from Widmann & Micheli[6]).

have been affected far more often than girls, reports suggest that the incidence of avulsion fractures is increasing significantly in girls[4] (Fig. 16.2).

Three stages of apophyseal avulsion have been noted. The first stage consists of non-displaced apophyseal injuries termed apophyseolyses. The second stage consists of acute avulsion fractures, and the third stage is of chronic non-union.[5] Patients with non-displaced apophyseal injuries respond well to rest and partial weight-bearing. Most displaced avulsion fractures with non-union are asymptomatic. However, certain cases will continue to cause pain with activity or with sitting and these may require excision.

Most authors concur that the conservative non-operative treatment with rest, partial weight-bearing and appropriate positioning of the extremity in order to minimize muscle stretch is indicated in the treatment of acute avulsion fractures.

Iliac crest apophysitis

Iliac crest apophysitis is an unusual traction apophysitis that originally was described in adolescent distance runners between the ages of 14 and 17 years.[6] Patients with iliac crest apophysitis have been involved in track-running programs. They present with gradual onset of localized tenderness to palpation and localized pain with resisted abduction of the hip. Both anterior and posterior iliac crest apophysitis syndromes have been described. Anterior iliac crest apophysitis has been attributed to overpull of the tensor fascia lata, the gluteus medius and the oblique abdominal muscles whereas posterior iliac crest apophysitis has been attributed to overpull of the latissimus dorsi or of gluteus maximus. Most patients respond well to 3 to 4 weeks of rest with complete resolution of symptoms and resumption of training.

Hip dislocation

Although hip dislocations are rare in children and adolescents, when this injury occurs it is commonly caused by mild to moderate trauma during athletic activities. Hip dislocation occurs in all age groups with an average between 7 and 10 years. Most dislocations are posterior, and physical examination is quite helpful in differentiating between anterior and posterior displacement. The posteriorly dislocated hip will be shortened, flexed, adducted and internally rotated whereas the anteriorly dislocated hip will be abducted, flexed and externally rotated. Complete neurological examination is mandatory prior to reduction since sciatic nerve injury may occur in association with hip dislocation. In older children, hip dislocation is associated with more severe trauma and associated other injuries. In addition, high-energy trauma associated with adolescent sports is correlated with late degenerative changes and radiographic abnormalities. Complications include soft tissue interposition, nerve injury, avascular necrosis, premature closure of the triradiate cartilage, recurrent dislocation and osteoarthritis. When the podiatrist has a high index of suspicion of any type of injury of the hip or pelvis, immediate referral to an orthopedist or emergency room is indicated.[7]

Slipped capital femoral epiphysis and Perthes' disease

Although slipped capital femoral epiphysis and Perthes' disease are not sports injuries, the sports medicine specialist dealing with adolescent patients must consider both of these conditions in a differential diagnosis in any skeletally immature patient with hip or knee pain and limp.

Slipped capital femoral epiphysis is a very common problem in adolescents between 11 and 15 years and it affects between 0.7 and 3.4 children per 100 000.[8] The disorder consists of chronic or acute disruption of the proximal femoral growth plate with a clinical presentation of pain, limp and limited internal hip rotation. Standard radiographs, i.e. anterior posterior pelvis including both hips and a frog lateral of both hips, are indicated. Both hips are included on initial and subsequent radiographs because of the high incidence of bilateral disease, which approaches 40%. The hips are classified as stable

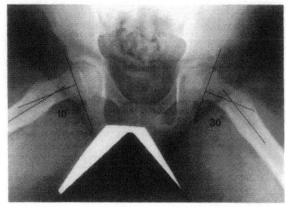

(A)

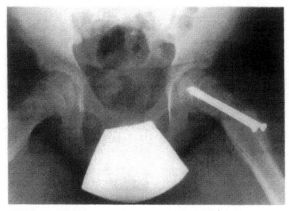

(B)

Figure 16.3 (A) Frog view of slipped femoral epiphysis with 30° slip angle (reproduced from Widmann & Micheli[6]). (B) Stabilization with a percutaneous screw.

or unstable based on the patient's ability to ambulate (Fig. 16.3A, B).

Standard treatment of both groups consists of single pin fixation, undertaken as expeditiously as possible. The major complication of slipped capital femoral epiphysis is avascular necrosis and chondrolysis. Both avascular necrosis and chondrolysis are associated with increasing severity of the slip and with reduction of the slip.

Perthes' disease is a poorly understood pathological process of avascular necrosis of the proximal femoral epiphysis. The diagnosis of Perthes' disease must be considered in the management of children with limp and restricted hip range of motion between the ages of 3 and 12 years and most commonly between the ages of 5 and 7 years. The disease affects boys approximately three times more frequently than girls. The etiology is unknown but the pathophysiology is consistent with avascular necrosis. Clinical examination will demonstrate restricted internal rotation and abduction of the hip, Trendelenburg gait and hip pain. In addition, there will be referred thigh or knee pain. The history is consistent with activity-related symptoms.[8] Goals of treatment include relief of symptoms, containment of the femoral head and restoration of range of motion. Return to athletic activities is restricted during the active phase of Perthes' disease until the patient is well into the healing phase in order to protect the revascularized epiphysis.

Quadriceps contusions and myositis ossificans

Muscle contusions are frequent injuries in the pediatric athlete, comprising up to 38% of injuries in large studies of pediatric athletes.[9] Although quadriceps contusion occurs in many athletic activities, the greatest number occurred as a result of football tackle injuries in Jackson & Feagin's landmark study.[10]

Myositis ossificans is an unusual complication of quadriceps contusion in young athletes sustaining moderate and severe injuries. Conservative management is the mainstay of treatment in myositis ossificans. Protection of the patient from re-injury is essential in preventing myositis. Most patients achieve normal function despite the appearance of heterotopic bone. Persistent symptoms after at least 1 year of observation and radiographic maturation of the lesion may warrant surgical excision in a small percentage of patients.[8]

KNEE INJURIES

Anterior knee pain in the child and adolescent may be difficult to classify based on physical examination. A system of classification based on etiology including primary trauma, malalignment or a combination of both appears to be a very reasonable approach.

Patellofemoral stress syndrome

The patellofemoral stress syndrome is an overuse injury of the extensor mechanism that results from repetitive microtrauma in susceptible individuals during the period of most active growth.[1] The syndrome results from a complex interplay of mild soft tissue imbalance without overt bony malalignment. With rapid growth, the tight lateral structures including the fascia lata and vastus lateralis exert lateral forces on the patella that are countered by the relatively weak vastus medialis. Patients typically present with pain as a result of activity, difficulty with prolonged sitting and a history of knee giveaway. Acute symptoms may follow abrupt increases in training programs. Physical examination reveals lateral patellar tightness without overt bony malalignment.

Initial treatment of patellofemoral stress syndrome in a young athlete consists of training modification, strengthening of the medial quadriceps and stretching of the fasciae lata and hamstrings.[1] Excessive foot pronation and secondary functional knee valgus with lateral patella maltracking and patellofemoral stress syndrome should be treated with biodynamic functional foot orthotics. Patients who fail with conservative treatment may benefit from a lateral retinacular release.

Subotnick has described the functional varus in running which predisposes to rapid excessive pronation and secondary valgus of the knee with lateral maltracking of the patella as a cause of patellofemoral stress syndrome. Likewise, he has further described the miserable malalignment syndrome, which typically presents with ligamentous laxity, anteversion in the hips, valgus in the knees and externally rotated, pronated feet. This further leads to a functional increase in the Q angle of the knee predisposing to lateral maltracking of patellofemoral stress syndrome[10] (Fig. 16.4A, B).

Osgood–Schlatter disease

Osgood–Schlatter disease and Sinding–Larsen–Johansson disease are two common overuse injuries to the extensor mechanism of the knee. Osgood–Schlatter disease results from repetitive

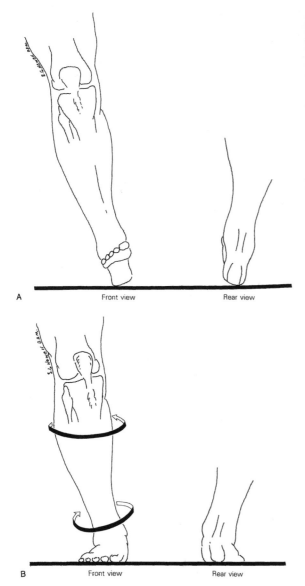

A   Front view   Rear view

B   Front view   Rear view

Figure 16.4 (A) Functional varus in running (reproduced from Subotnick SI, ed. Sports medicine of the lower extremity. 2nd ed. New York: Churchill Livingstone; 1999). (B) Pronation secondary to functional varus.

microtrauma at the level of the skeletally immature tibial tubercle. It occurs most commonly in boys and more commonly in athletes participating in sports involving kicking, jumping and squatting. Patients typically present with pain to palpation over the tibial tubercle with associated swelling and an exacerbation of symp-

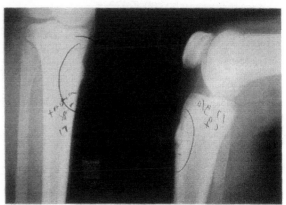

Figure 16.5 Osgood-Schlatter disease in a 17-year-old soccer player.

toms with resisted extension of the knee. Plain radiographs will demonstrate fragmentation of the tibial tubercle, as well as patella alta.

Osgood–Schlatter disease is related to the start of a second growth spurt in adolescence. Clinically, symptoms usually appear between 4 and 6 months after peak growth velocity.[8]

Conservative treatment of Osgood–Schlatter disease consists of pain relief with anti-inflammatory medication and physical therapy modalities such as quadriceps stretching and strengthening programs as required (see pp **290–291**). Brief periods of immobilization may be neces-sary in rare acute cases. Approximately 12% of patients will develop a distinct symptomatic mobile ossicle. This group of children will fail to respond to conservative treatment and will require early surgical intervention to excise the ossicle (Fig. 16.5).

Sinding–Larsen–Johansson disease

Sinding–Larsen–Johansson disease is a closely related overuse injury of the extensor mechanism resulting from a traction tendonitis of the proximal attachment of the patella tendon to the inferior pole of the patella. This syndrome represents a subset of broader classification of patients with 'jumper's knee' which includes adults who may or may not have distinct radiographic findings. Boys are affected more often than girls and the typical age group is between 10 and 13 years.

Clinical presentation is quite similar to Osgood–Schlatter disease with pain and swelling over the inferior pole of the patella and pain with resisted knee extension. Radiographs demonstrate calcification of the inferior pole of the patella that may coalesce over time and fuse to the patella or form a separate ossicle. Most patients respond well to conservative treatment as described earlier for Osgood–Schlatter disease, and should achieve full return to function between 3 and 13 months from the initial presentation. These uniformly excellent results in children contrast sharply with results of both conservative treatment and surgery in the older athletic population with jumper's knee.

Use of orthotics

Subotnick[12] has described the utilization of orthotics in the treatment of Osgood–Schlatter disease as well as in Sinding–Larsen–Johansson disease when biomechanical abnormalities of the foot are associated with maltracking of the patella and excessive stress on the extensor mechanism of the knee. Patients with Osgood–Schlatter disease have had relatively good results when abnormal pronation of the foot is controlled with orthotic devices. Similarly, patients with a high degree of functional valgus in the knee associated with foot pronation have also done well with orthotics. Patients involved in running sports, who have a valgus deviation of the knee and excessive pronation of the foot and who suffer pain at the inferior pole of the patella, may also respond well to orthotic management. However, those patients involved with jumping sports tend to fare less favorably with orthotic foot control.

Internal derangement of the knee

Adolescent patients may present to a podiatrist with internal derangement of the knee. This can be caused by such conditions as plica, meniscal tears and, in cases of severe injury, cruciate ligament damage. In addition, there may be damage to the medial collateral ligament of the knee with traumatic injury. These injuries require referral to an orthopedist.

FOOT AND ANKLE INJURIES

Adolescents are subject to a variety of acute and overuse injuries to the foot and ankle. Acute injuries include sprains and dislocations. Anatomical considerations explain the significance of higher incidents of physeal ankle fractures compared to sprains in skeletally immature individuals. The ligaments insert below the physes, and the open physes are weaker than the adjacent bone or ligaments. Physeal fractures of the ankle in children are classified both by the mechanism of injury and by the Salter–Harris system. Several fracture types deserve special attention because of the high incidence of associated complications including growth arrest with shortening of the extremity and angular deformity as well as joint incongruity. These high-risk fractures include Salter–Harris type 3 and 4 fractures as well as juvenile Tillaux fractures, triplane fractures and comminuted epiphyseal fractures. In a retrospective review of these high-risk fractures, the overall complication rate was 32%[11] (Fig. 16.6A, B).

Other less common injuries include sprains and osteochondral lesions. Overuse injuries include Sever's apophysitis, plantar fasciitis and stress fractures.

Sever's disease

Sever's disease describes apophysitis in the growth plate of the heel (Fig. 16.7A–C). This typically occurs in adolescent children in either the posterior or plantar portion of the calcaneal apophysis. Sever's disease is often secondary to running on hard surfaces and may occur at the beginning of the soccer season. Typically, the patients are just starting a rapid growth period and have tightness of the posterior structures of the legs. This tightness puts excessive pull on the calf muscles and on the Achilles tendon where it inserts into the posterior aspect of the calcaneus. This force is countered by a reciprocal pulling of the intrinsic foot muscles and of the plantar fascia. Subsequently, an excessive tension is created on the calcaneal apophysis resulting in pain and inflammation on the posterior and/or

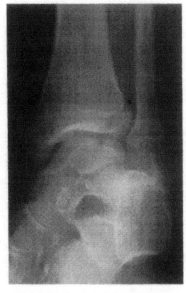

(A)

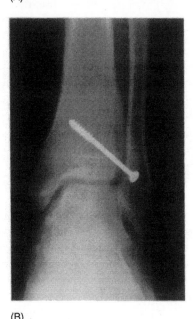

(B)

Figure 16.6 (A) Mortice view of ankle with Tillaux fracture. Juvenile Tillaux fracture with incongruity is seen best on mortice view (reproduced from Widmann & Micheli[6]).
(B) Open, reduced and fixated Tillaux fracture (reproduced from Widmann & Micheli[6]).

plantar aspects of the calcaneus. In addition, posterior calcaneal apophysitis may be complicated by a stiff, unyielding counter of the shoe rubbing

on the posterior aspect of the heel. Likewise, a child's shoe with too thick a midsole may predispose the child to plantar and/or posterior apophysitis.

Treatment consists of orthotic foot control with ⅛ inch to ¼ inch heel lift (Fig. 16.8). Stretching exercises are prescribed. Patients may need some form of natural or prescribed anti-inflammatory medication for short periods of time. Homeopathic medications have been described by Subotnick in treatment of various foot and leg problems in children.[12]

Navicular apophysitis

Navicular apophysitis (Kohler's disease) is an avascular necrosis of the navicular and may be a serious problem. It must be differentiated from stress fracture of the navicular, which is often difficult to diagnose without a computed tomographic scan of the foot. Stress fracture of the navicular if untreated may result in a serious problem with malunion requiring later bone grafts and surgery. Kohler's disease usually occurs in young children aged between 6 and 12 years. A cast and crutches are often necessary to prevent further stress to the area. Orthopedic abnormalities or imbalances should be corrected with appropriate orthotic foot control during the rehabilitative phase.

Os navicularis syndrome

Adolescents may present with complaints of avulsion fracture or hypermobility of the os navicularis, a secondary center of ossification of the navicular bone (os navicularis syndrome) (Fig. 16.9A, B) Likewise, such children may present with other overuse symptoms, e.g. medial shin splints, secondary to the excessive pronation of the foot. This occurs because the posterior tibial tendon may insert into the os navicularis and not into the main body of the navicular itself. Therefore, the muscle is unable to fully exert its primary force upon that bone. As a result, there is inadequate stabilization of the foot by the posterior tibial muscle, which predisposes to hypermobility and excessive pronation. In addition,

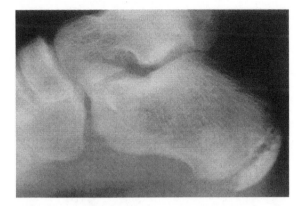

(A)

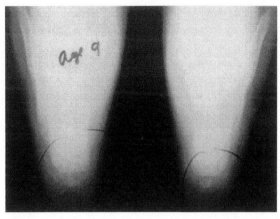

(B)

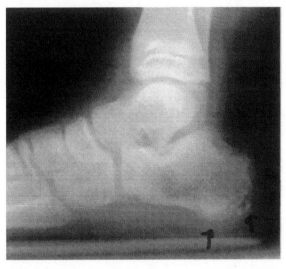

(C)

Figure 16.7 (A) Sever's disease in an 11-year-old female soccer player. The lateral calcaneal view demonstrates posterior and plantar apophysitis from shoe counter pressure and traction between plantar intrinsics and plantar fascia and the counter forces of the Achilles and triceps surae. (B) Calcaneal axis view demonstrates posterior apophysitis in a 9-year-old male soccer player. (C) Lateral calcaneal view in the same 9-year-old player as (B), demonstrating plantar and posterior apophysitis.

there will be excessive internal rotation of the leg and an excessive oblique pull of the muscles of the leg upon the tibia predisposing to shin splint syndrome. This usually occurs in the medial compartment of the leg and involves the posterior tibial muscle[13] (Fig. 16.10A, B).

Os navicularis syndrome is initially treated with orthotics with a wide medial flange and a deep heel-cup with adequate rearfoot control (Fig. 16.11A–C). In the event of persistent symptoms, a Kidner surgical procedure will be necessary in order to excise the os navicularis and to reposition the posterior tibial tendon in a more plantarwards direction. With excessive hypermobility of the foot, a Kidner–Young modification of the Pissini procedure is recommended in which case the posterior tibial tendon is reinforced by tethering it to the anterior tibial tendon.[14]

Stress fractures

In the skeletally immature athlete, stress fractures are a common type of overuse injury.

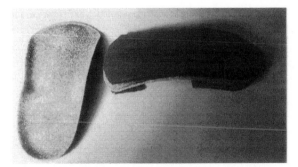

Figure 16.8 Birkenstock 'generic' orthotics with Spenco cover and posting for 'in office' treatment of calcaneal apophysitis and other foot-related injuries.

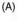

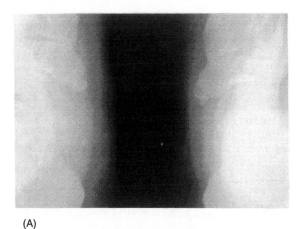

(A)

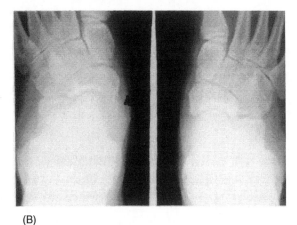

(B)

Figure 16.9 (A) Anteroposterior view of feet, demonstrating avulsion of secondary center of ossification of the os navicularis in a teenage female hurdler. She experienced pain at the fibrous union when running and jumping. (B) Os tibialis externum presenting with posterior tibial insertional tendonitis and pain over the ossicle which was worse when jumping and kicking while playing soccer.

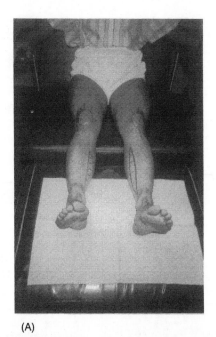

(A)

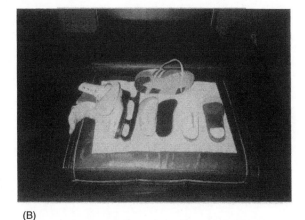

(B)

Figure 16.10 (A) Medial shin syndrome and patellofemoral compression syndrome in a 15-year-old female figure-skater and runner with hypermobile pronated feet, valgus knees and anteversion at the hips – the so-called 'miserable malalignment syndrome'. (B) Custom sport orthotic, and 'in-office' soft support system with medial wedge for ice-skate boots for the same patient.

Almost every bone in the lower extremity and pelvis is susceptible to stress fractures. The mechanism of injury is thought to be by excessive, repetitive forces acting across the bone. An association between certain sports and specific types of stress fractures has been demonstrated.[15] The difficult clinical presentation includes history of gradual onset of localized pain that is relieved by rest. Patients may also have localized tenderness and swelling. Continued activity may increase the severity of the pain and, in unfor-

tunate circumstances, the affected bone may go on to complete fracture.

In the foot, the most serious stress fracture is that of the tarsal navicular. The majority of these stress fractures are in the sagittal plane. They occur mainly in track and field athletes. Rapid

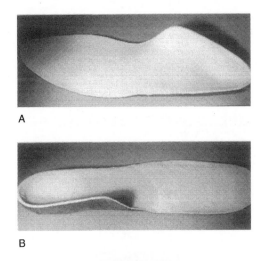

A

B

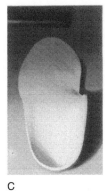

C

Figure 16.11 Orthosis with medial flange and deep heel-cup for os navicularis syndrome control.

forceful pronation with plantar flexion is associated with the injury.

Athletes with a history of vague, activity-related midfoot pain with associated tenderness over the proximal dorsal third of the navicular in the central portions – the so-called 'N' – should be suspected of having a navicular stress fracture. Plain radiographs frequently fail to demonstrate the fracture, thus radionuclide scanning is the investigation of choice to detect navicular stress injury. A computed tomographic scan should be performed in order to confirm the presence of the fracture.

The continuum of bony stress progresses from silent stress reaction to stress reaction and stress fracture. Computed tomography or X-ray changes are present as pain increases and the stress reaction of bone is converting to stress fracture. This may be 6 to 8 weeks after the first symptom occurs. At onset, there is frequently a history of increased intensity of activity or of changed activity. A minimum 6 weeks of strict, non-weightbearing, cast immobilization is the treatment of choice. Following removal of the cast, a further 6 weeks of physical therapy with gradual return to activity are required. Aquatic water therapy and water aerobic work out are beneficial. Surgery for non-union or delayed union is rarely required if initial treatment is appropriate. Surgical methods include internal fixation with curettage and grafting. The fracture is usually difficult to see at operation since the dorsum of the navicular is rarely disrupted. Therefore, the talonavicular joint must be separated by traction to pinpoint the fracture. Postoperative treatment requires 6 weeks of non-weightbearing cast immobilization. Historically, there has been a high incidence of delayed and non-union injuries.

Delayed union is often in the central portion of the middle third of the navicular However, recovery may be aided by the use of an external bone stimulator. A high index of stress reaction of bone or frank stress fracture in the dorsum of the navicular adjacent to the talonavicular joint in the middle third should lead the clinician to appropriate diagnostic and therapeutic intervention in order to prevent the complications of malunion. Decreased activity alone may alleviate the symptoms but will not allow osteoblastic activity or the fracture site to be bridged. Strict non-weightbearing for 6 weeks will give excellent results.[16]

Bone scans simplify early diagnosis of any suspected fracture. Such scans often reveal multiple foci of increased uptake correlating with abnormal stress. Plain radiographs will subsequently demonstrate periosteal reaction and may demonstrate complete fractures if progression occurs. The major diagnostic dilemma is in differentiating stress fractures from osteomyelitis and osteogenic sarcoma. The history will provide the most valuable information in this regard.

Initial management of stress fractures includes activity modification, non-weightbearing and, at times, cast treatment. Tibial diaphyseal stress fractures exhibit a unique tendency to proceed to non-union and complete fracture despite conservative treatment. Surgical excision and bone grafting of the tibial diaphysis have been successful in treating this condition.

Stress fractures of the leg often occur as a late result of continued overuse and inadequate treatment of stress reaction of bone or shin splint syndrome of the legs. This may take place in any of the four compartments of the legs but more commonly takes place in the posterior medial, or anterior extensor compartment of the legs. Treatment consists of activity modification, physical therapy and orthotic foot control when imbalances are present.[17]

COMPLEMENTARY MEDICAL TREATMENT

In adolescent podiatric sports medicine, any of the injuries may be treated with natural complementary medical modalities along with standard orthodox medical care.[18]

REFERENCES

1. Micheli LJ. Overuse injuries in children's sports: the growth factor. Orthop Clin North Am 1983;14:337–360.
2. Garvin KL, McCarthy RE, Barnes CL, et al. Pediatric pelvic ring fractures. J Pediatr Orthop 1990;10:577–582.
3. Fernbach SK, Wilkinson RH. Avulsion injuries of the pelvis and proximal femur. Am J Radiol 1981;137:581.
4. Sundar M, Carty H. Avulsion fractures of the pelvis in children: a report of 32 fractures and their outcome. Skeletal Radiol 1994;23:85–90.
5. Martin TA, Pipkin G. Treatment of avulsion of the ischial tuberosity. Clin Orthop 1957;10:108.
6. Fox IM. Iliac apophysitis in teenage distance runners. J Am Podiatr Med Assoc 1986;76:294–296.
7. Widman RF, Micheli LJ. Lower extremity sports injuries in children. In: Subotnick SI, ed. Sports medicine of the lower extremity. 2nd ed. New York: Churchill Livingstone; 1999;21–37.
8. Stanitski CL. Acute slipped capital femoral epiphysis: treatment alternatives. J. Am Acad Orthop Surg 1994;2:96–106.
9. Watson AW. Sports injuries during one academic year in 6799 Irish school children. Am J Sports Med 1984;12:65–71.
10. Jackson DW, Feagin JA. Quadriceps contusions in young athletes. J Bone Joint Surg Am 1973;55:95–105.
11. Speigel PG, Cooperman DR, Laros GS. Epiphyseal fractures of the distal ends of the tibia and fibula. J Bone Joint Surg Am 1987;60:1046–1050.
12. Subotnick SI. Sports injuries in childhood and adolescence. In: Subotnick SI, ed. Sports and exercise injuries: conventional, homeopathic and alternative treatments. Berkeley, CA: North Atlantic Books;1991;351–360.
13. Subotnick SI. Lower leg injuries. In: Subotnick SI, ed. Sports and exercise injuries: conventional, homeopathic and alternative treatments. Berkeley, CA: North Atlantic Books; 1991;213–235.
14. Volger HW, Subotnick SI. Surgical intervention in the foot and ankle. In: Subotnick SI, ed. Sports medicine of the lower extremity. 2nd ed. New York: Churchill Livingstone; 1999;505–605.
15. Subotnick SI. Podiatric considerations of specific sports (section 5). In: Subotnick SI, ed. Sports medicine of the lower extremity. 2nd ed. New York: Churchill Livingstone; 1999:645–739.
16. Khan KM, Brukner PD, Kearney C, et al. Tarsal navicular stress fracture in athletes. Sports Med 1994;17(1):65–76.
17. Bouche R. Exercise-induced leg pain. In: Subotnick SI, ed. Sports medicine of the lower extremity. 2nd ed. New York: Churchill Livingstone; 1999;277–298.
18. Subotnick SI. Complementary approaches. In: Subotnick SI, ed. Sports medicine of the lower extremity. 2nd ed. New York: Churchill Livingstone; 1999;747–765.

Appendices

Appendix I

Special investigations

Laboratory investigations may be required to make or to confirm a clinical diagnosis. Most hematological, bacteriological or radiological procedures are not unique to dermatology and will not be discussed. However, there are some which require an extra knowledge in order to obtain valid results.

1. MYCOLOGY SPECIMENS

An active area of the lesion, usually the outer border, should be selected. If the lesion shows signs of being contaminated with ointments it should first be cleaned using surgical spirit. Scrapings should be taken using a clean scalpel blade held at right angles to the surface. Care should be taken not to draw the blade longitudinally or a cut will ensure. A blade with a round end, e.g. a no. 15, helps to avoid the point causing damage. The scrapings should be collected in folded paper and should not be put in universal containers as the static makes it very difficult for the laboratory to remove them adequately. Black paper makes it easier to find the small scrapings. Commercial packs are available, although expensive, e.g. Dermapack.

Adhesive tape, e.g. Sellotape, may be used and it is particularly useful in awkward sites or when the patient will not stay sufficiently still to allow a blade to be used safely. The specimen may be posted to the laboratory taped to a slide or doubled back on itself, although the latter is more difficult to handle.

Swabs have little place in the diagnosis of dermatophytes although they can be used for moist areas where *Candida* is suspected. More rapid transport is required for these.

Nail samples may be obtained by scalpel blade scrapings from under the nail or from the dorsum, depending upon the type. A chiropody drill with vacuum extraction may be used. Nail clippings may also be sent. As proximal a specimen as possible should be obtained.

All specimens may be sent to the laboratory by ordinary post. Apart from the swab, they will not deteriorate within this time scale. The laboratory will normally carry out a direct examination and will try to culture a specimen within 3 to 4 weeks.

The practitioner can examine scrapings under a microscope on site. The specimen is placed upon an ordinary microscope slide and a drop or two of potassium hydroxide 10–30% added. A cover slip is added. Ideally the preparation should be left for approximately 20 minutes (much longer for nails) but warming the slide, although not boiling the potash, may speed it up. Slight pressure on the cover slip helps to squash out the preparation. In the optimum the keratin cells are single thickness and any hyphae may be seen traversing their boundaries. Spores may also be seen. The same technique may be used for other diseases, e.g. scabies, molluscum contagiosum.

Certain forms of fungi can be diagnosed using a Wood's light, which is an ultraviolet light from which most of the visible rays are removed by filters. Cheap hand-held battery types are available and have largely replaced the cumbersome machines of the past. The Wood's light's main use is in scalp ringworm which fluoresces when the light is shone upon it in a dark room. Care must be taken not to confuse the non-specific fluorescence of ointments.

2. BIOPSY

A skin biopsy is a common procedure and is not usually technically difficult. However, unless one or two points are remembered, the specimen may well be useless for diagnosis. There are two main types: (i) an elliptical biopsy and (ii) a punch biopsy. The elliptical biopsy traverses the margin of the skin lesion, thus allowing the pathologist to look at some normal skin and then progress to the abnormal skin. This zone may be vitally important in diagnosis and is, therefore, usually the preferred option. It must be remembered that a skin biopsy is an elective procedure and the aim is to obtain a specimen without causing any disfigurement. Therefore, it should be carried out in an aseptic manner in an appropriate area. The operator should scrub up, mask and gown, and wear sterile gloves. A suitable lesion should be chosen and a suitable line of excision should be planned, weighing up the importance of the specimen with the ultimate cosmetic result. Where possible, the long axis of the excision should be parallel to the line of one of the skin markings. Langer's lines were used in the past but it is perhaps better simply to try pinching the skin between the forefinger and thumb and see in which direction there is most 'material'. The area should be cleansed and the local anesthetic administered; usually 1% lidocaine is satisfactory. In very vascular areas lidocaine with epinephrine may be used but this should be avoided around the digits. In order to obtain satisfactory analgesia in thickened areas, e.g.

the palm or the sole, the addition of some hyaluronidase may help spreading and thus speed up the anesthetic effect.

Once the area is anesthetized, the ellipse should be cut out. It is best to use a D-shaped blade such as a no. 15. This allows the instrument to be held in a more pencil-like position and a more vertical cut through the skin will be obtained. It is best to try to make the cut in one firm movement in order to avoid ragged ends. The incision should then be extended to an adequate depth. The specimen of skin should not be removed with forceps as this procedure will traumatize cells and make them look abnormal and the pathologist may therefore be unable to determine whether there are malignant cells or not. A skin hook should be used to gently tease the ellipse out which is then freed from its base. The next vitally important point is for the specimen to be placed on a small square of blotting paper. This will stop it from twisting in the formalin and will allow the pathologist to view the correct orientation of all the layers of the epidermis and also their relation to the dermis. Once again, this is of the utmost importance in making the diagnosis.

Thereafter, the wound should be sutured depending upon the size of the area; deep vessels may require to be tied off and subcutaneous stitches may be required. The skin is then stitched in the conventional manner.

A quicker method of skin biopsy is to use a punch. Disposable skin biopsy punches are available in sizes varying from 2 to 6 mm. The punch is really a circular blade, rather like an apple corer. It is more difficult to get an adequate biopsy of a transitional zone and the orientation of the subsequent specimen can be much more difficult. However, they are very useful in biopsying a solid tumor or a large plaque. Once again, care should be taken with asepsis. Analgesia is obtained as before and the punch is rotated with some firm pressure until it has reached full depth. The small core specimen should again be treated gently and should be removed by means of a skin hook. When this is not available, gently teasing it out with a needle may be successful and then cutting the base. Under no circumstances should forceps be used or crush artefacts may be caused. Again, the specimen should be placed upon blotting paper and, after a few minutes, should be transferred to the formalin fixative. It is important that the specimen is on the blotting paper when it enters the formalin. If it subsequently floats off this does not matter. With the 2 mm punch, a stitch may not be necessary, although with the larger punches one or two stitches are usually required.

3. IMMUNOFLUORESCENCE

Immunofluorescence is used for detecting the location and the extent of substances in the skin, e.g. antibodies and antigens. It is of great use in the diagnosis of many skin conditions of which the most important would be the blistering skin conditions. The specimens are obtained by the same means as, and often in conjunction with, a conventional skin biopsy. It may therefore be possible to dissect the specimen either before removal from the patient or immediately thereafter. The specimen for immunofluorescence should be snapfrozen, which is usually achieved using dry ice or carbon dioxide snow, and then transported to the laboratory.

4. IMMUNOPEROXIDASE METHODS (IMMUNOENZYMES)

This technique depends upon the antigen on site in the skin being made to react with a reagent antibody to which has been attached an enzyme with peroxidase. The ensuing reaction may be demonstrated as dark brown deposits. Its great advantage is that it can be used on many fixed specimens and that a non-facing preparation can be obtained.

Appendix II

Examples of recognized human teratogens

Chemicals and drugs		Maternal disorders	
Aminopterin/ Methotrexate	Facial anomalies Microcephaly Mesomelia (short forearms) Talipes equinovarus Hypodactyly	Maternal cytomegalovirus infection	Microcephaly Mental deficiency Chorioretinitis Neonatal hepatitis
Phenytoin	Cardiac defects Limb defects Growth retardation Nail hypoplasia	Maternal diabetes mellitus	Cardiac defects Sacral agenesis Spina bifida
Sodium valproate	Facial anomalies Spina bifida Developmental delay Long, thin fingers and toes Hyperconvex finger nails	Maternal HIV infection Maternal phenylketonuria	Microcephaly ? Characteristic facies Growth failure Anencephaly Mental deficiency Microcephaly Cardiac defects
Thalidomide	Phocomelia Anomalies of teeth, gut and eyes	Maternal rubella	Cardiac defects Microcephaly Cataracts
Warfarin	Short digits Stippled epiphyses Hypoplasia of nails Nasal hypoplasia Mental deficiency		Deafness Mental deficiency Neonatal hepatitis Chorioretinitis
Alcohol	Intrauterine growth retardation Microcephaly Mental deficiency Cardiac defects Flexion contractures Characteristic facies	Maternal systemic lupus erythematosus Congenital toxoplasmosis	Congenital heart block Microcephaly Megalencephaly Microphthalmia Mental deficiency Neonatal hepatitis Chorioretinitis
Lead	Cognitive impairment	Varicella	Skin scars
Smoking	Intrauterine growth retardation ? Abnormal facies at birth		Limb hypoplasia Microphthalmia Cataracts Mental deficiency
Methyl mercury	Mental deficiency Microcephaly Spasticity		
Iodides	Goiter Neonatal hypothyroidism		

Appendix III

Autosomal dominant disorders

Condition	Presentation
Achondroplasia	Short limb dwarfism Microcephaly Frontal bossing Short stubby trident hand
Adams–Oliver syndrome	Aplasia cutis of posterior parietal region Terminal transverse limb defects
Apert's syndrome	Acrocephaly Syndactyly Hypertelorism Midfacial hypoplasia Mental retardation
Beal's syndrome	Contractural arachnodactyly 'Crumpled ears'
Brachydactyly syndrome	Short metacarpals Brachydactyly Short stature
Clouston syndrome	Nail dystrophy Dyskeratotic palms and soles Hair hypoplasia
Distichiasis–Lymphedema syndrome	Double row of eyelashes Below-knee lymphedema
Dystrophia myotonica (Steinert's syndrome)	Myotonia Severe neonatal hypotonia with talipes Frontal alopecia Cataracts Variable mental retardation
Ectrodactyly–ectodermal dysplasia–clefting syndrome (EEC)	Cleft lip/palate Ectodermal dysplasia Ectrodactyly (total or partial absence of fingers or toes)
Ehlers–Danlos syndrome	Neonatal hypotonia Blue sclera Hyperextensible skin Hypermobile joints Poor wound healing

Condition	Presentation
Epidermolysis bullosa simplex	Non-scarring intraepidermal blisters; prognosis good
Fibrodysplasia ossificans progressive syndrome	Short hallux Fibrous dysplasia with ossification of muscles and subcutaneous tissues
Freeman–Sheldon ('whistling face') syndrome	Microstomia/puckered mouth; grooved chin; flat mid face Talipes equinovarus/ulnar deviation of fingers
Greig cephalopolysyndactyly syndrome	Frontal bossing Polydactyly Syndactyly
Hereditary spherocytosis	Recurrent hemolytic anemia Splenomegaly Acholuric jaundice
Hypohidrotic ectodermal dysplasia (Rapp–Hodgkin type)	Hypohidrosis Oral clefts Dysplastic nails
Hypochondroplasia	Short limb dwarfism Near normal craniofacial appearance Caudal narrowing of spine
Huntington's chorea	Progressive involuntary movements (choreoathetosis) Dementia
Langer mesomelic dysplasia	Mesomelic (mid portion) Dwarfism Rudimentary fibula Micrognathia
Leri–Weill dyschondrosteosis	Short forearms Madelung's deformity Short lower legs

Condition	Presentation	Condition	Presentation
Marfan's syndrome	Arachnodactyly Pes planus Hyperextensible joints Lens dislocation Aortic aneurysm	Robinow (fetal face) syndrome	Flat facial profile Short forearms Hypoplastic genitalia Broad thumbs and toes Hypoplastic middle and terminal phalanges of fingers and toes
Nail patella syndrome	Absent/hypoplastic nails and patellae Limited elbow mobility	Spondylo-epiphyseal dysplasia	Short trunk Lag in epiphyseal mineralization Myopia
Neurofibromatosis (Von Recklinghausen's disease)	Multiple café au lait spots Axillary intertriginous freckles Multiple neurofibromas Hemihypertrophy Many neurological complications	Stickler syndrome	Flat facies Myopia Lag in mineralization of epiphyses
Oculodentodigital syndrome	Microphthalmos Enamel hypoplasia Camptodactyly of fifth finger Syndactyly of third/fourth toes	Treacher Collins syndrome	Malar hypoplasia Antimongolian slant of palpable fissures Defect of lower limb Malformation of external ear
Osteogenesis imperfecta type one	Fragile bones Blue sclera Hyperextensibility and/or odontogenesis imperfecta	Trichodento-osseous syndrome	Kinky hair Enamel hypoplasia Sclerotic bone Brittle nails with superficial peeling
Pachyonychia congenita syndrome	Thick nails Hyperkeratosis Foot blisters	Tuberous sclerosis	Facial angiofibromas Depigmented macules of skin Subungual fibromas Seizures Variable mental handicap
Pfeiffer syndrome	Turricephaly/brachycephaly Broad thumbs and toes Syndactyly Proptosis Strabismus Midfacial hypoplasia	Von Willebrand's disease	Decreased factor 8 (clotting factor) Decreased platelet adhesiveness

Appendix IV

Autosomal recessive disorders

Disorder	Presentation
Acromesomelic dysplasia	Short distal limbs Frontal prominence Low thoracic kyphosis
Ataxia telangiectasia (Louis-Bar syndrome)	Conjunctival and cutaneous telangiectasiae Café au lait spots Sclerodermatous changes Progressive neurological deterioration with involuntary movements Immune incompetence
Autosomal recessive muscular dystrophy	Pseudohypertrophic type of muscular dystrophy Progressive weakness affecting both sexes
Chondroectodermal dysplasia (Ellis–van Creveld syndrome)	Short distal extremities Polydactyly Nail hypoplasia
Cotten syndrome	Hypotonia Obesity Prominent incisors Narrow hands and feet Short metacarpals and metatarsals
Epidermolysis bullosa letalis	Blistering skin lesions from birth Secondary infection common Defective dentition Secondary nail dystrophy Prognosis poor
Escobar syndrome	Multiple pterygia Camptodactyly (flexion deformities of fingers) Syndactyly Talipes equinovarus Rockerbottom feet
Geleophysic dysplasia	Short stature Round face 'Pleasant, happy natured' appearance

Disorder	Presentation
	Short hands and feet Progressive multiple joint contractures
Hemoglobinopathies (sickle cell anemia and thalassemia)	Recurrent hemolytic anemia secondary to abnormal hemoglobin
Homocystinuria	Mental deficiency Arachnodactyly Pes planus Subluxation of lens Malar flush
Mohr syndrome	Cleft tongue Conductive deafness Partial reduplication of hallux
Mucopolysaccharidosis Types 1, 3, 4, 5, 6, 7	Variable effects of mucopolysaccharide storage in bone, viscera, skin and central nervous system
Phenylketonuria	Blond hair, blue eyes Mental retardation Eczema Mousey odor in untreated individuals
Radial aplasia/ thrombocytopenia syndrome	Absen/hypoplastic radius Associated ulnar hypoplasia and defects of hands and feet Severe thrombocytopenia
Rothmund–Thomson syndrome	Poikiloderma (marbling and hypoplasia of skin) Cataract Ectodermal dysplasia Small dystrophic nails and hyperkeratosis of palms and soles
Sjögren–Larsson syndrome	Ichthyosis Spasticity Mental retardation
Weill–Marchesani syndrome	Brachydactyly Small spherical lens Short stature

Disorder	*Presentation*
Werdnig–Hoffmann syndrome	Early onset spinal muscular atrophy Progressive weakness and lower motor neuron paresis Death in early infancy

Appendix V

X-linked disorders

Disorder	Presentation	Disorder	Presentation
Albright hereditary osteodystrophy (pseudohypopara-thyroidism)	Short metacarpals and metatarsals Rounded facies Hypocalcemia and osteoporosis		Deficiency of steroid sulphatase enzymes (less severe dominant type and more severe recessive type also described)
Child syndrome	Unilateral hypomelia Skin hypoplasia Cardiac defect	Oral-facial-digital syndrome	Oral frenula and clefts Hypoplastic alae nasi Asymmetrical shortening of digits and polydactyly of feet Fatal in utero in male
Duchenne muscular dystrophy	Pseudohypertrophic type of progressive muscular dystrophy		
Dyskeratosis congenita syndrome	Hyperpigmentation of skin Leukoplakia and nail dystrophy Pancytopenia	Oto-palatal-digital syndrome	Deafness Cleft palate Broad distal digits with short nails Hallucal nail dystrophy Syndactyly of toes
Glucose-6-phosphate dehydrogenase deficiency	Recurrent hemolytic anemia	Vitamin D resistant rickets	Genetic rickets resistant to large dose of Vitamin D Bow legs and waddling gait
Hemophilia A and B	Recurrent bleeding owing to factor 8 or 9 deficiency		
Hypohidrotic ectodermal dysplasia	Defective sweating Alopecia Hypodontia Eczema Nail dystrophy	X-linked agammaglobulinemia (Bruton type)	Recurrent pyogenic infection Bronchiectasis Eczema Increased incidence of malignancy
Ichthyosis	Scaling skin of scalp, neck, face, anterior trunk and limbs		

Appendix VI

Developmental milestones

Birth. When the child lies prone the head is turned to one side and there is flexion of the hips and knees so that the infant's legs are tucked under the chest. Head control is absent and there is general flexion of the upper and lower limbs. The walking reflex is apparent but is lost by the end of the first month. This reflex may be demonstrated by holding the child so that its feet are placed on a hard surface such as a table. This leads to a reciprocal flexion and extension of the lower limbs and simulates gait. This movement does not continue for very long as the activity of the hip abductors leads to one leg becoming caught behind the other.

1 month. The legs are less flexed and therefore they do not tuck under the chest as much as when in the prone position.

2 months. When prone, the child may now rise up onto the forearms and may extend the head to look forwards.

3 months. The hips are now extended in prone lying so that the pelvis can now lie flat on the supporting surface. The pelvis also lies flat when the child is supine. The child's heel can rest on the surface for the first time.

4 months. The head is now vertical when the child lies prone with forearm support. The child begins to roll and to flex and to extend the limbs when supine.

5 months. The child may now take a major proportion of the body weight when supported in standing. This may be said to be the first time, albeit passively, that dorsiflexion has occurred. The infant can also extend the upper limbs in prone.

6 months. The child can self-support on the hands when lying prone. The child begins to grab hold of the toes and to bounce up and down in supporting standing. This is brought about by reciprocal contraction of the flexors and extensor muscles of the lower limb. Rolling from prone to supine is now possible.

7 months. The child can sit unsupported but requires to keep the body weight well forward in order to avoid toppling over. The toes now reach the mouth and may be sucked. Rolling back to prone is now possible.

8 months. Sitting posture is now much more stable. The child can move from prone lying into prone kneeling with the hands and feet in contact with the floor.

9 months. The child begins to crawl and can stand momentarily with the help of nearby furniture.

10 months. Crawling and standing and holding on to furniture become easier.

11 months. The child can walk on hands and feet and in an upright position when held by both arms.

1 year. Supported walking progresses to the child being able to walk supported by one hand. The child can squat with a wide base of support.

15 months. The child can walk, kneel and stand up unaided. The child can climb stairs on all fours.

2 years. The child can climb stairs without help; two feet per step, and can run and jump.

3 years. The child can now run and hop and falls over less frequently.

4 years. The child can walk downstairs one foot per step.

5 years. The child is now able to skip on both feet.

Index

Page numbers in *italic* refer to figures and tables, those in **bold** indicate main discussion.